JMLB

JAZZTIME MORGAN FARM
NANCY & MIKE JEWELL
ROUTE 1
LIBERTY LAKE WA 99019

Keep Your Horse Healthy

ADVICE FROM A VETERINARIAN

M. Phyllis Lose, VMD

ARCO PUBLISHING, INC.
NEW YORK

Published by Arco Publishing, Inc.
215 Park Avenue South, New York, N.Y. 10003

Library of Congress Cataloging-in-Publication Data

Lose, M. Phyllis.
  Keep your horse healthy.

  Includes index.
  1. Horses. 2. Horses—Diseases. I. Title.
SF285.3.L67 1985   636.1'089   85-18504
ISBN 0-668-05712-2 (Cloth Edition)

Printed in the United States of America

10 9 8 7 6 5 4 3 2 1

Contents

Foreword

This book is a condensation of my lifetime of observing and caring for horses. It is organized alphabetically under several broad topics and presents certain selected and key facts not readily available to novice horse owners and caretakers. I hope it will be read and used by all who want to learn more about horses. Even professional horsemen will, I think, find some useful reminders in its pages. Most of the information has been gained in the school of my daily experience over more than 25 years as an equine veterinarian. Some of it is wisdom imparted to me by many old friends and, of course, by my teachers. I acknowledge my debt to them all.

Among equine veterinarians there seems to be a tendency to stay in the specialty for a dozen or so years, then to move into government service, a state agency, public health, teaching, or some other area of this widely diversified profession. But the sheer mystery of the horse has kept me in thrall all these years. It still does. And the profession itself becomes even more satisfying, as new techniques and new drugs come along. How I wish I could go back in time and have a second chance with some of those cases that were lost in the days when we worked without benefit of the latest lifesaving knowledge!

This book is intended to be more than a compendium of knowledge. It is a plea to horse owners and caretakers: that we try to understand our friend, the horse, that we guard its health and functioning through sound husbandry practices, and that we train it at a pace that keeps step with the individual animal's growing maturity and ability.

Not only are these standards humane; they are the most productive of desired results. They are what we should strive for. Please, let us try.

M. P. LOSE, V.M.D.

Introduction

January 1. A new year was born.

I began thinking of my 25 years—a quarter of a century—in the practice of veterinary medicine.

My beginning as a struggling country vet came to mind. I thought of the mares I'd helped get ready for breeding, the foals I'd delivered, the hunting horses I'd patched up, the race horses I'd operated on. So many of them, and—fortunately—how very few had been lost!

I wondered what I could do to preserve this great fund of happy and sad experiences. Then I had an inspiration. I would review my records; there were thousands of cases, certainly enough material for a book. Perhaps I could even be able to express the humility and pride I feel in having been sufficiently well trained to serve the needs of these silent patients.

So, I compiled a list of the diseases, syndromes (conditions known by a set of recognizable symptoms), and entities (conditions not yet classified as diseases) that plague today's horse.

While I worked my way through case history after case history, it occurred to me that there are characteristics unique to the horse, characteristics concealed from view of the average person who works with horses. These facts may be known, even taken for granted by a few people who learned from stories and demonstrations handed down from generation to generation. Otherwise, much of this knowledge seems to have vanished. Rarely is it found in current literature. Yet it is essential knowledge for the successful horse owner and trainer and is the key to understanding the horse's individuality and peculiarities.

For example, are you aware:

- that a horse's teeth continue to grow throughout his entire life?
- that his Eustachian tube contains a balloon-like pouch in which air or infectious matter may lodge or be entrapped?
- that his vision is such that a wide range of head and neck movement must take place in order for him to see efficiently?
- that the horse breathes only through his nose and is absolutely unable to regurgitate?
- that his stomach is only one-fifth the size and weight considered to be normal for other similar species?
- that he lacks a gall bladder?
- that he alone of all the species possesses chestnuts, or "night eyes," small, crusty tissue deposits on the inside of the legs, as unique to each individual horse as fingerprints are to humans?
- that the horse has a prehensile muzzle, a bundle of fibroelastic tissue capable of stretching eagerly to grasp tiny blades of grass and sorting so delicately through the contents of a feed tub that it can—and will—leave

1

aside one tiny pill or many grains of medicated powder mixed in feed? (The abundance of nerve endings in that small area of muzzle gives the horse a kind of "third eye" for protection. He cannot see that portion of the end of his nose, yet, by means of the tactile hairs, he can sense with great discrimination anything that approaches that area of the face.)

- that the horse is a highly selective eater? If he takes something foreign into his mouth, he suddenly stops chewing, opens his jaws wide, and expels the entire contents of his mouth, then, after a moment, quietly resumes eating.
- that the foal enters the world with absolutely no immunity against disease, but receives lifesaving antibodies in the first milk it drinks from its mother's teats?

Awareness of these and other oddities should make the perceptive owner or caretaker more sensitive to the horse and its mental and physiologic problems, more concerned with his horse's welfare and alert to the slightest sign of trouble.

Attentiveness is the key word in the code of horse husbandry. It begins with attentiveness to diet. Horses are herbivores; they subsist on a diet of grasses, herbs, and other forms of vegetation. But the horse is radically different from all other herbivores such as the sheep, the cow, and the goat. Those animals are ruminants and they possess four stomachs! No wonder their gastrointestinal tracts are infinitely superior to the horse's single undersized stomach!

The cow, sheep and goat can prosper on diets that are absolutely intolerable to the horse. Any feed that contains dust or mold threatens the horse with gastrointestinal involvement and probable illness. So when you buy hay make sure it is clean, green, leafy, and dust-free. Use your hands, your eyes, and—above all—your nose, to make sure it is top-quality *horse* hay (not cow hay). Perfectly clean, properly cured hay, or a combination of pasture and hay, provided free-choice, not only supplies necessary roughage, but can prevent boredom and subsequent development of stable vices such as cribbing, weaving, and wind-sucking.

Working animals that have extra energy demands require the addition of cereal grains (otherwise known as concentrates). Grain should be fed in small meals two or three times daily, with the quality and quantity adjusted carefully to the individual horse's physiology and work schedule. There is no such thing as a cut-and-dried feeding rule. An effective feeding program must be tailor-made to each horse's nutritional needs.

Ideally, only one person should be made responsible for feeding and that person should be familiar with each horse's eating habits and exercise schedule. A back-up person should always be on call to supervise feeding.

Wise, experienced barn managers know that a quick visual check of each animal at feeding time is a daily safeguard. If anything seems amiss, if your horse seems slightly "off," you should take the animal's temperature. This is a vital "first alert" procedure. A fluctuating body temperature is a sign of possible trouble. Realize, however, that body temperature is influenced by a number of factors such as age, size, breed, time of day, exercise, and grain intake. (For example, the smaller the animal, the higher the normal temperature.)

I particularly urge attentiveness in the matter of regularly scheduled veterinary visits to carry out a fixed routine of parasite control, preventive vaccinations, and routine boosters. If neglected, parasites can be insidious killers affecting the animal's intestinal lining and blood vessels. Progressive destruction of his vital organs leads to undefined illnesses and eventual death.

Recurrent respiratory infections are common to young horses and can lead to chronic upper respiratory disease. Regardless of the veterinary profession's multiple vaccines, it seems that some young horses have to develop their own immunity in a natural, non-drug-supported manner. Others can benefit from prophylactic treatment. But too often, common viral infections are compounded by secondary bacterial infections. A vaccination schedule can appreciably reduce these problems.

I would warn you, however, against unprofessional and promiscuous injections of nonspecific antibiotics. The result can be viral and bacterial resistance to these drugs, which sets up an unending vicious cycle.

In my opinion, respiratory disorders are always the result of infectious diseases or poor housing and careless stable management. Of all the respiratory diseases to which older horses are prone, heaves (pulmonary alveolar emphysema) is the most common. It is interesting to note that this incurable condition, so like asthma in the human being, is never seen in young horses. It takes years of exposure to dust and dirt, stress, and confinement in a stall with poor ventilation to produce this noninfectious respiratory problem.

The healthiest horses I have observed are those that were free to walk in and out of shelters at will. This living pattern for horses is contrary to my early training, but the results from such unrestricted housing are so astounding that I have happily made a radical adjustment in my thinking. Horses are healthier roughing it. Too much tender love and care can interfere with a horse's well-being and happiness.

I know many horse owners who believe that they really care for their animals. They tuck them up for the night (sometimes all day, too) in a warm, closed-up stall, bed them knee-high in straw, and provide hay from a hay rack stuffed full and hung high.

This luxurious arrangement courts disaster. Draft-free ventilation is absolutely essential. And, at the risk of disturbing fastidious owners, I recommend feeding hay on the stall floor to prevent inhalation of dirt and other irritating particles. Dirt ingested is far less dangerous than irritants inhaled. If it offends you to floor-feed, you may use a hay net, provided your hay is absolutely clean and dust-free.

A clean stall, aired out each day, is imperative to maintain your horse's health. Bedding that harbors dust must be eliminated. The beams, rafters, and sides of your stalls must be cleaned to get rid of cobwebs and dirt.

Filthy bedding, plus moisture, plus warmth in an unkempt stall have the effect of eliminating oxygen. In this atmosphere fungi and fatal bacteria flourish and the horse becomes prey to botulism and the foot infection called thrush.

A mere teaspoonful of botulism toxin will kill a thousand-pound horse. This disease causes weakness, then death; a related disease, tetanus, causes rigidity, then death. The microbes responsible in either case belong to the same family of spore-formers—the Clostridiums. They remain quiescent or inactive until the conditions just described are present, then they spring into action. The simple introduction of oxygen, by means of a well-cleaned, well-shaken-up, freshly bedded stall, changed daily (or even twice daily), breaks the deadly cycle.

That old adage, "No foot, no horse," is alive and well. A study of all breeds and their varying uses has shown the veterinary profession that 85 percent of all lameness originates in the feet.

Attentive care of the horse's feet is a daily necessity. Use a hoof pick after exercise and before putting up for the night to remove dirty packed materials and lodged foreign objects and to uncover possible punctures or lacerations. This routine also allows air to circulate around the frog and sole areas. Such daily care shows up the condition of the hoof and the need for dressing and balancing before a problem can become acute. If your horse is shod, daily inspection will reveal a loose nail, a shifted shoe, or sprung bars. This is the easiest way to prevent certain lamenesses and subsequent loss of productive time.

By far the most common foot infection I encounter is thrush, which is caused by fungi. A close second is gravel, which is caused by bacteria (not by gravel).

Again, I must say that cleanliness is the first line of defense. The evidence in favor of keeping stalls dry and clean at all times is irrefutable.

The art of detecting lameness continues to elude many horse people. Here is a simple guide.

A lame horse will elevate his body and stay on the sore leg for the shortest possible time. He then shifts his weight to the opposite side, dropping his body weight as he lands on the sound limb. He will stay on the good leg as long as possible and delay passing his weight to the sore leg.

Imagine yourself walking or jogging with a pebble in one shoe! You can easily visualize how you would shift your body with each step.

You can turn your back on a horse that is being jogged for soundness on a paved drive and hear the difference in the cadence of the hoof beats. Try it.

A method that invariably locates the seat of lameness was told me many years ago by an old farrier friend. I have used this method all my professional life and am happy to share it with you.

Evaluate the amount of pulsation in the lame leg by searching for the enlarged and engorged metacarpal artery. To find it, reach around the back of the horse's left front leg with your right hand placed just below the knee on the inside surface of the cannon area. Slide your index and third fingers forward so that they rest in the groove between the major (flexor) tendon group and the cannon bone. Reverse the process to check the other front leg.

If the opposite leg, the good leg, is normal, any pulsation you feel should be imperceptible. If the pulse in the lame leg is profound (very noticeable), or if a real difference exists between the two front legs, you can safely conclude that some form of pathology (inflammation) exists below the point of pulsation, that is, in the foot.

If you feel no extreme pulse or if you detect equal amounts of pulse in both front legs, you may safely conclude that the trouble lies above the area of pulsation, perhaps in a knee or shoulder.

In the case of rear leg lameness, place your fingers on the outside of the rear cannon bone, just below the hock. Slide your fingers backwards from the cannon bone into the indentation that separates the cannon bone from the posteriorly located tendons. The large pulsating metatarsal artery will be found in this groove. Then compare degree of pulsation with the other hind leg. The same conclusions can be drawn as with the front legs.

This diagnostic method has never failed me.

Care of the young foal's feet should begin when it is six weeks old. The foal's problem is not foot growth, but, rather, foot shape. During the early months of a foal's life, a persistent "point" forms at the front and center of the young toe. These points, considered of no great consequence by the uninformed, can seriously affect the foal's future soundness. Simply rounding off the center of the little toe with a blacksmith's rasp, done weekly (from six to eight weeks onward), allows the foal's foot to "break over" as nature intended, so that a straight and normal stride can develop freely.

If these young feet are neglected, the foal will be forced to break either to the inside of the foot, causing "toeing-out," or to the outside, causing "toeing-in." A defective gait results, and unnatural stress is thus forced on all joints of the young, vulnerable legs. Again, you see how a little bit of attentiveness makes a great difference in the horse's health and functioning.

Colic, azoturia, and founder are three common illnesses of distinct environmental etiology that pose a constant threat to the health of any horse. Colic is defined as pain in the abdomen; azoturia is a paralytic disease; founder is a crippling disease of the feet. Two of these illnesses, founder and azoturia, are entirely unique to the horse. Colic is, of course, universal in its occurrence among animals and humans.

The common denominator for all three conditions is the gastrointestinal tract, the home site of the initial physiologic reaction. Instantaneous physiological changes result in colic, slower and more complicated changes may result in founder or azoturia.

Any imbalance between the factors of food and exercise, or any abrupt change in daily routine can easily create discord in the horse's primitive though extensive (nearly 100-foot-long) gastrointestinal tract. The punishing effects can expand into the horse's massive musculature. In such cases, overall circulation may be radically disturbed, with subsequent alteration of the function of both the vascular and muscular system.

Sad to say, the physically fit, competitive horse, highly strung and highly tuned, is particularly vulnerable to azoturia if even minute variations are made in the usual daily schedule. (I'm sure this is why we often see horses being exercised by rain-drenched or freezing riders; there is reason behind such seeming madness.) The fat pony or obese family pet is not a likely candidate for this disease, but is very susceptible to founder and colic, illnesses that attack all horses regardless of age, sex, or breed. Azoturia is totally preventable, but it is quite incurable once paralysis develops. Founder, too, is preventable. It results from environmental abuse and lack of proper stable husbandry. With astute veterinary counseling, certain degrees of laminitis (inflammation of the horny fibers of the foot) can be avoided or controlled in 90 percent of founder cases.

With these facts firmly in mind, we must be sure to pay strict attention to the maintenance of a properly adjusted diet balanced against the demands of the animal's exercise program. I cannot emphasize this too strongly.

Our present day horse is strong, but he is not tough. He is a sensitive animal and he possesses a nervous system with which we have to reckon. Horses do show pain and they do indicate their states of mind—good, bad, or indifferent. I firmly believe that the horse's nervous system is the key to his potential; it directly affects his ability to eat, rest, and perform. You should place as much emphasis on caring for his peace of mind as you do on caring for his coat, feet, and stall. Compromise the care of his nervous system and you will inevitably end up with little, if any, of the horse's original potential.

Attention to the cleanliness of your horse is not only essential to his general good health, but contributes also to his state of mind and good humor.

By providing certain creature comforts to your sensitive charges, you can build a cushion against the shocks of work and discipline. Please do not look upon the act of grooming—brushing and cleaning the horse—as a tiresome chore. Conscientious grooming promotes healthy muscle tone, improves circulation and skin tone, and enhances the condition of the horse's coat. A glowing coat is a mirror of general good health.

As a child, I was confused by the term "strapping" a horse. Then one day I entered a well-run hunter barn and saw a horse cross-tied in the center aisle. A groom was slapping the horse's body with his open hands. He systematically covered every inch of the muscled areas. At the end of the groom's strapping, the horse's coat literally shone. And the animal had not resisted for a moment—he obviously enjoyed it. Only the exhausted groom needed a rest. If you doubt what I say, try the strapping method yourself. Then step back and admire your work.

And don't overlook the finer details of grooming. For example, your mare's mammary glands collect dirt and mud around and between the teats. Watch her reaction of pleasure as you bathe, cleanse, and carefully dry this tender, out-of-view area.

In hidden areas of the mane and tail you may find ticks, parasites, dandruff, and dirt. Brush and clean thoroughly every day.

Twice a month at least, cleanse the sheath of your gelding or stallion to clean away gummy deposits. Follow with a coating of olive oil to help maintain moisture in these tissues.

A stimulating bath of warm water with the addition of an antiseptic of your choice prevents coat and skin irritation in all horses. Use a metal scraper to remove excess water. Your horse will clearly show you that this is a pleasing reward after strenuous work.

Beware of leaving heels moist. Inflamed or "cracked heels" result. Dry around the fetlocks and bulbs of all four heels. This should be done religiously after every bath, when the horse has been out in wet weather, ice, snow, or mud, and when it has been on a chemically treated ring or track surface.

Fresh blankets or sheets are a real courtesy, both to horses and to personnel. Besides being unpleasant to handle, soiled blankets harbor bacteria and fungal infections. They should have no place in your barn.

I am happy to report that I have watched and talked with many trainers of young horses who exercise good judgment toward the animals in their charge. They do not allow themselves to be forced into hurrying or overtraining the equine youngsters. They insist upon proper feeding, rest periods, training sessions, and excellent hygiene, all on a regular schedule. In addition, they require that their charges live in peaceful and secure surroundings and receive kind but disciplined handling by all.

To be sure, the horse world has its share of abuses. Many a well-bred horse has been "washed out" by subjection to physical and emotional stresses for which he was not prepared. He suffers pain, shock, and exhaustion, and on the heels of these symptoms comes a systemic breakdown of the physiologic and psychologic functions. The condition is readily apparent. Typically, the horse is underweight and rough-coated. He stands motionless, almost stiffly planted, in a far corner of the stall, not at the door. He seems reluctant to move and ignores his filled feed tub and hay. He is the picture of depression and despair. Once the nervous system has been traumatized to this point the damage is done. There is no full return—although some do recover partially, given time and loving care.

I hope that instances of abuse—through ignorance, or worse—will become increasingly rare. I dream of a world of horsewomen and horsemen who fully realize that the only way with these equine pupils is to make haste slowly—laying down a strong foundation of training, and proceeding up the educational ladder without skipping any of the rungs.

Attentiveness is the key. We have as much to learn from our horses as they have to learn from us!

Abbreviations

The following abbreviations are used:
I.M.   intramuscular
I.U.   International Unit
I.V.   intravenous
N.F.   National Formulary
q.s.a.d.   quantity sufficient to make
q.v.   which see
U.S.P.   United States Pharmacopeia

COMMON DISEASES

abscess A circumscribed or "contained" accumulation of pus. An abscess is the result of an unsuccessful attempt by a pathogen (usually staphylococcus) to gain entrance to the body and a successful battle by the body tissue to surround and limit the infection. The pus, or purulent material, consists of dead leucocytes (white blood corpuscles) that have served their main purpose of containing the infection.

An abscess, regardless of its cause, moves gradually toward the skin surface, causing great swelling, heat, and pain. If untampered with, it eventually "points," with gradual thinning of the outer skin; finally it ruptures, discharging its contents. Nature sometimes does an admirable job of cleansing the area, with subsequent healing; however, if the abscess contains a "pocket" of tissue, incomplete expulsion occurs and a chronic state develops characterized by feeble drainage and retarded healing.

Lancing is the ideal treatment. It requires no local anesthetic, only a sterile scalpel. A stab incision is made to permit escape of the accumulated purulent material and establish drainage. The incision gives the veterinarian access to the inner surface of the cavity caused by the hot, putrid, trapped infection. Treatment consists of flushing with sterile saline solution, then packing with drains of antibiotics or sterile gauze soaked in Lugol's Solution.

The success of the treatment depends upon the timing. An abscess should never be opened or lanced before it is well pointed. It is ready to drain when an "onionskin" covering can be palpated. Incomplete drainage can cause a chronic condition to develop requiring repeated treatment and medication. Chronic abscessation has reportedly been the cause of founder.

Hot compresses, poultices, and in some instances systemic injections can aid in the pointing process. In my opinion, a horse doctor is the person best qualified to counsel, guide, and determine the ideal time of treatment and the preferred procedure.

Another dangerous and somewhat similar condition can develop in the uterus of the mare. Under certain circumstances, the uterus can collect and wall off a huge amount of purulent matter resembling the matter contained in an abscess, with the uterine wall serving as a container. This condition poses the same danger as does an abscess in any other kind of tissue. *See:* BRUCELLOSIS, FISTULA, POLL EVIL, PYOMETRA.

African horse sickness A highly fatal viral infection transmitted by biting insects, particularly the fly and mosquito. Extensive air transport of horses between countries has alerted the veterinary profession to the possibility of the

9

African horse sickness continued

disease appearing in North America. As yet, however, no case has been recorded.

It is a noncontagious seasonal infection characterized by high fever and widespread edematous swellings of the horse's head and neck primarily that progress to the lungs and heart, causing death.

allergy Hypersensitivity or reaction by the body to a foreign substance. Symptoms range from a mild dermatitis to an occasional wheal and erythema over the body of the horse. The foreign substance may have been eaten in the hay or grain, or ingested by the horse while out in the pasture. Simple steroids or antihistamines relieve the itchiness in quick order and make the animal comfortable. *See:* ANAPHYLAXIS.

STEROIDS

Injectable	Oral
dexamethasone (Azium)	dexamethasone (Azium powder)
hydrocortisone	
prednisolone	

ANTIHISTAMINES

Injectable	Oral
Antiphrine	Antiphrine granules
pyrilamine maleate	Phenergan tablets
tripelennamine	tripelennamine syrup

anhidrosis Complete suppression of the ability to sweat; commonly known as "dry coat." A horse from a relatively humid climate may develop this condition if it is moved abruptly to a hot, dry region. Although the cause is unknown, malfunction of the temperature-regulating mechanism in the hypothalamus (a group of nuclei at the base of the brain) is believed to be the factor. Although it is difficult to treat, rest and acclimatization and careful monitoring over a period of time may restore improved function.

anthrax A communicable disease caused by the bacterium *Bacillus anthracis* (commonly called splenic fever and wool-sorters' disease in human beings), characterized by high fever (septicemia) and a rapidly fatal course.

A spore-former and soil inhabitant, *B. anthracis* can resist dry climates, intense heat, freezing temperatures, and chemical disinfectants. The spores seem to survive all adversities.

Anthrax cases appear spontaneously after a wet, rainy period. Grazing horses, cattle, sheep, and goats easily become ill when the activated spores revert to the vegetative form.

Because this dreaded disease can invade all tissues of the body in animals and in human beings alike, infected carcasses are destroyed (incinerated) under authorized supervision in order to prevent the spread of the disease. Anthrax occurs worldwide, and although strict state and federal controls have eradicated the disease from the United States for the present, sporadic outbreaks are anticipated.

Penicillin, oxytetracycline, and other antibiotics are useful only in the early stages of anthrax infection. A vaccine has been developed for preventive therapy.

I envision the spore-forming micro-organism as an elusive enemy with the ability to change face rapidly and apply protective armor, living secretly among us until ideal conditions occur, when it abruptly pulls off the mask and attacks.

Other spore-formers and the diseases they cause are: *Clostridium tetani* (lockjaw), *C. botulinum* (botulism), and *C. septicum* (malignant edema).

arbovirus   A varied group of viruses that attack the central nervous system of horses, causing lethal encephalitis. For transmission to occur from the reservoir of wild animals and birds to the horse, special climatic conditions and a specific mosquito (vector) must act in combination. This infection carries 100 percent mortality, thus the horse is the last link in the chain of transmission. *See:* ENCEPHALITIS.

ARBOVIRUS GROUP

Disease	Vector
Eastern Equine Encephalomyelitis (EEE)	Freshwater swamp mosquito (*Culiseta melanura*) and swamp-dwelling birds
Western Equine Encephalomyelitis (WEE)	Mosquito (*Culex tarsalis*) and wild birds
Venezuelan Equine Encephalomyelitis (VEE)	Mosquito (*Culex melanoconium*); cotton rat (*Sigmodon Hispious*)
Japanese Equine Encephalitis (JEE)	Mosquito (*Culex tritaeniorhynchus*)

aspergillosis   A mycotic (fungal) infection caused by *Aspergillus fumagatus*, *A. nidulans*, and *A. flavus*. *A. fumagatus* is by far the most common fungal infection in the horse and is a cause of abortion in mares.

Fungal infections are a major challenge to both the veterinary and human medical fields. The fungi can establish disease anywhere in the world and represent a serious threat to future livestock.

Mycotic infections have an affinity for the respiratory tract and can create a resistant pharyngitis, laryngitis, or sinusitis. They are especially found to invade and establish chronic infections in the guttural pouches. Fungi in the trachea, bronchi, and lungs are difficult to treat but the expense and effort are warranted since some cases do recover. Mycotic pneumonia is usually lethal in the horse, however.

When aspergillus attacks the gravid uterus and fetus, abortion results; when aspergillus invades an empty uterus, sterility results.

Diagnosis is best achieved by tissue section, cultures, and cytologic washings. With identification, sensitivity tests can be run and the practitioner be informed of the drug of choice.

Fungus-caused abortions characteristically occur later in gestation as a result of destruction, interference, and reduced efficiency of the diseased placenta. The fungi probably enter through the cervix and uterus and proceed to infect the fetus through the chorioallantois and amnionic membranes. A fungus-related abortion is identified easily by the gross lesions found extensively throughout the fetus and all placental membranes.

Unfortunately, fungal infections are increasing faster than the pace of research and development of effective drugs to counteract them. Antimycotic drugs are few in number, very costly, and in most cases their effectiveness is

aspergillosis continued

questionable. Although it is well known in the veterinary profession that abuse, overuse, and incorrect use of antibiotics can actually foster the growth of some fungi, still the irrational practice continues. Often, a persistent and resistant bacterial infection finally responds to treatment with a clean culture after massive antibiotic therapy, only to be followed by a flourishing growth of molds and fungi.

Consult your veterinarian for advice regarding the long or protracted use of antibiotics. *See:* ANTIFUNGAL AGENTS (CHART), PAGE 226).

azoturia A metabolic muscle discord produced in the physically fit horse. Overproduction of lactic acid and other metabolic wastes serves to overload and stress not only the circulatory system but the liver and the kidneys as well. Unpredictable degrees of paresis, or irreversible paralysis, characterize azoturia.

Any time within the first minute, up to the first 15 minutes of exercise, the characteristic sweat will begin at the base of the ears and spring forth simultaneously all over the body. This symptom will be accompanied by overt pain, muscle stiffness, and increasing inability to move. Such signs *always* occur during exercise and outside the barn, usually in cold weather. Interestingly, the amount of vigorous exercise has no effect upon the development of symptoms.

The alert rider or driver will recognize a change in the horse's attitude and gait. Pain and abundance of sweat associated with the short period of work should be noticed immediately and all work stopped instantly.

Many years of study have shown us that a special group of circumstances must be present for azoturia to develop. A biochemical muscular discord is triggered by exercise of any form that is preceded by a short rest period; usually the victim has been on a high-carbohydrate diet, and is a heavy working horse of the draft or athletic type. The process involves the large muscle masses, which store glycogen for use during exercise. Through habit muscles continue to store glycogen even during rest periods. When exercise is suddenly renewed, an abundance of glycogen is released, creating biochemical imbalance at the cellular level. Varying degrees of muscle destruction result, with large amounts of lactic acid, metabolites, and myoglobin clogging and overloading the vascular system. All of this overload eventually moves to the kidneys for elimination. The blood vessels and kidneys cannot adjust rapidly enough and are subsequently incapacitated.

Urination is painful and what scanty urine appears is tinged red to dark brown in color, due to the presence of myoglobin. This is why for so many years azoturia was incorrectly thought to be kidney disease. The musculature is the primary site of the disease and the kidneys are involved only secondarily through their function of eliminating all the products of muscle destruction.

Should the symptoms present themselves, *stop* the animal immediately, cover with blankets or coolers, and summon veterinary assistance. Do not walk the horse; do not move it one unnecessary step. Allow only the few steps necessary to walk onto a van or trailer or into the stable. Each stride only serves to aggravate an already dangerous situation.

Veterinary treatment will vary depending on the practitioner, but usually it consists of tranquilizers, sedatives, sodium bicarbonate I.V., electrolytes, diuretics. Serum enzyme studies carried out by the nearest laboratory will help predict the course of the disease.

Supportive treatment is of paramount importance. Depending upon the amount of paralysis, a sling for support may be used. Hand massage over main muscle masses, together with the application of a heating pad, is sometimes helpful.

Unfortunately, the outcome is predetermined by the amount of muscle destruction and degree of paralysis, and is also dependent upon whether the horses becomes recumbent (down). The course of disease can vary from two hours to two or three days.

The prognosis is guarded to poor if the animal shows signs of paralysis. If the horse can remain on its feet, the prognosis is then guarded to fair.

Be aware that the symptoms of azoturia and colic are similar. You can always differentiate between the two by remembering that the onset of symptoms of azoturia (or any related myopathy) always manifest itself *outside* the barn and at the *beginning of exercise*. Colic symptoms usually develop *inside the barn* while the horse is *at rest*.

A few additional comments will help you to understand azoturia in lay terms.

1. A broodmare or a young developing animal is never afflicted.
2. A malnourished horse is never afflicted.
3. A nonworking horse is never afflicted.
4. A horse that is never fed large amounts of expensive feeds will never be afflicted. (Azoturia is known as the disease of the rich man's horse.)

To think more positively and "preventively," remember that azoturia is commonly experienced by well-fed, heavily muscled, physically fit work horses or competing animals. Invariably, this disease is associated with ignorance and poor husbandry practices.

To avoid its occurrence, remember:

1. Once a horse has begun a rigid training schedule, you must maintain a steady, carefully supervised balance between exercise and food intake.
2. Exercise daily regardless of weather, a lost shoe, or the absence of a rider or driver. Back-up personnel are essential. No excuses permitted.
3. Adjust food intake with each minute change in physical exertion. If you anticipate less work, *reduce the quantity of concentrates (grain) by 50 percent of normal;* substitute a hot bran mash.

Remember, the fitter the horse becomes, the more vulnerable it is to the ravages of azoturia and the more essential the exercise-diet balance becomes.

If a horse survives an attack of azoturia, an expected sequel to this disease is a condition called *femoral* or *crural paralysis*. The odds of a survivor developing this condition are around 40 to 50 percent.

A severe and permanent hind leg lameness suddenly develops. The horse abruptly refuses to bear weight and has difficulty, even at the walk, advancing the limb. A constantly flexed position of the hind leg when standing is characteristic of this paralysis.

azoturia continued

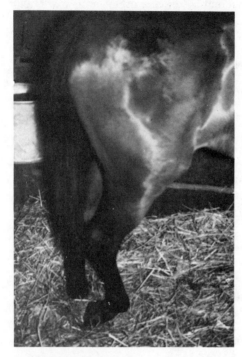

Femoral Paralysis, sequel to azoturia

If muscle tissue was damaged during azoturia, this infringes upon and injures the femoral nerve, subsequently causing paralysis of the muscle group that it innervates.

Treatment is futile and the prognosis is dim.

botulism   *See:* POISONS.

brachygnathia (parrot mouth; overshot jaw; buck-toothed)   An abnormal shortness of the lower jaw (mandible), which allows the upper incisors to grow downward unopposed; the upper jaw (maxilla) thus seems longer, simulating a parrot mouth. Falsely appearing as an overgrown, or "overshot," upper jaw, the maxilla is in fact quite normal! The deformity is in the lower jaw, which suffers a growth aberration of congenital origin, making it undersized and abnormally short.

A jaw condition affecting the upper jaw, also of the congenital origin, is called *prognathia*. This is the same abnormality as in brachygnathia, but affecting the maxilla. It is an abnormal shortness of the upper jaw, causing the lower jaw to appear overly long, or "undershot" (sow mouth).

Both jaw conditions result in dental irregularities, altered mastication, and the potential for gastrointestinal upsets.

An animal with one of these jaw abnormalities is unable to grasp short grasses when grazing, so it can't be treated as a mere member of a normal group. Its survival and health depend upon a favorable environment and the availability of food.

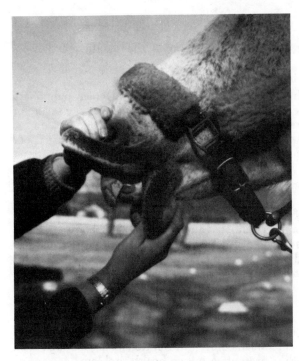

Parrot Mouth (Brachyg-
nathia)

   Constant watchfulness and frequent dental care make it possible for such a
horse to serve well, however. There is no treatment. What little help we can
render consists of running a sterilized horseshoer's rasp horizontally across the
long, overgrown, sharp points of the upper incisors of the parrot mouth, or the
lower incisors of the undershot jaw. Done twice a year, this prevents painful
penetration of lip tissue by the razor-sharp "fangs."
   Dental conditions in the horse are usually well hidden from sight. Before
purchase, you are well advised to carefully lift the horse's lips and look into the
mouth—even if it's a gift horse!

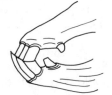

Sow Mouth,
mandibular prognathism

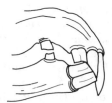

Parrot Mouth,
mandibular brachygnathia

brachygnathia continued

Better still, ask your veterinarian to examine the mouth for signs of abnormality.

bracken fern poisoning *See:* POISONS.

broken wind An old-fashioned term for "heaves," or alveolar pulmonary emphysema. Most often seen in the older horse, it can develop after a severe or neglected case of infectious respiratory disease. More often seen in long-standing, chronic cases due to poor husbandry conditions (dust, poor ventilation, stress, inadequate or unclean housing). *See:* HEAVES, PULMONARY ALVEOLAR EMPHYSEMA.

brucellosis A contagious disease primarily affecting cattle, sheep, and goats, caused by bacteria of the *Brucella* group and noted for causing abortion, orchitis, and increased incidence of infertility.

Although cattle are commonly afflicted and horses to a much lesser extent, the disease presents two such diverse groups of symptoms that it is hard to believe that they are caused by the same micro-organism. (The micro-organisms and their targets are: *B. abortus*—cattle, horses, rarely goats; *B. melitensis*—goats; *B. suis*—hogs.)

In cattle, brucellosis is called *Bang's disease,* after the doctor who first isolated the causative factor. In a bovine population the affected animals become systematically ill and inefficient in reproduction, but the disease does not always stop there; it can directly affect human beings, transmitted mainly through meat and milk consumption. It thus presents a public health problem.

All cases of this very serious infection must be reported. State-mandated control measures include continuous blood testing and a rigidly enforced vaccination schedule in *all* cattle. These are necessary evils, if the disease is to be eradicated.

With much less frequency, brucellosis is seen in the horse with totally different characteristics from the bovine form. For some reason, these micro-organisms show an affinity for two areas of the horse's body. One is the poll, at the location of the supra-atlantal bursa (between the ears). Here bursitis develops accompanied by an infection called "poll evil." The second area is the withers, site of the supraspinous bursa. An infected condition here is called "fistulous withers." Brucellosis micro-organisms frequently are isolated from these deep, well-established infections, and the abscesses are resistant to treatment.

With the advent of antibiotics, incidences of these two undesirable infections are rare these days. However, any infected area involving either the poll or the withers in any horse, or in any barn, should alert you to the possibility that the fearsome brucella micro-organism might be present. The risk is appreciably increased if the horse grazes near beef cattle or is stabled in or near a dairy barn. If there is any question of brucellosis, call your veterinarian, who will undoubtedly take a routine diagnostic blood sample and submit it to the laboratory for evidence of a brucellosis antibody titre. When cleansing and treating the area as directed by your veterinarian, wear gloves to protect yourself. Warn all others to stay away from the animal until the blood test results are known.

Brucellosis in the equine, once identified, can be successfully treated with antibiotics. A properly timed vaccination with Strain #19 has proved to be a satisfactory follow-up measure when the micro-organism is discovered in a horse member of the barn.

Early in the twentieth century, "hunchbacked" people were a common sight and seemed indiscriminate as to age group. It is now thought that they were suffering from the long-standing effects of undulant fever, a human manifestation of brucellosis.

Rarely is this crippling deformity seen today. Credit must be given to both state and federal health agencies for a successful program of regulatory control.

It was also common for bovine veterinarians to develop undulant fever in its various forms. As a child I knew three practitioners who learned to live with the intermittent attacks of fever, pain, and weakness by using the then-new antibiotics; these three doctors managed to live well into their eighties. Today, I know of no veterinarian who has this incurable infection.

buck-tooth   *See:* BRACHYGNATHIA.

canker   A chronic hypertrophy (increased tissue production) of the tissues of the foot creating a characteristic fetid odor. Unlike thrush, it involves not only the frog, but the entire sole and wall, and may result in separation of the horny tissue from the sensitive laminae.

Canker is most often seen in draft breeds, with the hind feet commonly affected. No specific cause has been identified, but it is thought to be husbandry-related, since the affected animals usually stand in straight stalls with a build-up of bacteria-laden bedding, soiled with urine and feces, under the hind feet.

Treatment consists of surgical removal of the putrid material from the foot followed by the application of pressure bandages saturated with an antibiotic solution or healing powder.

We see little canker today, now that draft horses have largely been replaced by motorized vehicles. In former years, however, when these big horses were confined in standing stalls of questionable cleanliness or tied in one position, canker was a common source of pain, lameness, and incapacity to work. Old-fashioned veterinarians routinely supervised the farrier's crude removal of excess tissue in the feet, followed by bandaging the entire sole and foot with a pack soaked in a 10 percent formaldehyde solution. As a youngster, I saw horses so much improved by this severe treatment that they were able to return to work; it seemed to work faster than today's less severe methods. But when I ponder how they used strong iodine with formaldehyde in those days, I wonder that the sensitive areas of the foot (coronary band and heel area) were not irreparably damaged.

Currently we treat and inhibit canker so that the horse is usable, but we cannot completely cure the condition once it is established in the foot tissues.

circling disease   *See:* LISTERIOSIS.

colic   A nonspecific term defined as a pain in the abdomen.

Who among us shares the burden of the 100-foot length of intestine that belongs to our friend, the horse? Anything that causes interruption of peristalsis (normal intestinal movement), or even a slowing or hastening of the intestine's contents, can cause mechanical colic by exerting pressure on the intestinal wall.

colic continued

It certainly presents a challenge for the veterinarian to determine the affected site in the gastrointestinal tract, the cause, and the appropriate treatment.

The types of colic are synonymous with their cause: chill, circulatory, gas, heat, impaction, mechanical, sand, and stress.

Other causes may be interrelated: enteroliths, fermented ingesta, parasites, and poisons. Neglected sharp teeth can also be a factor in colic.

Associated vices: bolting grain, cribbing, temperament, and windsucking.

Colic is a frequent companion, acting as a symptom, in other specific conditions: azoturia, myopathies (muscle disorders, such as eclampsia), founder (acute or chronic), poison cases, and high fevers from any cause. In fact, colic symptoms can be seen in almost any systemic disorder.

Obviously a horse can fall victim to colic for many reasons and from various causes, but please note that, excluding some genetic cause, an inseparable factor in freedom from colic is the daily basic, fundamentally sound husbandry provided by the owner or caretaker. *See:* CONSTIPATION, IMPACTION.

colic mixture *See:* TURCAPSOL.

colitis X An often fatal disease of rapid onset and unknown etiology. Characterized by profuse diarrhea, sweating, abdominal pain, rapid heart rate, and weakened pulse rate, followed inevitably by shock syndrome. Death ensues shortly.

The cause is yet to be documented, but we strongly suspect that a special set of circumstances must be present for colitis X to develop. A common denominator does exist. The victim usually is an athletic horse that at some point, from a week to ten days after recovering from an illness (usually respiratory infection with high fever), is through ignorance subjected to some form of physical stress and exhaustion (competition, exercise, or vanning). With stress, sudden symptoms of colitis X appear and the awesome challenge of treatment presents itself! All veterinarians have learned to recognize this syndrome!

An indwelling I.V. catheter is established in the large jugular vein and taped into place around the neck, and the prescribed replacement fluids are started flowing and kept flowing for 24 to 48 hours on a round-the-clock basis. The profound fluid and electrolyte loss due to diarrhea and sweating must be matched (via I.V. injections and the nasogastric tube) or the affected animal will dehydrate and succumb. Steroids are used to combat stress as well as massive dosages of sodium bicarbonate to neutralize the acidosis normally caused by any illness.

Even with all stops pulled out, once the symptoms are established, the losses far outnumber the survivors.

constipation Condition characterized by bowel movements that are infrequent, hard and/or dry in consistency and texture, and expelled with difficulty.

Constipation should be suspected if a horse, in an extremely clean, dry stall, shows low-grade intermittent pain (colic), coupled with a history of dullness and lethargy.

Treatment by the owner:

1. Offer a wet bran mash.

2. Give 6 ounces of heavy white mineral oil by means of an oral syringe.

3. Hand walk periodically until the veterinarian arrives; if the horse begins to roll, walk it continually until help comes.

The veterinarian will undoubtedly inject a pain killer (analgesic) or a smooth-muscle relaxant (Dipyrone), and then carefully examine the horse. A cathartic added to a large volume of heavy-grade white mineral oil will be administered via stomach tube. If impaction is diagnosed, the doctor may choose to perform a rectal examination to determine the location of the sluggish intestinal contents and the general condition of the intestinal wall. Administration of an electrolyte solution I.V. to restore lost fluids and essential minerals is a very popular treatment in constipation and impaction cases; the added fluids seem to benefit the immobile area.

Veterinary program of treatment:

1. Analgesic and/or tranquilizer to reduce anxiety and discomfort

2. Rectal examination for diagnosis and prognosis purposes

3. Stomach tube—used for possible release of any gas trapped in the stomach and for administration of cathartics, laxatives, emollients, electrolytes, sodium bicarbonate, and replacement fluid

4. Electrolytes intravenously to treat dehydration in protracted cases through restoration of fluids

5. Enema—helpful in some cases to restore some degree of peristalsis; should not be done too often since it can irritate the intestinal and rectal mucosa

I have found that some constipation (impaction) cases can persist in spite of treatment for from 24 hours to four or five days. Surgical intervention is sometimes, though not frequently, the only alternative for saving the life of an extensively impacted horse. This is a veterinary judgment. I have found that vigorous fluid therapy and intravenous electrolyte replacement have dramatically affected and profoundly shortened recovery periods in some of my difficult constipation cases. Oral, rectal, and intravenous routes of treatment usually bring a response.

Whether it is simple constipation or serious impaction, the condition definitely reflects poor husbandry practices. To prevent this malady, provide:

1. Regular exercise

2. Balanced diet, including wheat bran mashes

3. Adequate hay and water

4. Salt lick at all times

5. Parasite control

If your horse suffers repeated bouts of intestinal discomfort, please discuss this with your veterinarian. It is not normal; seek advice. *See:* D-S-S.

crural paralysis *See:* AZOTURIA.

cryptorchidism A failure of the testicles to descend normally into the scrotal sacs, being retained instead in the inguinal canal, inguinal ring, or abdomen. In monorchidism, only one testicle is descended, which usually appears quite large. The individual in this case is fertile.

When both testes are retained, the animal is sterile and can appear as a gelding although not behaving as one, especially in the company of other horses.

cryptorchidism continued

A retained testicle is always defective in development, appearing smaller, softer, and obviously imperfect in comparison with the normally descended testes. This testicle cannot produce spermatozoa, but it is capable of producing the hormone testosterone, responsible for sexual aggressiveness (libido). At times, undescended testes can secrete excessive amounts of male hormones which can stimulate nervousness, irritability, and increased libido resulting in a subtle but hazardous problem of tractability and management.

A horse that exhibits descent problems to any degree—no matter how superb an individual he may be—should never be used for breeding purposes, since this condition has been well documented as an inherited characteristic. Most breed registries prohibit the use of these defective individuals as breeding stallions and candidly encourage castration, which is the expedient and prudent solution. If properly performed it not only relieves the horse of discomfort, and perhaps of gait problems, but it also precludes the possibility of reproducing this genetic characteristic. It has been my experience that a stallion with this problem never seems to reach his full potential in the competition world until after castration.

Don't be hasty in judging testicles as retained until after 18 months of age, for they have been known to appear suddenly and be as "normal as blueberry pie."

Injections to aid the descent of testicles have varied rates of success. Small doses of chorionic gonadotrophic hormone, administered over long periods of time, have been reported as helpful, though only moderately encouraging.

There exists an unscrupulous practice, that of removing the one visible testicle of a monorchid horse while leaving the retained testicle covertly in place. The horse is then a false gelding; it appears as a gelding, but it has a potential for aggressiveness and unpredictable behavior, possibly presenting a danger to all involved. This practice is unethical; I consider it almost criminal.

To diagnose a possible cryptorchid, there are four steps:

1. Thorough external physical examination of genital organs: scrotum, inguinal canal, inguinal ring
2. Rectal examination of complete pelvic area for evidence of retained testicle
3. Injection of human chorionic gonadotropin (HCG) intravenously to provoke a response from the hidden gland in the form of increased testosterone levels within 15 minutes of the initial injection
4. Exploratory surgery to retrieve the testis.

No treatment for cryptorchidism, other than total castration, has ever been successful in my equine practice. After castration, all these horses are normal, well-adjusted, useful individuals.

Cushing's syndrome   A condition caused by a pituitary gland tumor resulting in subsequent enlargement of the adrenal gland. Found in older horses, and more frequently in mares.

Diagnostic symptoms are hirsutism (an abnormally heavy coat with long, wavy hairs), muscle wasting, excessive thirst and urination, and profuse but intermittent sweating.

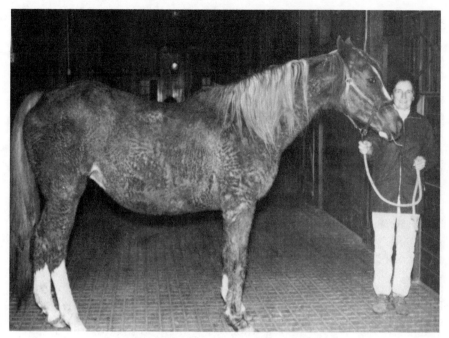

Cushing's Syndrome, also called hirsutism

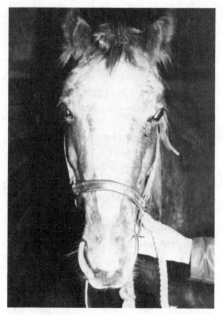

Wavy Coat and Swollen Eyes

Cushing's syndrome continued

It is believed that this strange failure of the animal to "shed out," without regard to season or temperature, may be the first clinical sign of the tumor's presence. Such horses characteristically grow long, wavy coats.

No practical approach to successful treatment has yet been found. (In human beings, surgical removal of the adrenal glands and radiation treatment of the pituitary gland have become almost routine since the 1960s.) Prognosis is poor.

diarrhea An abnormally frequent discharge of watery fecal matter from the bowel. Changes in the character and consistency of fecal material should never be discounted. Diarrhea in adults is caused by parasitism, infections, or mechanical means (e.g., diet, eating manure). A complete physical examination and a fecal analysis is important to identify the cause (i.e., protozoal, fungal, or bacterial). *See:* TRICHOMONIASIS.

eclampsia There are two types: *grass tetany*, seen in work horses, and *lactation tetany*, seen in broodmares. Both involve a mineral deficit (magnesium and calcium), and are characterized by muscle spasms and sweating. Any stressful circumstance imposed upon a horse that is living on a diet of lush grass can produce eclampsia with its clinical symptoms of rigidity and tremors.

Grass tetany is not often seen today in our light breeds of horses. It was most commonly observed in the era when heavy draft horses were used, and it received its name "tetany" from its overt symptoms. The term "railroad disease" was coined to describe a condition developed by these large-muscled, soft breeds that were taken from their grass pasturage and abruptly loaded onto trains where they often stayed for days under unnatural conditions. More died than we will ever know.

Muscle spasms, tremors, sweating, and heavy breathing signal an attack of eclampsia in a work horse that is removed from a grain diet and turned out to pasture. It is caused by a sudden decrease of calcium and magnesium levels in the blood when these large animals are fed on rough pasture only. Rapid treatment with calcium and magnesium replacement (usually I.V.) brings about a prompt recovery.

Another form of eclampsia, lactation tetany, is seen in broodmares shortly after foaling. It is due to lowered blood calcium (hypocalcemia). Symptoms are muscle rigidity, uneasiness, and inability to rise after parturition accompanied by profuse sweating and great anxiety. These mares will panic if not promptly treated. Physical support and mild sedation are suggested.

Treatment of 20 percent calcium gluconate I.V. reverses the distress and brings about a quick recovery.

emphysema (heaves) Distention and loss of elasticity of lung tissue, accompanied by inability to empty the lungs of air. Expiration then is possible only by the combined effort of the abdominal muscles and the diaphragm. *See:* PULMONARY ALVEOLAR EMPHYSEMA.

encephalitis (sleeping sickness) A viral inflammation of the brain tissues caused by arboviral infection. There are several forms of arboviruses that attack horses; all produce similar symptoms and require vectors (flying, biting, and sucking insects) to transmit the usually fatal diseases. Encephalitis, then, is infectious, but not contagious; it can be transmitted only by an insect carrier under favorable conditions.

Arboviruses winter over in wild animals, especially in birds (pigeons and pheasants), who serve as reservoirs. Mosquitoes feed on the birds and, after an incubation period, bite the horse, which ultimately contracts encephalitis and promptly succumbs. These same mosquitoes also bite humans, who similarly are "dead-end hosts." The disease is equally fatal in people.

The four types of equine encephalomyelitis are: Eastern (EEE); Western (WEE); Venezuelan (VEE); and Japanese (JEE). Eastern is the most lethal form and Japanese the least lethal.

It is interesting that while we have an effective vaccine against equine encephalitis, as yet, in spite of numerous human deaths each year, we have *no* vaccine for preventing the disease in humans. *See:* ARBORVIRUS.

encephalomalacia (moldy corn poisoning, fodder disease) Softening of the brain cells caused by a neurotoxic agent. Encephalomalacia is sometimes listed under *mycotoxicosis,* a lethal toxicity produced by a fungus or mold.

Cows, goats, and sheep can tolerate some mold, but horses none at all. Mold in any form found in feed, hay, or straw can be fatal if ingested by a horse. Moldy corn or fodder are common sources of the deadly neurotoxin.

Early but well-developed symptoms are muscle tremors, weakness, constipation (colicky), and—most telling—the inability to swallow; the animal cannot eat or drink. As the disease progresses, other salient symptoms are walking in circles, depression, and lowered head position. Icterus (yellowing of the membranes of the eyes and mouth), combined with head pressing, usually in the corner and against the wall of the stall, are characteristic symptoms caused by the destructive action of the neurotoxin on the liver.

Treatment is very unsatisfactory even when heroic measures are applied. Every supportive therapy should be offered: nutrients and activated charcoal or emollients via stomach tube; fluid replacement orally or I.V.; electrolytic and acid-base I.V. therapy.

With any case of poisonous-substance ingestion, the sobering truth is that the outcome is decided by the initial amount of poison ingested! Unlike human medicine, where victims of poisoning are saved by immediate measures, veterinarians cannot apply stomach pumps and other emergency procedures in time because they usually do not see their poison cases until hours after the ingestion occurs, or until irreversible symptoms appear and are first recognized. Death usually occurs in from three to four days regardless of treatment. Necropsy shows liver changes and encephalomacia (brain tissue reduced to almost liquid consistency).

Prevention is the only hope. Eliminate all evidence of mold. Never permit a horse's nose or mouth to come near *any* substance that even remotely smells like, is suggestive of, or appears to resemble *mold!*

epistaxis (nosebleed) Hemorrhage from the nose has many causes and can have its source at many locations within the entire respiratory tract. Nosebleed is most often seen immediately after a race or during the following cooling-out period. Endoscopic examinations immediately post-race have confirmed the presence of lung bleeding in as many as 60 percent of race horses in the United States.

After years of research, the latest available information points to lung hemorrhage as the most common source of blood, although every area, from the

epistaxis continued

nose to the pharynx and guttural pouches and on through the larynx, trachea, and into the bronchi, has been investigated and suspected as the site of hemorrhage in race horses. How to treat bleeders successfully remains questionable; to date, no treatment has proved specific.

1. A detailed blood analysis is worthwhile to determine whether defective fibrinogen or a decreased number of platelets (thrombocytes) is present in such horses. Some trainers nebulize horses with thromboplastin prior to racing. (*Nebulize* means to break up a liquid into a fine spray or vapor that is directed through a hose into the horse's nostrils for therapeutic purposes.) Thromboplastin is found naturally in the blood and is thought to aid in coagulation.

2. Daily therapy of rutin and vitamins E and C (ascorbic acid) may be helpful. Rutin, a flavonoid found in buckwheat, seems to increase capillary resistance.

3. Rest after hemorrhage is certainly indicated to permit the ruptured tissues to heal.

4. Protecting the horse from extreme cold or intense heat during physical exertion is suggested. Competing during times of moderate temperature and allowing longer healing periods between races is certainly sensible in cases of known bleeders.

5. Lasix, a diuretic, has been used extensively on consistent bleeders with some evidence of improvement. However, there are no scientific data to prove that the use of Lasix is beneficial.

Horses that suffer varying degrees of lung hemorrhage with each major exertion and without external evidence (no bleeding from the nose) are called "silent bleeders." These individuals commonly compete poorly, require protracted periods to cool out and fully recover, and are definitely at risk. *See:* LASIX.

eye   The eye of the horse is subject to traumatic injury and infectious disease.

Excluding injuries to the eyelid, cornea, or other structures, the most common eye problem found in the horse is recurrent uveitis, an inflammation of the uveal tract located in the structures that surround and incorporate the ocular globe. The uveal tract comprises three vital components of the eye: the iris, easily visible to the naked eye; the ciliary body, hidden under and behind the iris; and the choroid coat, a midlayer that encapsulates the entire eye between the outer sclera coat and the retina, the sensitive inner surface of the globe.

The uveal tract is hypersensitive to trauma and systemic diseases. It vigorously responds to irritants with fullblown inflammatory changes—tearing, blinking, cloudy cornea, closed pupil, softening of tissue tone.

The horse seems very vulnerable to two major known causes of uveitis, the diseases *leptospirosis* and *onchocerciasis,* the former caused by a spirochete and the latter by microfilariae (worms)—both parasitic.

The illustration of the eye outlines the uveal tract, the site of the inflammation popularly known as "moonblindness."

The efficiency of the tear ducts in draining away excess fluid often is compromised. Respiratory infections cause additional production of exudates and tissue debris and often result in blockage or incomplete patency of the nasolacrimal canal, causing typical symptoms. An overflow at the inner corner of the eye, close to the third eyelid, produces an irritating stream of tears that stains the horse's face and causes loss of hair.

Treatment consists of flushing the ducts with isotonic saline solution and establishing an open tube for normal drainage. The flushing is followed with instillation of a mild, soothing ophthalmic ointment. Precise yet tender care is essential.

See: LEPTOSPIROSIS, ONCHOCERCA CERVICALIS, RECURRENT UVEITIS.

fainting *See:* SYNCOPE.

femoral nerve paralysis *See:* AZOTURIA.

fever versus normal body temperature The normal body temperature of an individual horse is judged according to its sex, size, weight, and age. Other considerations are time of day, amount of exercise, and time elapsed since the last meal. Some mares normally show a mild increase in body temperature during the estrus period.

An old and accurate rule of thumb: The larger the animal, the lower the temperature and slower the heart rate.

Foal	101°–101.5°
Yearling	100°–100.5°
Two-Year-Old	99°–100.5°
Adult	98°–99.5°

fistula *See:* BURSITIS.

founder *See:* LAMINITIS.

galls (girth sores, saddle sores) Caused by friction between the horse and an ill-fitting harness or saddle, such sores are the obvious result of improperly adjusted or badly constructed equipment; poor riding is often an aggravating factor.

Symptoms are swelling, heat, and tender areas found directly under the saddle. Rest and the application of cooling agents (poultices, cool packs, fuller's earth, or hosing) are indicated.

If a horse suffers repeated episodes of galling on the withers or back, not only swelling, heat, and pain result, but actual necrosis (tissue death) as well. A "sit fast," a small, hard cutaneous callus, develops which can only be removed surgically, requiring a long period of recuperation. White hairs on the withers are evidence of a previous saddle sore.

It is my opinion that saddle galls and sores of any kind reflect ignorance and neglect by the people in charge.

gangrene Following necrosis (dying of cells in a live body), gangrene develops by the invasion of saprophytic bacteria (bacteria that live on dead cells) into the necrotic or dying tissue.

Inflammation is present; a red zone develops between living cells and dead tissue as the necrotic area steadily sheds away or sloughs off. A characteristic odor is evidence that gangrene exists.

Call your veterinarian immediately. No wound should be so neglected that necrosis and gangrene are able to develop.

glanders (farcy) A highly contagious and fatal disease of both horses and humans. In the horse it is characterized by ulcers in the respiratory tract and weeping nodules on the legs and lower abdomen. *Pseudomonas mallei* (malleomyces mallei) is the causative micro-organism.

glanders continued

Acute symptoms are high fever and profuse mucous nasal discharge, with the skin nodules and ulcers appearing later in the disease. After an incubation period of two weeks, the animal falls sick with bronchopneumonia. Those cases that survive usually become carriers and can only be detected and diagnosed by the use of a blood test or the mallein test.

P. mallei is easily destroyed by sunlight and heat, but it can remain viable for long periods in damp and dirty areas. Disinfectants such as benzalkonium chloride, mercuric chloride, and iodine are effective. Surprisingly, phenol (carbolic acid) and Lysol are not useful.

Cutaneous glanders (farcy) is the form found on the skin of the hind legs and lower abdomen; it can be the result of direct infection or be secondary to pneumonia.

Oral ingestion of contaminated grain, hay, or pasturage is thought to be the main route of transmission. The purulent discharge from the nose and the leg nodules is very infectious, as are the feces and urine.

Diagnosis is based on a blood test (complement-fixation), or on an intradermal injection into the skin of the neck or an injection into the conjunctiva of the eyelid. Reactions to the injections, when read by an experienced veterinarian, indicate whether or not the animal is a carrier. All carriers should be destroyed and the premises thoroughly disinfected after imposing a quarantine.

Glanders is one of the oldest known diseases of horses and was found worldwide for many years. Through great effort, sacrifice, and expense, glanders has been eliminated in the United States and in most other countries, but be aware that it has *not* been eradicated! All must be alert that a carrier could be imported and introduced at any time. Obviously, this disease is high on the inspectors' list of "ones to watch." All imports are routinely quarantined and subjected to blood and mallein tests before they are allowed to enter the United States.

Euthanasia is indicated, because treatment is unreliable and usually results in the animal being a "carrier." The hazard that glanders presents to other horses and to public health precludes any attempt at treatment.

If this seems an extreme solution, consider the following story.

While attending the school of veterinary medicine, I became friendly with my professor of medicine. Formerly dean of a veterinary school in Austria, he had fled from the invading Nazis and come to the United States. He was a sincere and enthusiastic teacher with a great depth of knowledge to offer.

One day, when his equine lectures turned to the subject of glanders, the professor's face became somber, and he began to relate a true story about this dreaded disease. (Understand that glanders is particularly insidious because it can appear as a simple, noninfectious skin disease, requiring no precautions against transmission or infection.) The professor told of how he had once taken a test-tube specimen from a horse with ulcerative weeping nodules on the hind legs. The sample was delivered by messenger to the laboratory assistants. A few days later, as the professor waited for the results of the culture, he heard that the delivery boy was very ill. Then, he heard that the two laboratory men also were sick. All three died within ten days. Tears filled the professor's eyes as he finished his story. He himself had not been taken ill, but he lived with the guilt of having fatally exposed the three innocent people. This was the first time in my veterinary medical education that I understood the debt we owe to the courageous men and women who preceded us in dealing with diseases capable of causing death to both humans and animals.

This incident took place in the 1920s in Austria, well before the disease was fully recognized and years before the advent of antibiotics. Today we have effective broad-spectrum antibiotics capable of destroying and containing the spread of this once life-threatening infection. Ulcerative lymphangitis and epizootic lymphangitis both simulate glanders, but glanders, to repeat, has not been eradicated. Veterinarians must keep a watchful eye for suspect cases and constantly make differential diagnoses.

Through the efforts of regulatory medicine, through its constant surveillance, quarantining, and testing, supported by the government, the United States is kept comparatively free of many deadly diseases. But with international boundaries being crossed with ever greater frequency and speed, the job of the people in regulatory medicine has become more difficult than ever. We owe them our full cooperation.

granulation tissue The basic tissue that fills the gap in a wound after normal tissue injury, progressing during the periods of regeneration and repair. Granulation tissue consists of fibroblast cells, loose connective tissue, and an abundance of capillaries. This produces a bloody and reddish granular mass devoid of nerve tissue. If healing progresses without infection, the angry tissue will then shrink, turn pale, and form a scar (cicatrix).

The horse is notorious for producing granulation tissue in any open wound, but especially in leg wounds, and it seems that excessive amounts will develop in a healing wound if formation of the tissue is allowed to continue uninhibited. What is known as "summer sore" is excessive granulation tissue.

When faced with a wound on a horse—one perhaps that was sutured and has dehisced, one that was initially impossible to suture, or one that was just plain neglected—first recognize that it must heal by *secondary intention*, which means that granulation tissue must fill in the gaping area and then, if all goes well, some epithelial tissue might attempt to cross over the scar bed.

In the cases of a wound irritated by an infection or contamination, granulation tissue will begin to form in the deficit area, but it will appear very red, moist, and irregular in shape. In this situation, first exclude the presence of fever or the need for antibiotic injections, then "hose" the area with intermittent warm and cool water for 30 minutes two or three times daily. Warm water is well known to promote the production of granulation tissue. If possible, between hosing periods, apply warm-water bandages to the area. By using water and keeping the area warm with bandages, in a matter of five to seven days, you should see beautiful pink healthy granulation tissue filling the gap or indentation.

As soon as healthy pink granulation begins and establishes a firm bed, even with the skin edges, *stop the hosing and cease all water*. Begin daily application of caustic powder under dressings. Caustic powder not only burns away excessive granulation tissue, it also irritates and indirectly stimulates the wound edges into activity, so that the epithelial layer may begin some degree of closure.

granulation tissue continued

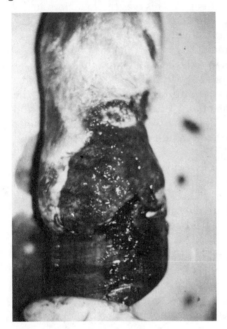

Excessive Granulation Tissue   **Excessive Granulation Tissue**

Lightly rub the wound surface with a sterile gauze sponge each day before applying caustic powder with a sterile dressing.

Of course, the ideal situation is to have your horse's wound sutured and thus healed by *first intention,* but in the situation described above, you must do what you can.

It is very gratifying to see how this old and proven regime can aid in healing the wound, minimizing the scar, and improving the appearance of the entire leg. *See:* CAUSTIC POWDER.

grass tetany   *See:* ECLAMPSIA.

grease   A chronic dermatitis in the heels of heavy work horses with long pastern hairs. Most commonly found in the hind legs and thought to be caused by filth, debris, and dirty bedding. "Grease" is not often seen today. This condition can be painful and if untreated can cause the development of a crusty type of skin.

Treatment consists of hygienic and sanitary practices along with heel scrubbing and application of antibiotic ointments. *See:* MANGE.

guttural pouch infection   The guttural pouch is a large sac interposed in the Eustachian tube that connects the middle ear with the pharynx. On each side of the pharyngeal wall is a flap-like valve that opens wide with each respiration, admitting air into the Eustachian tube and guttural pouch. The function of the guttural pouches is not fully understood, but it is thought to have a bearing on equilibrium and even on hearing.

Guttural pouches frequently become infected and inflamed and sometimes distended with fluid, pus, chondroids, or just plain air. Pharyngitis, laryngitis, and all forms of infection can easily gain access to the Eustachian tubes through the orifices in the sidewalls of the pharynx. Microbes, dust, and debris can ascend the tubes and enter the sacs, then become walled off inside, giving rise to infection. *Streptococcus equi* (cause of strangles) frequently is found in these areas. Mycotic (fungal) infections flourish in the guttural pouches and are not only difficult to diagnose and treat, but are quite destructive to the surrounding tissue. Most veterinarians are aware of the serious threat posed by mycotic infections.

Symptoms of guttural pouch infection are (1) lowered head carriage, especially during grazing or after hard strenuous exertion, and (2) a one-side nasal discharge of mucus, sometimes with a blood-tinged exudate. External swelling, difficulty in swallowing, and sore throat are nonspecific symptoms.

Diagnosis can be confirmed by a fiberoptic endoscopic examination that allows viewing the entire area inside the upper respiratory tract. Evidence of swelling, inflammation, and, in some cases, discharge in and around the entrance to the Eustachian tube is diagnostic.

Treatment consists of guiding a small tube with an angled tip into the small pharyngeal opening, under direct view through the endoscope (the scope makes it possible to see precisely where the catheter tube is directed). Medicine is then flushed through the catheter into the pouches and therapeutic drainage is next stimulated, sometimes producing dramatic results. Cultures can be obtained at this time for the purpose of identifying the causative agent (bacterial, fungal, or air).

When air is trapped in the guttural pouches, the condition is called *tympanitis,* or *tympany*. It sometimes happens that a young foal that has been whinnying and screaming due to stress or fright suddenly has its guttural pouches so distended with air that its face and neck are physically distorted. Although it is a painless condition, the foal will seem distressed and uncomfortable. The distension is caused by a one-sided valve-like action seen in the underdeveloped Eustachian-tube opening in foals. The back pressure exerted from within the pouches only serves to seal the opening, thus preventing the air from escaping. When a tiny catheter is admitted, air escapes in a great rush. For an individual with recurring tympany, surgical removal of the one-way valve-action flaps is indicated. This allows air to move freely in and out of the Eustachian tube and guttural pouch.

Surgery also is used to treat the enlarged, pus-filled guttural pouches sometimes seen in adult horses. Relief can be achieved by surgically lancing the huge infected sacs and draining the purulent material, which usually is caused by the bacterium *Strep equi* or, in more serious cases, by mycotic infections (aspergillosis). The incision site is in the jowl area called Viborg's triangle. The surgeon must have an expert knowledge of the horse's anatomy in order to locate and enter the deeply situated guttural pouch. The engorged pouch is somewhat elevated and permits drainage without impinging upon the vital nerves, vessels, and glands that are densely arranged in this area.

The incidences of guttural pouch surgery have been steadily reduced with the development and availability of improved antibiotics. Of course, another factor in reducing the number of highly infectious respiratory diseases has been the prudent and regular use of respiratory vaccinations. Preventive medicine is infinitely superior! *See:* VIBORG'S TRIANGLE.

heaves (broken wind)   A disease or condition in horses characterized by a difficult expiration of the air trapped in the lungs and often accompanied with an enlargement of the lungs and heart in long-standing cases. *See:* PULMONARY ALVEOLAR EMPHYSEMA.

hematoma   Escaped blood from a ruptured vessel confined in a mass of fluctuating swelling under the skin; found usually in the large muscles.

Trauma from a kick or bite is the common cause of hematoma development. Although most hematomas are painless, they sometimes do create a cumbersome mechanical inconvenience. It is upsetting to the owner to see a large fluctuating swelling hanging from the horse's body. Most owners are disappointed when I explain that there is nothing I can do to reduce the mass and that quiet rest is indicated.

No matter how ugly or disfiguring a hematoma may be, intervention is not indicated—except perhaps to prescribe a coagulant along with inactivity. Infection is only a minimal concern, since there is no break in the skin surface. After 14 days, during which the massive blood collection "organizes," or becomes firm, the animal can safely be exercised; the hematoma will gradually "wrinkle" and slowly disappear by resorption.

Aspiration (withdrawing the contents with a syringe and needle) is strongly contraindicated for two reasons:

1. When blood is withdrawn, the leaking vessel continues to pour blood into the skin sac until the pressure of the skin wall equals the blood pressure of the faulty vessel. All bleeding then ceases and coagulation can occur.

2. A puncture through the skin is necessary when aspirating blood, which automatically creates a portal of entry for micro-organisms. Infection then becomes a true threat.

Please abide, keep your patience, and allow a hematoma both time and rest!

Aside from the regular hematoma just described, I continue to see, with increasing frequency, what are termed "calcified hematomas." These are small calcium masses found in and around joint spaces and tendon sheaths which can only be discovered and identified by taking X-rays of the suspected areas. It is believed that this condition reflects a chronic state whereby calcium settles out into small blood masses in these critical areas. It is believed further that the tendency is the result of inexpert placement of needles, most likely during the intra-articular or intrasynovial injections. The presence of calcified hematomas should cause red faces among some equine practitioners.

hernia (rupture)   The protrusion of an organ or tissue through the wall of the abdomen in the horse.

Types of hernias seen in young horses consist of umbilical, inguinal, and scrotal, all of which are congenital in origin and fortunately lend themselves well to surgical correction.

Occasionally, a hernia in the abdominal wall is seen, not of congenital origin but caused by physical trauma. Here again surgery is indicated.

An "incisional hernia" is one that develops after surgery where the suture lines did not adequately secure the tissues as intended. This requires surgical intervention and reapposition of the tissue layers.

I have repaired literally thousands of hernias, especially on foals, and find

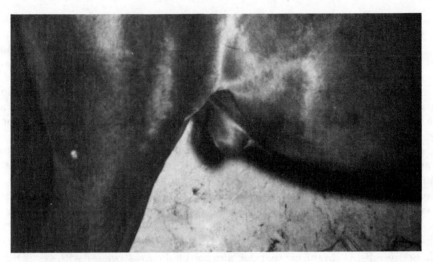

Umbilical Hernia

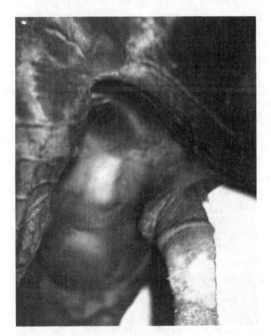

Scrotal Hernia in Stallion

the surgical procedure satisfactory in every respect and certainly superior to the various nonsurgical procedures for correcting hernias (belly bands, pressure tapes, taped skin, blisters over the area, wooden clamps tied with cords, etc.). Although the expense to owners is somewhat more than they would pay for one of the haphazard arrangements, most are more than happy to co-operate when they are assured of a healthy, sound, "hernia-free" foal.

hernia continued

A word of advice concerning hernias: Please consult your veterinarian, who is best equipped to assess the seriousness of a hernia, whether any abdominal contents are enclosed, and the degree of urgency for correction. In certain cases, hernias can present a potential hazard: if the abdominal ring opening is enlarged (larger than two fingers); if the contents are intestines; if the contents are irreducible (that is, if they do not move back into the abdomen upon manipulation); and if there is any possibility of strangulation. All these factors will be weighed and determined by your veterinarian; do listen. But do not listen to lay advice or lay treatments. Your young animal deserves better! *See:* HERNIORRHAPHY.

hirsutism Excessive growth of wavy hair in older individuals. Increased thirst with excessively large volumes of urine accompany the long wavy coat. *See:* CUSHING'S SYNDROME.

hydrophobia *See:* RABIES.

hypothyrodism In the horse, this condition has been associated with dermatitis of unknown or mysterious causes, obesity, laminitis (founder), and chronically lame, tender-soled horses. Any chunky built, lethargic, obese horse or pony, or any horse of the "easy keeper" type should be suspected of hypothyroidism. Although not popularly accepted, a breed predisposition definitely exists (Quarter Horses, Morgans, the draft breeds, ponies, and pet horses of all kinds).

A protein-bound iodine blood test (PBI$_2$) is used to reveal the functional status of the horse's thyroid gland. This simple blood test, a comparatively recent development, has greatly helped the practitioner to uncover the benign cause of skin problems, laminitis, and obscure, inexplicable foot tenderness. Even cases of infertility benefit by adjustments in the thyroid-gland activity.

Symptoms in the young (usually acute): slow or reduced skeletal growth and delayed ossification; joint changes; flabby muscles; dry coat; poor condition, unthrifty, and underdeveloped.

Symptoms in the adult (usually chronic): lethargy; excessive body fat; no muscle tone; rough coat; slowed metabolic rate; tendency toward laminitis attacks; intermittent lamenesses; low PBI$_2$ (1.5–2.0 meg percent; normal 4.0 meg percent).

Hypothyroidism is of unknown etiology, although hereditary predisposition is suspected.

Treatment calls for thyroid extract orally on a daily basis, as prescribed by your veterinarian. This can bring about a pleasant change.

CAUTION: Once you start administering the medicine, never allow it to run out or abruptly cease giving it. Aim for a gradual reduction of the daily dose over a long period of time and under the supervision of your veterinarian.

It has been my experience to find, over the years, a large number of good-looking, well-kept horses (usually gentle-natured and overweight) with a history of undiagnosed intermittent lameness in both fore feet. Under close examination of the feet and legs, I find evidence of minute touches of laminitis, much to the owner's surprise and dismay. Radiographs, in some cases, show a slight posterior rotation of the os pedis (coffin bone), but almost *all* these animals show a low PBI$_2$ as determined by a laboratory blood test.

When I diagnose this condition, I suggest the following measures:

1. Dress the feet at 45°; concave the sole to prevent sole pressure and apply a smooth, lightweight but wide-web shoe.

2. Reduce grain intake by one-third and exercise the horse regularly.

3. Administer a daily dose of a thyroid compound (dosage and directions as per your veterinarian).

The results of this approach have been very rewarding. And since the condition is so often overlooked, I hope that this report will be noted by those who may have, or may know of, similar cases. *See:* IODINATED CASEIN, LAMINITIS, THYROXIN.

impaction A form of colic; a blockage or semiblockage of the intestinal tract causing low-grade intermittent pain. Impaction means that the horse is superconstipated. Contrary to other forms of colic, it is characterized by a normal heart rate, normal pulse rate, normal respiration rate, even a subnormal body temperature, and also by a persistent pain in the gastrointestinal tract that can become acute at times. The horse has periods of quiescence followed by sessions of restlessness when it will get down in the straw and stretch out. Episodic inappetance and general unhappiness should alert you that impaction could be developing.

A sobering bit of knowledge is that impaction actually requires many days to build up before the symptoms finally appear. Your horse can be in the early stages of impaction development with an impending illness and yet be symptomless. Eventually pain sets in and then so do the symptoms.

The horse is weakened by its reduced intake of food and water, the intestinal mass dries out, and poison can be absorbed through the compromised gut wall. Now toxicity and infection are a real threat!

The pain is more acute if the sluggish mass is located in front of the caecum and colon than when the ingesta is located in the caecum and colon. Rectal examination in the adult horse can confirm the diagnosis and determine the location of the usually large, firm intestinal mass. The severity of pain and discomfort and the expected duration of the blockage are directly related to the size, consistency, and location of the impacted material.

At this time, your options are either to van the horse immediately to a hospital for surgical intervention, or to continue conservative or routine treatment.

The latter treatment consists first of injectable sedatives and analgesics; among the safest and most effective are methampyrone (Novin, Dipyrone), xylazine (Rompun), and flunixin meglumine (Banamine). Coupled with the drugs are enemas of warm soapy water or detergents that have a surface-reducing property. The stomach tube is used to administer mineral oil, glycerine, colic medicine, and other agents to soften the mass. Generous amounts of fluids and electrolytes given intravenously shorten the period of illness dramatically.

If after a period of time your efforts have failed to move the intestinal stasis, your veterinarian may then choose a harsh drug to stimulate the peristalsis in the intestines. This injection is usually a parasympathetic drug; it causes pain and discomfort in the animal about ten minutes after it is administered, and with intestines already under stress, it also creates a danger of intestinal rupture and death.

impaction continued

I have been placed in this position only a few times in my practice and the decision is awesome. My patients fortunately pulled through the ordeal, although it left them pretty exhausted.

To forestall impaction, be alert to the causes: change in weather; change in diet; change in exercise; decreased water supply; decreased salt supply; parasitism, including vascular parasitism; age and debility; neoplasms (tumors). *See:* CONSTIPATION.

infectious anemia (equine infectious anemia, EIA, swamp fever)   A reportable viral disease affecting horses, mules, and donkeys.

The natural transmission of infectious anemia requires a specific set of circumstances. There must be: an infected and acutely sick horse or a carrier horse suffering a febrile period; a swampy or wet, warm, and humid atmosphere; an adequate number of bloodsucking and biting flies or culex mosquitoes. When all these circumstances come together, an epidemic can result. The causative virus is quite resistant to heat and sunlight and can live inside a carrier animal indefinitely. If an animal survives the acute form of the disease, it then becomes a chronic carrier *for life*.

Symptoms are intermittent fever with anemia, followed by weakness and weight loss, along with the development of edema on the ventral (under) side of the abdomen and in the legs (the condition called "stocking-up"). Blood-serum virus titres are higher during clinical symptoms and acute attacks. This is the time—that is, during a febrile (fever) period—that the virus-infected blood can be transmitted to a susceptible horse by biting and bloodsucking insects.

No amount of managerial cleverness can prevent this devastating disease. Prevention is nil, and there exists no vaccine or prophylactic drug. In most cases, state law mandates destruction of the afflicted animals in order to remove the threat to healthy animals. It has been suggested that an infected horse represents an "end product" and that its blood-serum titre never reaches the degree of infection capable of being transmitted to another horse via a vector. This concept, although never documented, encourages people to resist the euthanasia of carrier horses.

In lieu of euthanasia, some state regulations allow the affected animal to live provided the owner assumes responsibility for a very rigid regime. The animal must live inside a screened-off area and be constantly sprayed with insecticides during the insect season. Occasionally, this mandatory unnatural confinement is workable, but in other cases it actually encourages owners to choose humane destruction for their horse.

For long, veterinarians had only the symptoms to rely upon and could only suspect the presence of the deadly viral disease. Uncontrollable fevers, profound anemia, and generalized weakness usually led to fatalities. Autopsy findings were inconclusive. One or more horses, usually pastured together in warm weather, would become hosts of the virus, and the disease would run rampant and uncontained regardless of treatment. With no diagnostic test, the situation was desperate and mortalities ran high.

Finally, in 1970 Dr. Leroy Coggins developed the laboratory test called AGID (agar-gel immunodiffusion) for detection of the blood-borne viral disease.

This made it possible to confirm the diagnosis and to uncover the horses that carried a concealed reservoir of the virus. Today certification of a negative Coggins test is mandatory for all horses crossing state lines and for those being entered in competitions. By preventing exposure to EIA, the Coggins test has saved thousands of horses.

At the same time, the Coggins test leaves room for argument for those who would resist euthanizing an animal. They ask, up to what blood level titre is a horse in fact noninfectious, not a threat to other horses? What level is necessary for this individual to present a hazard? Much more information is needed to answer these questions.

It is a very emotional issue for owners. And the answers will not be forthcoming until much money is spent on the needed research. For the time being, as a veterinarian who has witnessed the ravages of the disease, I must accept euthanasia as the truly humane approach.

influenza A respiratory disease of viral origin in the horse. To date, two causative viruses have been identified: Type A-equi 1, first identified in Prague in 1956, and Type A-equi 2, discovered in Miami in 1963.

Symptoms are a dry, persistent cough, fever, and watery nasal discharge. Highly contagious, influenza can spread rapidly through the entire barn or herd. With its brief incubation period of three to four days, the sickness seems to explode, with few individuals escaping its effects.

Veterinary attention is required to control fevers and associated dehydration, preventing secondary and perhaps more serious infections from developing and thus complicating the illness. If treated so as to prevent secondary invaders, and if properly contained, influenza can be kept to the status of an inconvenience.

Prevention is the best treatment. For this we rely on the vaccine Fluvac, which contains inactivated A-equi 1 and A-equi 2 viruses. This safe and useful vaccine must be administered as directed. The first intramuscular injection does not produce detectable protective antibodies; however, the second injection, given preferably at five weeks, *does* produce a satisfactory immunization. Boosters should follow on a yearly basis. It has been learned that the blood titre, or immune bodies, "wane" faster than was first expected. Thus, an active horse should receive boosters at more frequent intervals. Individuals that are competing or traveling should receive boosters as often as every three months. Seek the advice of your veterinarian. *See:* VACCINATION.

intestinal flora The wide variety of bacteria and other microscopic forms of life found in the intestinal contents.

Beneficial bacteria play a vital role in the digestive process and coexist with pathogens that need only the right environment in order to produce disease. Daily oral antibiotic therapy, for any reason, can conceivably alter the balance of "good" versus "bad" bacteria in the gut and indirectly cause disease.

For example, it is well documented that fungi grow well in the absence of certain bacteria. With the preventive bacteria killed off by promiscuous doses of oral antibiotics, there is a real possibility of a full-blown fungal disease developing in the gastrointestinal tract.

As a veterinarian, I prefer the parenteral route (injections) and thus avoid *intestinal flora continued*

massive oral doses of antibiotics—unless, of course, there is no other means of treatment.

Intestinal flora can be disturbed not only by antibiotics, but also by indiscriminate use of worm medicines—usually manifested by intractable diarrhea.

Originally antibiotics were added to livestock's mixed feeds as a growth stimulant. This succeeded somewhat in ruminants (cows, sheep, goats), but never in the equine.

When using any oral preparation, first stop, read the label, and consider the possible effects on the beneficial intestinal flora. *See:* DIARRHEA.

isoerythrolysis   *See:* NEONATAL ISOERYTHROLYSIS.

isoimmunization   *See:* NEONATAL ISOERYTHROLYSIS.

kidney stones   *See:* UROLITHIASIS.

laminitis (founder) The words *laminitis* and *founder* strike fear in all horsemen's hearts, for they conjure up visions of pain and perhaps crippling and chronic lameness in a beloved horse.

Laminitis is defined as an inflammation of the laminae of the feet; although the foot changes that result are highly visible, they are not the cause of founder. The condition can exist in *acute* and *chronic* forms affecting all four feet, but more often the fore feet are more vulnerable than the hind feet.

For various reasons not fully understood, an excessive amount of blood is suddenly pumped to the horse's extremities and becomes entrapped, as the venous circulation is seemingly unable to remove the flux of blood from the feet. Excessive blood congested in the small and rigid hoof area causes not only

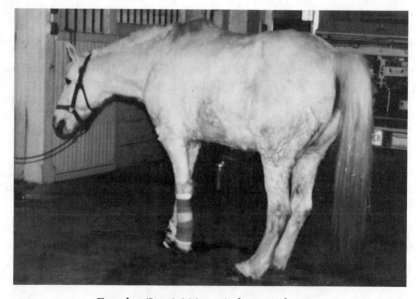

Founder (Laminitis), typical postural stance

excruciating pain, but also permanent damage to the foot tissue. Blood trapped between the sensitive and insensitive laminae causes the tissues to separate. After the acute symptoms subside, irreversible and sometimes crippling foot changes appear.

The primary initiating site of founder is thought to be the intestines. When an enterotoxemia (passage of bacteria from the gut into the circulation) occurs from one of many possible causes, a yet ill-defined substance is produced which is subsequently released into the circulatory system. This substance, suspected to be a form of histamine, signals all blood vessels, especially those of the horse's limbs, to enlarge in diameter. The enlarged vessels allow a great volume of blood to flow unimpeded into the extremities, resulting in a distressed horse with very painful feet.

Any stressful condition primarily involving the gastrointestinal tract can trigger the syndrome: overeating or drinking large amounts of water while still hot or nervous from exertion; ingesting unsuitable hay or grain; gorging feed. Excessive or abusive treatment that affects the horse's nervous system, and/or physical exertion beyond the point of exhaustion are other potential causes of acute founder. Other causes are use of drugs contraindicated in the equine and perhaps harmless drugs with erroneous dosages.

Poor husbandry practices and accidents that occur through ignorance are the most common causes of acute founder. Recently, another cause of acute and refractory laminitis has appeared stemming from the injudicious use of corticosteroids (*see below:* STEROID-INDUCED LAMINITIS). This form of laminitis is gradually receiving recognition and may, therefore, be reduced in incidence through education.

A typical case of acute founder begins when a horse escapes its confines, gains entrance to the feed room, and gorges itself. Quickly call your veterinarian! Your horse will most likely be sedated and tubed with a cathartic to move the ingesta through the gastrointestinal tract, hopefully before the trigger release of histamines that initiates laminitis. A heavy-grade mineral oil can prevent further absorption of the damaging toxins in the intestines.

As preventive measures, some people treat with an anti-inflammatory drug (phenylbutazone) and place the horse's feet in ice even at the first suggestion of laminitis. Cold constricts blood vessels and somewhat reduces the volume of blood flow.

You should abide by your veterinarian's assessment and judgment. Blood samples may be drawn to test for the enzyme level of SGOT (serum glutamate oxaloacetate transaminase). This test is used as a barometer, since high levels indicate severe involvement, and it is thus a great aid in treating and in making the prognosis.

Other causes of founder are hypothyroidism, grass founder, and fractures and accidents that cause acute pain.

In *fracture* cases, it is not uncommon to see founder or degrees of laminitis develop in the opposite supporting leg, since body weight is shifted on to that limb.

Hypothyroidism, whether congenital or acquired, is believed by some veterinarians to be the culprit in repeated low-grade attacks of laminitis. This is referred to as "touches" in the horse world. Usually, no dramatic symptoms are noticed, but insidious tissue changes are occurring intermittently in the feet.

laminitis continued

In *chronic* (low-grade) founder, breed predisposition seems to be a factor. Morgans, Saddlebreds, ponies, and work breeds are especially at risk.

Eighty-five percent of all fat ponies show founder rings on their feet from subclinical low-grade intermittent fever attacks. The majority of attacks are silent although perhaps detectable by perceptive, knowledgeable horse people.

Symptoms of chronic laminitis include varying degrees of soreness, development of concentric hoof rings, and, with time, some blood in the form of tinges or splotches appearing in the sole tissue of the bottom of the foot. If the attacks are severe, then simultaneous foot changes occur; the sole drops due to a ventral shift of the os pedis (coffin bone).

Treatment for chronic laminitis:

1. Blood test for protein-bound iodine (PBI_2) to determine thyroid activity; low thyroxine levels are expected. Daily doses of thyroxine orally are begun immediately. This medication must be prescribed and supervised by your veterinarian. Thyroxine is a drug that must not be withdrawn abruptly, once instituted.

2. Radiographs (X-rays) of the feet may reveal various changes in the position of the os pedis. Corrective foot dressing and shoeing will be helpful. Foot deformities are always more dramatic in acute founder cases, although chronic laminitis, if unchecked by treatment, can be compared to the drip of water on a stone in its destructiveness over time.

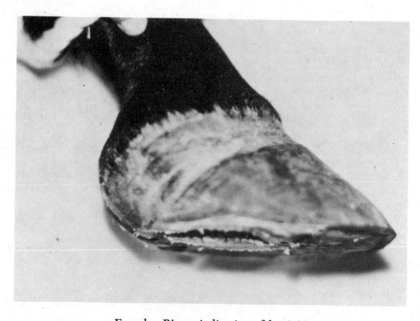

Founder Rings, indication of laminitis

With a program that provides normal foot balancing, no sole pressure, and a wide-web shoe, as well as oral daily medication, most of these horses will slim down, firm up, and become serviceably sound and quite useful.

CAUTION: A vicious cycle can be present in horses with hypothyroidism. Unfortunately, most affected horses are retired pets and ponies. Owners of these horses have a tendency to virtually starve their charges in an effort to reduce the visible fat. This is a mistake.

The deprivation produces weakness and anemia, and focal deposits of fatty tissue seem to worsen or become exaggerated. Now, with lowered carbohydrate intake, the animals are even more susceptible to founder!

This can be avoided by feeding an obese animal a small amount of grain or corn daily with thyroxine powder added. The results will be gratifying! Lumpy areas over the body seem to smooth away and cresty necks slim out, and there are signs of renewed vitality, co-operative attitude, and good health.

Either iodinated casein or thyroxine powders are indicated in cases of low-grade chronic founder. Rely on your veterinarian's preference for oral medication. But, either way, for successful results, provide skilled attention to the care and balancing of the fore feet, abide by the reduced grain intake, and feed the iodine/thyroid preparation prescribed by your veterinarian.

This regime should convert the hypothyroid individual to one that is relatively normal and serviceable—and, more important, one that is comfortable and pain-free.

Grass founder is a form of laminitis well known to fox-hunting people and farmers with draft horses. It usually occurs in physically fit hunters and draft horses that are suddenly turned out on lush grass after a hard winter of hunting and early spring rains. A solid diet of rich grass (no grain and no hay) results in a dramatic gastrointestinal upset, causing a form of enterotoxemia with laminitis resulting. Over the years this pattern of husbandry has foundered untold numbers of fine horses with permanent crippling foot changes. Although the mechanism is not fully understood even today, a small daily addition of carbohydrates to the grazing animal's diet can prevent the devastating entity of grass founder.

(As a child, I remember seeing farmers throw a few ears of corn out into the deep nutritious grass, but I never knew why they did it. Years later, as a doctor of veterinary medicine, I learned that carbohydrates would prevent founder in grazing animals who had just changed their roles from work to rest and their diets from high amounts of cereal grains to nothing but rich, lush pasture. It is interesting to see how people will keep up a traditional practice, not necessarily knowing why, but just because they saw their elders methodically carry out certain chores.)

True founder can occur under any stressful condition and is found frequently in neglected broodmares (postparturient) with retained placentas. *See:* POSTPARTUM PROBLEMS IN THE BROODMARE.

Steroid-induced laminitis is a new form of founder, quite destructive and refractory to the usual treatment used to buffer or dilute the ravages of other forms of laminitis. For years the cause of this form of laminitis eluded everyone and remained a mystery until a common denominator was recognized.

laminitis continued

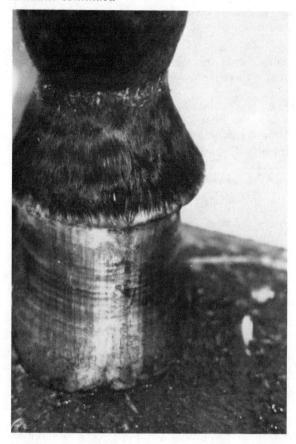

Advanced Founder, separation at coronary band with potential shedding of hoof

Each case had a history of being treated with an injectable steroid preparation eight to 12 days prior to onset of founder symptoms. This seemingly unrelated act, easily overlooked, caused an unfortunate number of horses to suffer the awful consequences. These cases were nonresponsive to known treatment and, unfortunately, some deaths occurred before the etiologic culprit was identified. (Indeed, these drug-induced cases of founder, when compared with other founder cases, were so characteristically refractive to all treatment that I could almost diagnose the cause by the lack of response to treatment.)

Not all steroids cause founder. It depends upon the drug, the dose and route of administration, and the veterinarian's judgment. By all means, as an owner, do not permit promiscuous use of steroid therapy in the treatment of your horse. Some horse families seem hypersensitive to steroids. Other species, including humans, can tolerate these drugs in multiple uses, many more than in horses. I know of no specie, however, other than the equine, that suffers from the entity called "founder." *See:* METHIONINE.

laryngeal hemiplegia (roaring)   The term *roaring* is descriptive of pathologic noise produced on inspiration during physical exertion. The characteristic high-pitched whistle can best be heard while the horse is under tack during a steady gallop. It is easily identified, even by the uninitiated. Because the respiratory noise is generated during inspiration only, a rhythmic pause is heard between each sound as air is expired inaudibly.

Degeneration of the recurrent laryngeal nerve, located on each side of the larynx, is the underlying cause of laryngeal hemiplegia. The two nerves are somewhat dissimilar to each other, although each controls one-half of the intrinsic laryngeal muscles responsible for tissue tone, stability, function, and position. It is well documented that impaired innervation causes flaccid tissue tone resulting in a sagging of tissue surrounding the tracheal opening at the larynx. This diminishes the amount and quality of inspired air.

When paralysis or paresis (partial paralysis) occurs, the vocal cord with its closely associated arytenoid cartilage becomes atonic and subsequently falls across the tracheal opening.

During exercise, the amount of oxygen available falls short of the demand by as much as 50 percent in the horse with a one-sided paralysis. Weakness and distress result, in addition to the outrageous noise emitted during this exertion.

The left side is more often affected. Reason suggests that this has to do with the anatomical course traversed by the left nerve, which differs markedly from that of its counterpart on the right side of the neck. The left nerve passes backward and around the aorta (largest artery of the body), then under the bronchial lymph nodes, and on up the trachea. Constant vibration and pulsation from the intimate contact with the large artery is believed by some to be the cause of the increased incidence of left-side paralysis.

Although all breeds of horses are susceptible, laryngeal hemiplegia is recognized more often in competing Thoroughbreds, Saddlehorses, and Standardbreds. Interestingly, whatever their breeding or bloodlines, roarers are commonly large, long-necked individuals.

No one, however, has satisfactorily advanced the true etiology of the degenerative process of the recurrent laryngeal nerve tissue. We know the effects, but *not* the cause. Other suspected causes of nerve degeneration include: infections, especially respiratory infections, such as strangles; local trauma; and hereditary predisposition.

Laryngeal hemiplegia is to be differentiated from other breathing conditions and diseases that also cause a variety of symptoms and respiratory sounds during exercise. The following entities all cause discomfort and distress, and interfere with performance:

1. Pharyngitis—through inflammation, moisture, and thickening of the membranes—can cause an audible respiratory noise. Moist in character, this noise can be heard distinctly on both inspiration and expiration.

2. The so-called high breather, or high blower, produces a guttural sound heard during both inspiration and expiration. The condition is associated with certain breeds noted for their heavy jowls and necks and commonly occurs while the animal is under unnatural restraint or nervous stress. It is probably caused by an elongated soft palate (*see:* PALATE).

laryngeal hemiplegia continued

3. Nasal nares can cause a fluttering sound due to thickened soft tissue. This is not considered pathologic.

4. A snorting sound, or nose-blowing, is a nervous condition found in normal horses. It has been misinterpreted in the past as pathologic.

5. Tumors, cysts, or polyps, if of considerable size, can be responsible for respiratory stenoris (pathologic noise). Also, excessive tissue folds or flaps in the pharynx can at times cause a sound that simulates some other conditions.

6. Do not confuse a "windy" horse with a roarer. Roaring is an upper respiratory condition, whereas a "windy" horse is suffering from pulmonary alveolar emphysema, or heaves, a lung condition (q.v.).

When examining a horse for the presence of laryngeal hemiplegia, it is essential to: (1) gallop the horse under tack—longeing will not suffice; (2) examine outdoors, not inside the riding hall; and (3) avoid examining on a rainy or windy day.

Before the advent of the endoscope, veterinarians were at a disadvantage when presented with a respiratory case that had vague symptoms and a poor performance history. They had to rely on history, symptoms, and palpation to determine which respiratory condition, out of a possible dozen entities, was the actual one concealed inside the horse's head.

With the modern fiberoptic endoscope, veterinarians now can examine visually the entire respiratory tract, entering even the guttural pouches and continuing down into the lung space. This instrument is entirely flexible, capable of going around corners, and incapable under any circumstances of injuring a horse's tender respiratory membranes. To prove a point, few horses even resist its use. With the endoscope, an accurate diagnosis is highly probable. Samples can be obtained and treatment can even be administered under its guidance and use.

Surgery is the only successful treatment for laryngeal hemiplegia. There are two distinct surgeries available today; some surgeons combine the procedures, believing that they work synergistically.

A *ventriculectomy* is a proven procedure performed on a standing animal or on one under general anesthesia. The lining of the ventricles (the small sacs found very close to the vocal cords) is strategically stripped *and* removed in order to produce scar tissue after healing. This has the effect of enlarging the tracheal opening. However, because the arytenoid cartilage is still sagging into the opening from above, a second procedure may be in order. In this case, a *laryngeal prosthesis* (synthetic material permanently implanted) is surgically placed somewhat above and in back of the larynx, to retract the sagging arytenoid cartilage and thus enlarge permanently the opening to the trachea.

The success rate of a simple ventriculectomy ranges around 50 to 60 percent of cases. Although the laryngeal prosthesis requires a general anesthetic, the success rate is a gratifying 90 to 95 percent.

leptospirosis   A contagious disease of animals and humans caused by the spirochetes *Leptospira pomona*, *L. icterohemorrhagiae*, and *L. canicola*, among others. In horses, it is an insidious destructive disease more prevalent than recognized.

Essentially water-borne, leptospires survive best in stagnant water or surface water in any form.

Although rarely seen in the horse, acute symptoms consist of high fever, depression, lack of appetite, and perhaps icterus (yellowing of mucous membranes). A blood test taken at this time will reveal a neutrophilia (marked increase in white blood cells).

Antibiotic therapy has little value during the acute initial stage, other than to suppress secondary infection. Supportive treatment—fever reduction, fluid replacement, and nursing care—is indicated. A bacterin has been developed for leptospirosis in cattle, but it is of questionable value in the horse.

Since acute clinical cases are seldom seen, the disease is most often recognized by the overt aftereffects of the leptospires' silent attack. There may be early undetected abortion in pregnant animals and/or an assortment of eye lesions. Mares abort unnoticed and are then found empty at a later date. Uveitis appears months after the acute infection as periodic ophthalmia, popularly known as moonblindness. The currently acceptable term for this eye disease is *recurrent uveitis* (q.v.).

Interestingly, I have found that massive doses of penicillin and dihydrostreptomycin administered in combination during an ophthalmic attack are quite effective and, as an added bonus, I have noted a reduction in the severity and number of recurrent attacks.

Since leptospires localize in kidney tissue once a horse is exposed to the infection, spirochetes are shed in the urine for several months to years after the acute stage has subsided. Varying amounts of kidney tissue damage can be sustained and possibly go undiagnosed.

Leptospirosis is spread not only by horses' urine; the main offender is rat urine. Rodents with infected urine can readily contaminate a grain or water supply, so great emphasis should be placed on eradication efforts. Clean up wet, dirty areas and beware of streams flowing through pastures from adjacent farms, especially farms where there are hogs and cattle. Leptospirosis is a major disease problem for swine and bovine breeders and is thought to be transmitted basically through drinking water that has been contaminated with infected urine.

Leptospirosis should always be suspect when there are unexplainable abortions coupled with uveitis eye cases. To confirm the diagnosis, two blood samples taken seven to ten days apart will provide a definitive answer. A positive serum titre of antibodies is conclusive that the horse has been exposed to the disease leptospirosis.

Since treatment with drugs is quite unsatisfactory, it appears that good care, cleanliness, and hygiene are the only valid treatment for this chronic destructive disease.

listeriosis Originally thought to affect only cattle, this entity has been appropriately called "circling disease." Affected animals constantly walk in a treadmill fashion, perpetually circling with a dazed expression. Listeriosis is caused by the bacterium *Listeria monocytogenes*, a facultative anaerobe (a class of bacteria that thrive in the absence of oxygen, but can survive in its presence). Listeriosis is a poorly understood disease that is only rarely seen in horses. It attacks the central nervous system and resembles viral encephalitis with its nervous-system symptoms. An attack of listeriosis produces abortion in mares,

listeriosis continued

septicemia (blood poisoning) in foals, and a generalized weakness with throat paralysis that prevents swallowing or eating. Death usually occurs in one week.

Antibiotics are quite ineffective and no vaccine is yet available to prevent the disease.

Incidence of listeriosis is much greater in Europe than in the United States. This disease is transmissible and often fatal in human beings.

lockjaw   *See:* TETANUS.

lymphangitis   *Ulcerative* lymphangitis is a disease characterized by lesions confined to the hind legs that spread via the lymphatic system. Ulcers and nodules are typical and are caused by *Corynebacterium pseudotuberculosis;* most areas are resistant to treatment. Incidence of this form of lymphangitis has been greatly reduced.

Epizootic lymphangitis is caused by the fungus *Histoplasma farciminosum.* Symptoms are usually lung infection, enlarged hind legs with nodules interspersed along the thickened cords of the lymphatic vessels, and nasal and

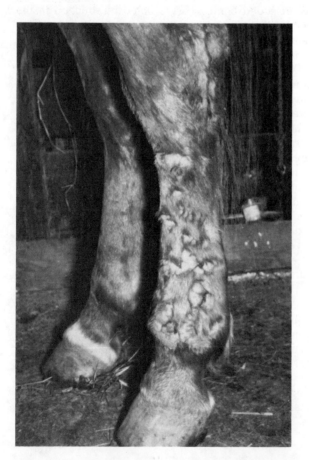

Ulcerative Lymphangitis

eye discharges. The nodules subsequently form abscesses with a yellow, oily-like pus discharging from ulcerated craters. Lesions can be found not only on the limbs in the form of abscesses, but also around the eyes and in the inguinal and thigh areas. This fungus seemingly follows the course of vessels, either blood or lymphatic.

The pulmonary infection, with its nasal discharge, is thought to be the main method of transmission, since the disease is highly infectious and spreads rapidly. There is no satisfactory treatment, and fatalities are consistently high.

Control measures call for insect and rodent control, good hygiene, and disinfection of all equipment, barn, tack, and boots. Burn all dressings. Incinerate carcasses and quarantine the premises and paddocks for six months. This is a dreaded disease requiring the sternest efforts at eradication.

Bacterial lymphangitis is manifested by an elevated body temperature, enlarged hind leg (usually only one), and generalized discomfort. It ensues after a minute break in the skin or a pin prick allows accidental entry of a nondescript bacterial invader into the lymphatic vessels and nodules of the hind leg.

Antibiotic therapy, pain killers, and cold-water hosing will alleviate the discomfort. Cold-water supportive dressings will help maintain tissue integrity and the shape of the hind leg. These attacks, once begun, run about five to seven days and persist in recurring every four to five months.

Chronic cases respond to diuretics, supportive bandages, and adequate exercise. Chemotherapy has merit in human and small-animal cases only but is inconsistent in the suffering equine. Just recently, immune deficiency has been suspected as an underlying predisposing cause common to all known forms of lymphangitis.

malignant edema An acute and often fatal wound infection caused by *Clostridium septicum*. Characterized by high fever and local areas of extreme swelling, usually large and edematous (will pit under pressure).

Treatment consists of antibiotic therapy systemically and local treatment of wounds and swellings. Establish drainage by hosing, cold packs, and poultices to reduce local heat and swelling.

Prevention can be achieved by hygienic practices, the use of disinfectants, and a general recognition of the need for an aseptic environment.

C. septicum is often found in surgical wounds, especially deep, dirty, and neglected areas. Postcastration incisions, accidental lacerations, the umbilical cord of neonatal foals, and the reproductive tract in postparturient mares are ideal sites where *C. septicum* can easily become established. This micro-organism is closely related to the cause of tetanus (lockjaw).

mange *See under* PARASITES.

melanoma Although this tumor is classified as a malignant neoplasm in humans, it is considered benign in horses. Melanomas are found principally in gray horses, occasionally in bays, and seldom in other colors. Considered rare in horses under six years of age, these tumors are found consistently in over 85 percent of gray horses older than 16 years. Jet black in color, rounded, and somewhat freely movable, melanomas can be identified easily. They occur usually in a chain of firm nodules on the under surface of the tail and in small masses around the anus and in the perineal region. I have seen many melanotic lesions located also in the parotid (jowl), supraorbital area (eyes), and along the jugular furrow in the neck.

melanoma continued

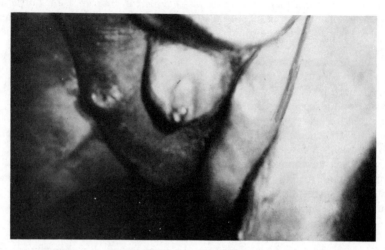

Melanotic Mammary Gland Tumor

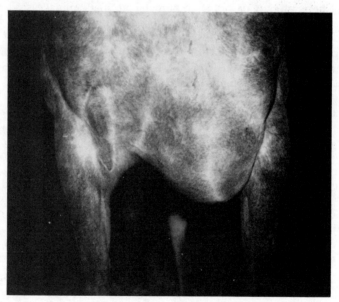

Melanotic Tumor of Pectorial Area

Surgical removal is the only treatment when an isolated tumor is present. As this neoplasm grows, it characteristically pushes the adjacent tissue aside, differing greatly in this from malignant melanomas, which relentlessly invade and destroy adjacent normal tissues.

mesentery   The mesentery is a serous membranous fold attached to the dorsal wall of the abdomen (backbone) and suspending the small intestine in its large fold. It also encloses and conveys all nerves and vessels to the area.

This fan-shaped fold of peritoneum that supports the small intestines is the notorious site of fatal colics caused by various intestinal disorders. Severe colic signs often indicate the need for surgical intervention, if only for exploratory purposes. The veterinary surgeon routinely inspects this vulnerable area for evidence of a twist or a tear in the curtain-like membrane. Loops of small intestine frequently are found hanging or strangulated through a torn aperture in the mesentery, requiring surgical reduction, replacement, and repair.

If surgery is embarked upon without delay, these mechanical displacements can easily be corrected and the prognosis is good for satisfactory recovery. If tissue destruction from impaired circulation has occurred, however, then surgical resection of the intestines (removal of dead tissue) can be attempted, although the prognosis for recovery is then guarded. In any event, with these means at our disposal, we should give the horse every opportunity to live.

Occasionally, the large vessels traversing the folds of the mesentery and carrying blood to the small intestine can become occluded by parasitic larvae and their by-products. (Horses do not suffer from arteriosclerosis, the "rusty pipe" syndrome seen in humans.) This parasite-related occlusion compromises the blood supply and circulation to the intestinal tissue. With repeated attacks, the horse falls victim to pain, depression, and illness. Proper diagnosis and surgery is the only hope for correction.

Monday-morning disease   *See:* AZOTURIA.

monorchidism   *See:* CRYPTORCHIDISM.

moonblindness *See:* LEPTOSPIROSIS, RECURRENT UVEITIS.

myopia   (nearsightedness)   Nearsightedness is not uncommon in the equine and is not considered an unsoundness unless the degree of nearsightedness is extreme. Myopia is inherited and can only be diagnosed by the astute use of an ophthalmoscope.

A complete ophthalmoscopic examination is a routine part of every soundness examination, particularly in prepurchase situations. Although myopia is found with some frequency in the horse, when present, it is considered a significant factor recordable on the report that is ultimately presented to the prospective purchaser.

Horses, as yet, cannot be fitted with contact lenses to correct this eye condition, although I do not rule out the possibility in the near future.

As a horse doctor, I am often called upon to examine horses' eyes, and, contrary to all information regarding myopia, from my standpoint a favorable common denominator exists here: Some of the finest jumping horses I have ever known have been nearsighted!

myositis   Tying-up, Monday-morning disease, and azoturia all refer to forms of myositis that are related physiologically, although they differ widely in the severity of symptoms, treatment, and prognosis. The distinction depends directly upon the size and weight, breed, temperament, and degree of abuse inflicted upon the animal.

Work or draft horses of heavy musculature are commonly affected by the *myositis continued*

extreme degree of myositis called azoturia (q.v.), or Monday-morning disease; paralytic symptoms are diagnostic.

Race horses and performance horses of all kinds commonly suffer varying grades of myositis called "tying-up." Symptoms are pain, stiffness, and irritability.

The differentiating salient factor is the amount and size of the skeletal musculature involved.

Tying-up symptoms may be as subtle as a reluctance to move or turn, shortened stride, or a poor attitude during and after performances. If untreated, this progressive muscle metabolic imbalance will produce exaggerated symptoms unmistakable to anyone: anxiety, sweating with lather forming quickly, rigid muscles, tense attitude, rapid and deep respirations, paresis with subsequent paralysis, and recumbency or prostration. *See:* AZOTURIA.

Mild myositis recognized early and treated promptly can be managed quite well with little disruption of the patient's training schedule.

To confirm the diagnosis and evaluate the amount of muscle involvement, a blood test (serum glutamate oxaloacetate transaminase, or SGOT), can be drawn for muscle enzyme levels; serum levels indicate the amount and degree of myositis taking place.

Treatment consists of selenium and vitamin E injections combined with oral preparations. Rest, together with an adjustment of the dietary and exercise schedule regulated by the trainer, usually results in resumption of training within one week.

Before resuming full training, however, a blood test to check muscle enzyme level is recommended as a means of determining readiness.

navicular disease   *See under:* LAMENESSES.

palate   The palate divides the oral cavity from the nasal cavity and consists of two parts, a hard palate and a soft palate. The hard palate is the rigid, ridged roof of the mouth beginning at the upper incisor teeth and continuing back to about the level of the last molars. It then continues as a soft musculomembranous curtain which separates the posterior oral cavity (mouth) from that of the pharynx above, except when swallowing.

The unusually long structure of the soft palate is responsible for the horse being dependent for survival on nose breathing. The horse is absolutely unable to inhale any air through the mouth, no oxygen at all!

A new entity has been recognized in competition horses called *elongated soft palate*. In this condition the epiglottis becomes entrapped when the horse attempts to swallow during great exertion, usually during a race. The tracheal opening is occluded by the soft palate, which is pushed upward by the trapped epiglottis. Oxygen flow is reduced dramatically and the horse stops running abruptly!

To correct this condition there is a surgical procedure called "soft palate resection." It has merit and has helped some horses, but great caution must be exercised in judging the amount and area of tissue to be resected. *See:* LARYNGEAL HEMIPLEGIA.

Potomac fever   The name given to a mysterious disease first recognized in 1979 among horses living in the riverine locale near Washington, D.C. The disease spread to other states, and in 1984 approximately one-third of 148 afflicted horses died in Maryland and Virginia alone.

Researchers knew that the disease was transmitted by insects and that the highest incidence was to be expected in coastal areas during warm weather. For some time they were misled in their investigations by the assumption that the associated diarrhea was the main symptom.

A five-year nightmare for veterinarians and horse owners ended in November 1984 when Dr. Ristic from the University of Illinois identified a rickettsia organism as the cause of Potomac fever. The disease has been renamed equine monocytic ehrlichiosis. Veterinarians will soon, through serologic tests, have a suitable diagnostic means and specific treatment—or, better yet, a vaccine to prevent the disease.

In my practice I have treated numerous diarrhea cases that had no specific diagnosis. The symptom of diarrhea was treated with inconsistent results. I ponder now how many of these idiopathic diarrhea cases might have been equine monocytic ehrlichiosis.

parathyroid There are four parathyroid glands in the neck area of the horse. An upper pair is located in the tissue above the thyroid gland, and a lower pair is less specifically located on the lower portion of the trachea.

These endocrine hormonal glands, with their secretion called *parathormone*, act in harmony with the thyroid gland and vitamin D to maintain calcium stability in the entire body.

Fortunately, primary disease of the parathyroid glands has not been reported. This is quite a contrast to the increasing prevalence of hypothyroidism found in the horse.

An entity called *fibrous osteodystrophy*, a type of defective bone formation, is thought to occur in young horses through improper diet. A diet containing too much phosphorus relative to the calcium intake is suspected as a cause of this disease. It is a matter of too much or too little. Anything that upsets the critical ratio between calcium and phosphorus can cause a gamut of clinical symptoms.

For about eight years I was the farm veterinarian of a large breeding establishment that housed 300 broodmares and six stallions. In my first few years there, we found several yearlings in each crop of 30 or 40 that developed crooked legs, contracted tendons, and enlarged ankles with development of torque forces in the limbs. Some of the better-bred individuals, the ones worth many thousands of dollars, were victims of this entity. Everyone was upset including the owners, who worried about their financial investment. But I was especially upset, since it was my job to find the cause of this crippling condition in these well-bred young horses.

I looked to diet. Nothing but the best, the heaviest, the richest, the highest in total digestible nutrients and protein content was good enough for this farm!

With the owners' consent, I halted *all* supplements, fed only the finest heavy Canadian oats and the best quality alfalfa or alsike clover hay (both have high nutritional value), and not one case developed thereafter. I carried this one step further and applied it to the broodmares and not one contracted foal appeared after this dietary change.

We, as Americans, are killing ourselves by our diets and, believe me, we are killing our animals in the same manner.

parrot mouth *See:* BRACHYGNATHIA.

peritonitis An inflammation of the peritoneum, a layer of tissue that covers the visceral organs and lines the abdominal cavity. An infection in this membrane can cause death, as was common in horses prior to the advent of antibiotics.

Peritonitis can result from punctures or penetrations into the abdominal cavity that admit pathogenic bacteria, either from the escape of intestinal contents through a break in the intestinal wall, or from a generalized systemic illness.

The development of peritonitis is usually secondary to some other condition, and it is usually fatal once established. Symptoms are an elevated body temperature, rigid stance and tense muscles, and severe mental depression. Mucous membranes are congested, heart rate is accelerated, blood pressure is reduced, and diarrhea is usually present. Fevers spike to 105° and above! These horses refuse to eat but commonly drink water. A grave sign of peritonitis is when a horse prefers to "lap" water and insists upon submerging its mouth in the water pail.

Blood counts reveal an elevated white-cell count, mainly leucocytes. Peritonitis progresses with dehydration, loss of body condition, and deterioration of body function. Death comes almost as a blessing!

Years ago, the word *peritonitis* was synonymous with death. Today the number of peritonitis cases has been greatly reduced, thanks to medical advances and wonder drugs. Prevention is the only method, as no satisfactory treatment exists. *Once established,* the entity still means death!

pneumonia An inflammation of the lung tissue with a tendency for the alveoli (air sacs) to fill with exudate. Pneumonia is usually secondary to other conditions and signals an alert for medical attention. It is chronic and progressive in adult horses, but usually acute in young foals.

Symptoms of pneumonia are inappetance, elevated temperature, nasal discharge, and shallow breathing. With the use of a stethoscope, a skilled practitioner will hear an accelerated heart rate, moist rales in the lung tissue, and increased bronchial and tracheal sounds.

Causes of pneumonia are many. Among the viruses, equine influenza virus A Equi-1 and -2, equine rhinopneumonitis virus, and equine viral arteritis virus are the most common causes of pneumonia, but there are many others. Bacterial invaders, such as Streptococcus, Staphylococcus, Pasteurella, *E. coli*, Salmonella, and Actinobacillus, all cause their share of pneumonia, if given the opportunity.

Treatment consists of the antibiotic of choice, systemic enzymes, supportive fluid therapy with electrolytic and oxygen therapy if required. Therapy should be continued for at least 48 hours after the temperature has returned to normal. All horses suffering from pneumonia should be allowed at least one month convalescence before they return to training. A blood count should be taken prior to any decision to resume activity. Blood count values will indicate the degree of recovery or reveal insight as to the status of the horse's health. Irreparable damage can be sustained if the horse is subjected to stress too soon after an illness. *See:* COLITIS X, SEPTICEMIAS.

poll evil *See:* BURSITIS.

proud flesh Excessive granulation tissue formed in a wound or laceration as it attempts to heal. The formation of proud flesh is characteristically found on the limbs of horses suffering from poorly managed wounds or lacerations. Wounds on the extremities have a tendency to overheal, especially in the equine.

When treating wounds and as healing progresses, the first concern is control of excessive granulation tissue. Limiting the amount of granulation and fibrous tissue deposition helps reduce the size, extent, and deforming properties of the scar tissue.

I treat proud flesh first by surgical removal of excess tissue followed by cauterization. Use of electrocautery or a caustic powder shrinks the capillaries and stimulates peripheral areas to produce epithelial tissue. At this stage of healing, avoid water, cleanse only with alcohol, and bandage to keep the area dry and free from air, irritants, and secondary infection.

Warm weather seems to promote the formation of proud flesh; close attention is necessary in getting a wound to heal properly. *See:* CAUSTIC POWDER, GRANULATION TISSUE, HABRONEMIASIS.

prussic acid *See:* HYDROCYANIC ACID POISONING.

pulmonary alveolar emphysema (heaves, broken wind, chronic alveolar emphysema, chronic bronchitis)   The newest label for this disease is currently *chronic pulmonary obstructive disease*. This respiratory disease is seen in adult horses over five years of age. It develops quietly in notoriously insidious fashion, and can become advanced before the inexperienced horse owner recognizes that a problem even exists. Once lung-tissue changes have occurred, however, the disease is clinically obvious, with quite explosive symptoms.

Early transient symptoms are an occasional cough, whitish mucous nasal discharge, and a slight shortness of breath. As these symtoms steadily progress, the cough becomes persistent and exhausting and the horse has difficulty breathing (dypsnea). There is generalized weakness due to poor exchange of gases (oxygen inspired and carbon dioxide expired). Eventually, the abdominal muscles actively begin to aid breathing, specifically assisting during expiration. This is the cause of the well-known "heaves line" in the flank of the horse, so easily observed in advanced cases. In my opinion, however, detection during the initial stages requires a skillful eye.

Heaves is a disease in which the lungs lose their elasticity; some alveoli (small air saccules) rupture and coalesce, causing weakening of lung tissue and respiratory inefficiency. The lung soon loses its ability to empty air trapped in and around the air saccules, and the amount of oxygen available to the blood and tissues is reduced. In a "heavy" horse, air is inspired easily in a passive manner; expiration is where the difficulty arises. The abdominal muscles are brought into play to pump the air out of the lungs with each expiration. This is followed by a total relaxation of all muscles, the source of the resulting "thump" so characteristically seen in heavy horses.

To better appreciate the breathing difficulties of a "heavy" horse, place your ear close to the animal's nostril and listen to the air being pushed out of the lungs forcefully and rhythmically on expiration. In contrast, observe the intermittent and effortless inspiratory sound as air is admitted.

There are many causes of this disease, some definitive and others suspect:

1. Respiratory infection of viral or bacterial origin (strangles)
2. Parasites (ascarids in young animals and lungworms)
3. Environmental factors—the largest category—including housing (stall

pulmonary alveolar emphysema continued

and barn), bedding, dust and dirt, poor ventilation, some feeds (concentrates and hays), air pollution (air-borne irritants, smog, and hazardous sulfates)

With each and every one of these alleged causes, an allergic response is triggered in the horse that plays an important role in the development of the disease. Attacks of heaves are seen more often in hot, dusty, or humid weather and in horses housed well and fed hay.

There is no cure for heaves once it has developed. It is possible, however, by good management and control measures, to produce a dramatic change, minimize symptoms, and prevent further lung destruction. Arrange for the affected horse to spend more time outside (weather permitting) than inside the stall. A run-in shed is preferable to stall confinement. Provide the most favorable possible environment. Clean up all sources of dirt and dust; allow good ventilation; change bedding from straw to large wooden chips (dampened with one gallon of mineral oil per 100 square feet), Staz-Dri™, peat moss, or similar material. Stable air can be dehumidified, if necessary, with sacks of calcium chloride hung from the ceiling. During the grass season reduce hay intake to nothing and then, with a change in seasons, feed alfalfa cubes or pellets, or even beet pulp to supply needed roughage; avoid hay wherever possible. Small amounts of timothy hay or orchard grass, when fed, should be shaken well outside, dampened down, and then forked into the stall. Allow the horse to eat from the floor; avoid the use of a hay rack as irritants can easily enter the nasal cavity and subsequently create havoc through irritation.

Medicines are useful in heaves, but they are only secondary in this environmentally related disease. Palliative treatment (corticosteroids and antihistamines) may be used in the acute stage of heaves to reduce inflammation, strangles, and relieve stress. Your veterinarian may want to check your horse for ascarids and lungworms first and then place it on a daily dose of sodium iodide powder, an oral expectorant that acts to dry excessive moisture in the respiratory tract and quiet respiratory irritants.

Regularly scheduled wormings and respiratory booster (against influenza and rhinopneumonitis) are strongly recommended to avoid undue respiratory infections and stress.

If you, as an owner, can endure this rigid regime, your "heavy" horse may surprise you by not only surviving the initial attack of heaves, but by continuing as a workable and happy animal. This can happen only if you persist in absolute control of your horse, however.

purpura hemorrhagica   A condition in which blood leaves the vessels and escapes into the tissues, lodging under the skin in huge swellings. It is a very old disease of horses with a 50 percent mortality rate. Modern medicine has not yet found the true cause of this condition, although one consistent correlation has been that all cases of purpura have just recently recovered from a bout with either *Strep equi* (strangles) or Influenza viral infection.

One school of thought believes it involves an allergic reaction. A hypersensitivity created by the streptococcus protein may exist in the animal's body and require only a simple response mechanism to cause extravasation of blood and fluid out of vessels.

Symptoms of purpura are so dramatic they are diagnostic even to nonprofessionals or lay people. Characteristic swellings develop gradually but relentlessly all over the body and limbs, slowly progressing to the neck, head, and mouth area. An emergency situation can develop quickly if breathing is impaired by edema. In this case, a tracheotomy is essential. These distorting and disfiguring edematous masses pit on pressure and are painless on palpation yet remarkably cool to the touch.

Appetite as well as heart and respiration rates are normal, and body temperature can even be subnormal at times. Small spotty hemorrhages appear on the mucous membranes and areas of the tongue tissue.

Treatment consists of daily antibiotic therapy, steroid injections, and antihistamines for the allergic aspect. At the same time, provide "super nursing" care: keep the horse comfortable, keep it eating and drinking, give gentle twice-a-day massage of the masses, bandage the lower legs for warmth and support, and hand walk very slowly to aid resorption of fluids (ten-minute periods, three times daily). This approach will greatly enhance the affected patient's chances for recovery.

rabies (hydrophobia, lyssa) An ages-old, worldwide, and highly fatal viral disease. With all mammals susceptible, rabies represents an important public health problem.

The rabies virus is carried in the salivary glands of infected animals and is spread exclusively through bite wounds. Reservoirs of the virus may be carried by skunks, foxes, and quite commonly bats, and transmission is chiefly through dogs, cats, and wild species.

The horse can be classified as a dead-end host for the rabies virus. Because of its nonpenetrating bite and its preference for kicking rather than biting when it attacks, the horse is less likely than other species to spread the disease.

Symptoms are extreme restlessness, irritability, excitability, and expressions of aggressive meanness. Tremors, rigidity, and muscle spasms occur initially, together with increased heart and respiration rates. Violent chewing on foreign objects, out of character for the animal, is a behavioral symptom strongly suggestive of a rabies infection.

The presence of microscopic negri bodies in the brain tissue is the only postmortem finding diagnostic of the viral disease of rabies.

Commercial vaccines for horse immunization against rabies are available, but the advisability of their use is a decision for your veterinarian.

A rabies vaccine for human protection has recently been developed. This is a medical milestone and one for which all should be grateful.

recurrent uveitis (moonblindness, periodic ophthalmia, recurrent iridocyclitis) Equine recurrent uveitis is the most common intraocular disease of horses, causing an inflammation of the uveal tract encompassing the globe, affecting as much as 10 percent of the horse population. Adult horses of all sexes are equally affected. The first attack is usually the most severe, with intermittent and irregular subsequent attacks appearing to be less intense and less destructive to the intraocular tissue.

Clinical symptoms are overt and quite diagnostic: tearing; red and swollen eyelids with discharges; excessive blinking; sensitivity to light; pupillary constriction; and reduced intraocular tone.

recurrent uveitis continued

In spite of many decades of research and dedicated efforts directed toward finding the cause or causes of recurrent uveitis, we still do not know the etiologic agent. Although a great amount of knowledge has been compiled regarding this destructive eye disease, with many treatments evolving from this information, the last chapter has yet to be written.

Suspected causes are: (1) deficiency in vitamin B_{12} (riboflavin), (2) leptospirosis, and (3) onchocerca cervicalis.

Treatment usually consists of:

1. Efforts to reduce the inflammation in the uveal tract of the globe

2. Mydriatics or eye ointment (atropine sulfate) to dilate the pupil and help to prevent damaging adhesion formation (adhesions that form due to inflammatory changes will bind the iris to the lens, creating an additional vision problem)

3. Corticosteriods locally and orally to reduce the inflammation; beneficial when combined with antibiotics (polymyxin, neomycin, and chloramphenical)

Tissue changes caused by the inflammatory process seem to be the major damaging factor of an ophthalmic attack, so all efforts should be directed toward reducing inflammation.

Ideal treatment for an acute attack, to be applied simultaneously:

1. Chloromycetin I.V. for five days

2. Chloramphenical ophthalmic ointment six times daily for ten days

3. Atropine sulfate ophthalmic ointment ten times daily for ten days

4. Local injection of methylprednisolone into both the upper and lower eyelids; intraconjunctival injections

5. Protection from light, dust, irritants, and air flow.

Eye lesions, present in the globe after the initial attack, are in the form of specks, spots, or precipitants. Adhesions form in the anterior chamber, on the iris and lens capsule, and in the posterior chamber. The lesions, which can be seen via the ophthalmoscope, vary according to the intensity of the attack and the adequacy of treatment.

Prompt attention and treatment can minimize the development of long-lasting lesions and thus salvage the vision and usefulness of the animal. An experienced horse person can easily detect the presence of a chronic eye condition simply by standing in front of the horse and viewing both eyes simultaneously for evidence of asymmetry. The affected eye will be flatter and smaller and will clearly exhibit reduced intraocular tone and fluid.

Horses commonly suffer from recurrent uveitis and rarely from glaucoma (very common in humans).

versus

Glaucoma	Recurrent Uveitis
Rare in horses	Common in horses
Increased intraocular fluid	Reduced intraocular fluid
Increased intraocular pressure	Reduced intraocular pressure
Dilated pupils	Constricted pupils
Corneal edema	Corneal edema
Constant blinking	Constant blinking
No conjunctival changes	Inflammation of conjunctiva

The Eyeball of the Horse

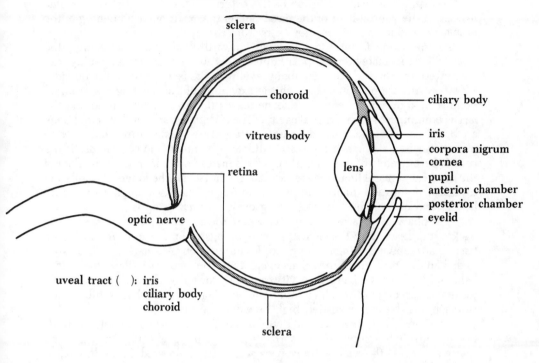

uveal tract ( ): iris
ciliary body
choroid

Ocular Globe

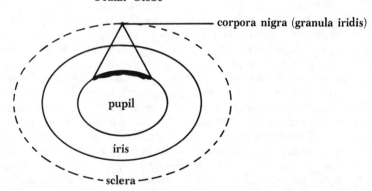

As glasses are impractical for horses and no one needs a horse with reduced vision, it behooves us to prevent eye disease!

respiratory tract   Familiarity with the mechanics of breathing and swallowing in the horse is essential knowledge for every responsible horse person. Therefore, through my fiberoptic endoscope, I would like to take you on a guided tour of the horse's respiratory tract.

respiratory tract continued

Inserting the scope into one of the external nares (nostrils), we see just inside, on the ventral floor of the nasal cavity, the small pinkish opening of the nasolacrimal duct which empties tears from the eye above.

As the scope is introduced slowly upward along the nasal cavity, the blood-filled turbinate bones appear immediately above it; the sinus openings can be viewed here on the side wall about level with the facial crest on the outside. All structures are pink in color with the exception of the startling red ethmoid bone seen above, just before the scope leaves the nasal cavity and enters the large communicating pharyngeal cavity. (The turbinate bones and ethmoid bone are both located on the roof of the nasal cavity and are the structures that bleed so profusely when a stomach tube is misdirected by inexperienced hands. If the tube is permitted to digress slightly upwards instead of remaining on the floor of the nasal canal, nasal hemorrhage results. The horse has the longest coagulation time of all domestic animals, and, once a nosebleed starts, although it appears to be the end of the world, the bleeding eventually *will* stop.)

The pharynx is a large, roomy area where the two nasal passages meet in the back of the head. The Eustachian-tube openings, seen in the form of oblique tissue flaps (about 1½ inches long) are found on each pharyngeal wall, located high and far back near the pharyngeal roof. Beyond each flap, there is a balloon-like protrusion into the cavity caused by the guttural pouch, a distensible sac that is part of the Eustachian tube. The opening to the esophagus (tube to the stomach) can be found nestled high between the sacs.

The "floor" of the pharyngeal cavity is the structure called the soft palate. It is a smooth, flat membrane that separates the pharyngeal cavity from the oral cavity below. At the back of the soft palate, centrally located, is the larynx, or opening to the trachea (windpipe).

In its symmetrical shape and its size, the larynx is designed for respiratory efficiency. It has a pair of arytenoid cartilages forming an arch over and down each side, and two vocal cords of equal size and shape, each one enclosing a ventricle saccule. At the base of the larynx, centrally located, is the large apical-shaped epiglottis. Cartilaginous in texture, with its identifiable scalloped border, the epiglottis represents a major structure in the upper respiratory tract.

The primary function of the epiglottis, as it rests its tip on the soft palate, is to protect by closing over the opening to the trachea (windpipe), especially during the swallowing process. Severe choking or even pneumonia can result if a minute amount of ingesta or fluid accidentally enters the windpipe.

Deglutition—the swallowing mechanism—is antiquated in the horse. After mastication by the molars, ingesta to be swallowed are carried to the back of the tongue, where tongue muscles forcibly elevate the soft palate, pushing the epiglottis up and over the tracheal opening. Passing upward, the food then enters the esophagus situated high in the pharyngeal cavity. This unwieldy process seems even stranger when we see how it interacts with the mechanics of breathing.

Air flowing into the nasal cavity, and from there into the pharynx, must proceed downward to enter the trachea. Food and air seem to "crisscross" in the pharynx. It is an anatomically bewildering arrangement.

The soft palate is remarkably long in the horse, extending snugly under the epiglottis, moving upward only when swallowing. This is the primary reason why a horse is a unique nose-breather and cannot under any circumstances inspire air through the mouth. This disadvantage has caused the death of some horses. Every caring horse person should be aware of this fact.

rhinopneumonitis   Caused by the intracellular virus, Equine herpesvirus 1, and manifested as respiratory disease, abortion, or neurologic symptoms.

In young horses, the notorious rhinopneumonitis virus causes a mild transitory upper-respiratory-tract infection that disappears just as quickly as it appears, with no great aftermath or damage to livestock. A few isolated coughs and runny noses are all that is noticed.

This same virus in broodmares causes abortion or the arrival of weak, comatosed foals. Mares do not suffer respiratory symptoms, in fact, they exhibit no symptoms at all when the devastating virus enters their systems. This insidious virus has an acute affinity for placental tissue which it invades, establishing its infection and thus interfering with fetal nutrition and other placental functions. Even though the rhinopneumonitis virus can be present in placental and fetal tissue for undetermined periods of time, abortion in the mare is the first symptom seen. Aborting broodmares receive an acquired immunity to the virus for an undetermined period.

Treatment of respiratory symptoms in young animals is not necessary unless the condition is complicated by secondary invaders.

All young animals should be vaccinated at four months of age, receive a booster in one month, and another every third month until two years of age. Adult horses should receive boosters depending upon environment. A broodmare should receive a booster before departing the farm to be bred and then receive an injection on her fifth, seventh, and ninth month of pregnancy. I strongly recommend the use of the killed rhinopneumonitis vaccine called *Pneumobort K* (Fort Dodge Laboratories). Do not, for any reason, use a live or modified live vaccine on pregnant mares.

Farm managers, especially those on large breeding establishments, should take the necessary steps to assure vaccinations of all young stock and thus minimize the degree of virulence and the presence of the abortive virus on the premises. Masked as a respiratory virus, it can destroy an entire crop of foals through abortion. Prophylactic vaccinations on a tight schedule can prevent and/or contain the disease.

This virus was responsible for the devastating "abortion storms" witnessed in Kentucky some years ago. Not one mare, but an entire barn of broodmares would dramatically abort, usually all in one night. Damage to the placenta, caused at intervals of infection early in gestation, was not manifested until perhaps the eighth or ninth month, when sudden abortions appeared.

Thanks to the newer vaccines and a better understanding of the "forked tongue" virus, we no longer see abortion storms in breeding farms. However, a recent phenomenon thought to be associated with rhinopneumonitis infection has appeared on the equine veterinary medicine horizon. Inexplicable and nondescript neurologic symptoms have been reported in cases known to have been exposed to the infection. Treatment is strictly supportive and nonspecific with no known cause. Prognosis is always guarded in neurologic entities. Again, research is sorely needed.

retained testicles   *See:* CRYPTORCHIDISM.

roarer   *See:* LARYNGEAL HEMIPLEGIA.

rope burns   In 90 percent of cases, rope burns are avoidable and inexcusable. They are sustained in two ways: when ropes ill-applied for restraint purposes (no hobbles) inevitably tighten, or when a tethered horse panics, usually because a leg has become caught in the rope. In either case, during the horse's struggle, the rope tightens and rubs in a saw-like fashion, literally burning hair and skin away.

Most rope burns occur on or around the legs, especially the pastern area, and result in a very painful, swollen leg with large weeping concentric rings of denuded skin. The swellings tend to cover or mask the rings of destroyed tissue, and not until the swelling subsides can the extent of damage be evaluated. It is unfortunate when the burn extends deep enough to invade the underlying sheath of the flexor tendon, since then the potential for infection and prolonged healing becomes great. A horse doctor can best determine the status and thus the course of treatment.

If a rope burn occurs and you see even one drop of yellow viscid oily material, this is synovial fluid, and its appearance means that the tendon sheath has been penetrated. Hastily notify your veterinarian! Hose the area profusely and apply sterile dressings only, preferably laden with some antibiotic healing ointment or oil (e.g., Furacin®, carbolated Vaseline®, vitamin A-D-E ointment).

Your veterinarian will undoubtedly institute a regime of antibiotics and a tetanus booster, and request from you a daily temperature chart.

Rope burns are accidents that should be *prevented*, not treated! It is not in a horse's nature to tolerate tethering, as is done successfully with other species. The few horses I have ever known to endure tethering were sick or debilitated animals, not healthy, normal individuals. Do not abuse your horse in this demeaning fashion.

When restraint is necessary, leather hobbles, kept soft and clean and applied properly, will never burn a horse. In the absence of hobbles, soft ropes of large diameter applied by someone who is skilled and considerate, can achieve the necessary restraint without injury to the horse. I would strongly urge caution here! Never attempt to restrain a horse physically without a general anesthesia or a drug injection to induce sleep. *See:* KNOTS.

rupture   *See:* HERNIA.

salmonellosis   A severe intestinal disease in animals, as much dreaded today as it was many years ago.

Salmonella typhimurium is the most commonly reported infection, with *S. enteritidis* a close second. Both are also known to infect other animals.

S. enteritidis notoriously attacks foals from four to six weeks of age causing profuse diarrhea, high fevers, and life-threatening dehydration. Colic is inconsistent. Mortality can reach 50 percent in untreated or poorly managed cases. This infection is known to be rodent-related and is spread by rat feces that get into horse feed and are subsequently eaten.

S. typhimurium also is spread by ingestion of contaminated material (feed, bedding, etc.).

S. abortus-equi causes abortion in broodmares, usually from the fourth to eighth month in gestation, and is curiously limited to the equine. The mare may or may not show signs of illness, but the aborted fetus with its placental membranes reveals characteristic dirty gray thickened plaques, truly diagnostic of salmonella infection. Although this infection apparently disappeared 15 to 20 years ago, it may just be under cover, so watch for its re-emergence!

Diagnosis requires blood samples and cultures: samples for culturing from an aborted mare's reproductive tract; samples for culturing by rectal swabs in young and adult horses; and blood samples from all involved. Even then, the salmonella micro-organism is elusive and insidious. A positive result is positive, but a negative can still be a positive!

In aborted mares, treatment consists of a series of medications to the reproductive tract with the antibiotic of choice. Insistence on a clean reproductive tract with a negative culture before breeding is imperative! This action protects the mare and the stallion.

In affected foals and other horses, oral administration of a combination of appropriate antibiotics and intestinal protectives is essential for calming the irritated intestinal mucosa. Fluid therapy, with antibiotic injections for fortification, is indicated. A blood transfusion, properly cross-matched and prepared, can be a lifesaving treatment for some foals.

Once the dreaded infection is on the premises, control measures are paramount. Hygiene practices, including disinfection of all stalls and aisleways, are essential. A thorough scrubbing of the stable area and removal of all organic material should be followed by an efficient flushing with an iodine-based disinfectant (Povodone).

Great emphasis should be placed on the proper elimination of contaminated manure and even of any feces-stained equipment (brooms, forks, wheelbarrow, etc.). The method and location of its disposal can determine the ultimate outcome—continued spread of the disease or containment of the infection. A great hazard to all animal health on the farm is the carrier animal. This is the one who suffers through the disease and recovers and now represents a built-in reservoir of infection. These "carriers" present a real threat to the next crop of foals or to any new member of the farm. The culprit can be the farm dog or cat just as easily as the ever-present birds, insects, and rodents.

If farm animals prove positive, they are destroyed rather than treated because of the threat of contagion. Salmonellosis is a bacterial infection, not a viral infection. Pets seldom become ill with the species that affects the equine; they do, however, mechanically carry the "bug" from one barn to another or from one farm to another.

Your veterinarian is equipped to manage and provide consolation for you in this unpleasant situation. Veterinarians who have experienced salmonella outbreaks tend to 'abandon routine treatment and suggest the production of a bacterin. A culture sample taken specifically from the site of the infection is developed in the laboratory for the involved barn and its infection. Although far from being the total answer, the routine prophylactic use of these old-fashioned bacterins can prevent some problems.

sarcoid   A sarcoma-like lesion in the skin, not known to invade internal organs.

Only the name sounds similar to the serious neoplasm called sarcoma. This cutaneous benign tumor appears on the head, shoulder, legs, and ventral abdomen as a nodular mass. Varying in size from 8 to 10 centimeters, the primary mass usually is attended by a cluster of smaller nodules nearby. With time and growth, the epithelial covering thins and bursts, and an ulcer develops which is vulnerable to invasion of secondary infections.

sarcoid continued

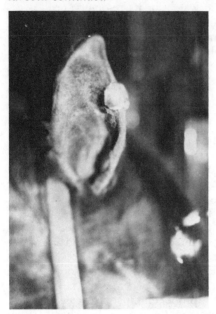

Sarcoid, tumor on ear

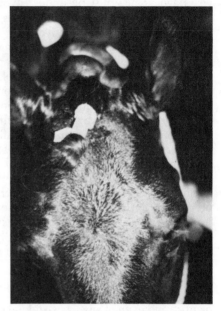

Sarcoid, tumor between ears

The cause is thought to be viral in origin, with bacterial infection establishing itself at a later period. A bovine papilloma virus has been under suspicion as a causative agent although laboratory tests for sera antibodies have to date been inconclusive.

As a practitioner, I have found a correlation between sarcoid prevalence in a horse and the animal's previous relationship with bovine companions.

Treatment is unsatisfactory. Surgical removal is the only method and this at times can be frustrating. A postoperative growth inevitably recurs, always somewhat larger in size and angrier in consistency. I have had success with the cryogenics technique (freezing the tumor), and I believe that this will be the future treatment of choice.

NOTE: Do not confuse a raw and irritated sarcoid with that of a summer sore (habronemiasis). *See:* CRYOGENICS, HABRONEMIASIS.

scrotal hernia　*See:* HERNIA, HERNIORRHAPHY.

shivering　A chronic neuromuscular disease of unknown origin. Hardworking horses, usually draft breeds, are commonly affected, although it has been observed in some light horses. With the reduced number of draft horses in the United States—and those that remain seldom being subjected to hard work—shivering is rarely seen.

Symptoms are unique and quite diagnostic. When the horse is asked to back, the muscles of the hind legs tremble and shake and the tail elevates with a series of jerks. These symptoms are not observed in any other reported condition.

Work seems to aggravate the shivering and rest appears to alleviate the symptoms. Symptoms reappear, however, with resumption of work.

Trauma, hereditary factors, and neural lesions caused by strangles, influenza, or other infectious diseases have all been blamed as the cause of shivering. To date the cause is unknown and there is no valid treatment to propose.

silent bleeder   *See:* EPISTAXIS.

sinuses   There are five pairs of paranasal sinuses in the horse, namely, the frontal, sphenopalatine, ethmoidal, posterior maxillary, and anterior maxillary sinuses. They all communicate, with the exception of the anterior maxillary sinus.

When sinusitis or infection is present and drainage is required, a trephine placed in the frontal sinus to establish irrigation as well as trephinization into the posterior and anterior maxillary sinuses are usually sufficient measures. Daily flushing with antibiotics and enzymes is indicated treatment. Sometimes injectable antibiotics are indicated to reinforce local therapy. The incidence of sinusitis has dramatically reduced since the advent of antibiotics. *See:* SURGERY, TREPHINING.

strangles (distemper, shipping fever)   A highly contagious and quite destructive disease whose very name conjures up dread among horse people. Caused by the troublesome *streptococcus equi* micro-organism, strangles is characterized by enlarged, pus-filled abscesses in the horse's lymph nodes and glands, principally in the upper respiratory tract.

A severe infection can spread to internal organs, with abscessation forming throughout the body; persistent untoward symptoms ensue with wavering illness for months and even years. This peculiar chronic form, called "bastard strangles," is believed to develop as the result of an interference with the horse's immune response to *Strep equi* infection. In the absence of normal antibody formation, the *Strep equi* escapes from the lymph glands and ultimately spreads throughout the body.

Penicillin is effective in the control of high fevers in *Strep equi* infections, but, unfortunately, it also attacks and destroys the *Strep equi* cell wall precisely where the antibody response occurs. Early use of penicillin injections has been incriminated as one of the causes of the "bastard strangles syndrome."

Symptoms of strangles are high fever, reluctance to eat or drink, depression, and swollen lymph glands around and under the head and neck regions. This infection is very contagious and is spread through ingestion of contaminated feeds and inhalation of air-borne droplets.

Young animals are supersensitive to *Strep equi.* These totally unprotected young horses, lacking the specific antibodies earned only by experiencing the disease or by receiving injections of a seldom-used bacterin, readily succumb to the slightest exposure to *Strep equi.*

Veterinary attention is imperative to contain the disease, treat the ill animals, supervise nursing care, and, when necessary, surgically lance the huge painful abscesses to relieve pressure. All personnel should now be on "red alert" against spreading the disease! The purulent material escaping from an abscessed

strangles continued

gland is loaded with *Strep equi* and, through carelessness of barn personnel and the movement of pets and rodents, the contaminated material can spread throughout!

Isolation of the animal combined with strict hygienic practices will restrict contagion and greatly reduce the chances of involving other horse members of the farm. These measures are essential.

Treatment consists of good control measures and nursing care mainly, as well as administration of antibiotics when required for spiked fevers.

There is available a *Strep equi* bacterin produced by Fort Dodge Laboratories that has merit when used with discretion by your veterinarian. It is our only means of stimulating antibodies for protection against this disease, and although it can cause muscle irritation and sometimes abscessation in the injection site, I, for one, am thankful for its availability. Used by a veterinarian who is skilled in determining dosage and in precisely placing the injections, it can result in satisfactory production of immune bodies.

CAUTION: Healthy horses *only* should be vaccinated, since this bacterin is known to be associated with some peculiar postinjection reactions.

Once the *Strep equi* micro-organism gains a foothold in a group of horses, it will continue to appear intermittently and worry the farm manager and veterinarian for months or longer.

Control of this unpleasant and difficult infection on a horse farm consists chiefly of regular vaccinations, rigorous isolation, and strict hygienic practices.

streptococcal infections There are two main species of streptococcus micro-organisms that have continued to cause the horse degrees of distress for many years. *Streptococcus zooepidemicus* and *streptococcus equi* are the infamous two.

S. zooepidemicus is noted for causing abortion in mares and is the causative agent in purulent wounds and abscess formation.

S. equi is equally conspicuous as the causative micro-organism of strangles in all its various forms. It can also cause a bacterial meningitis in horses. *See* STRANGLES.

swamp fever *See:* INFECTIOUS ANEMIA.

syncope A fainting or swooning. I cannot remember seeing a horse actually swoon or faint! I have, however, seen horses lose consciousness through traumatic physical blows, or when accidental stress was applied to the respiratory tract.

Indeed, stress on the respiratory tract can present itself faster than these words can be read, and just as fast a horse's life can hang in the balance.

While watching a loungeing session, I witnessed an inexperienced person allow the chain portion of the line to slide from the noseband area down over the horse's sensitive soft nostrils. The chain tightened and locked into position as the fearful horse struggled for air. With its mouth wide open, the horse threw itself violently to the ground. It quickly collapsed from lack of oxygen and surely would have died were it not for a courageous groom who managed to free the chain. Although the horse was understandably depressed and subdued, he recovered uneventfully.

The horse is solely a nose-breather. Please protect horses' nostrils from appliances, obtuse bits, and overstraps, or any undue restriction or restraint.

tetanus (lockjaw)   A highly fatal infectious disease caused by the micro-organism *Clostridium tetani*. This micro-organism requires an area of reduced oxygen in which to produce a deadly toxin that subsequently invades the central nervous system. It thrives in puncture wounds, deep, dirty, and contaminated areas, or in hidden necrotic tissue, well away from atmospheric air. Tetanus spores, resistant to sunlight and most chemicals, live naturally inside the horse's gastrointestinal tract and are passed with the feces, finally coming to rest in the manure pile. Also incriminated as a source of tetanus spores is rich, organic soil.

A change in environment can spontaneously activate the spore into an organism capable of producing the destructive exotoxin called tetanospasmin, which affects the central nervous system. This results in the first clinical manifestations of the disease called tetanus, or lockjaw.

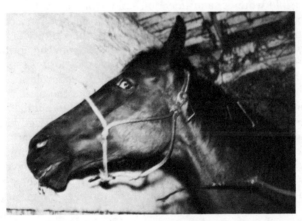

Tetanus (Lockjaw), evidence of prolapsed nictating membrane of eye, also called third eyelid

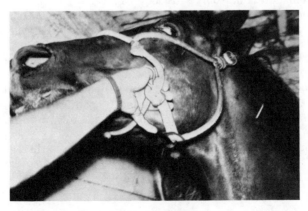

Tetanus (Lockjaw)

tetanus continued

Symptoms are stiffness of the neck, inability to swallow, and sagging third eyelids, giving the horse the appearance of being very sick.

A method that helps diagnosis early in the disease is to clap your hands suddenly and loudly. The horse will immediately react with almost uncontrollable muscle spasms and rigidity, confirming the diagnosis. After a few hours, the horse develops an erect tail, fixed ears, and a "sawhorse" stance, characteristic of tetanus.

Incubation time can range from 48 hours to several months.

Note that the term *spore* denotes the inactive form of specific pathogens or disease-producing bacteria. Spores, therefore, can exist either in the living tissue or out in the environment, remaining dormant for years. When suitable conditions are present for activation of the spore, it quickly produces its exotoxin and the disease—lockjaw—declares its unmistakable symptoms.

Treatment, once clinical symptoms are evident, consists of vigorous local flushing of visible wounds, and injections of antibiotics and tetanus antitoxin.

Massive doses of tetanus antitoxin can be administered in a dramatic effort to save an animal suffering from lockjaw. To me, the validity of this approach seems questionable. I have seen horses become ill from the antitoxin and few ever recover from lockjaw (tetanus) once a positive diagnosis is established. As is true in so many illnesses, nursing care plays a foremost role in any recovery.

Concerted efforts should be undertaken to make the patient comfortable, with emphasis on control of muscle spasms. The animal needs quiet surroundings. Tranquilizers and smooth-muscle relaxants used in combination provide some relief, if only for short periods of time. If necessary, a sling (q.v.) can be implemented for body support to prevent additional injury.

Supportive therapy is essential in the form of intravenous fluids, electrolytes, and mixtures of gruel administered via the stomach tube. Constipation and inability to urinate are two common problems encountered in lockjaw.

Although we have a very effective and economical vaccine against this fatal disease, tetanus continues to plague horses around the world, with a mortality rate of over 85 percent. It is seldom, if ever, successfully treated, so prevention through vaccination is our only satisfactory route.

Foals should be given their first vaccination at four months of age, a booster one month later, and a booster annually thereafter. Basically, the same recommendation holds for all horses. In the event of an injury, especially one sustained in the foot or lower leg, a booster is indicated. These areas are more subject to contact with manure and subsequent contamination.

Every horse on this earth deserves an annual tetanus vaccination!

trichomoniasis   An intestinal disease caused by the protozoal agent *Trichomonas*. *T. equi* and *T. fecalis* are the two species known to cause this severe disease.

Symptoms are a high fever and sudden onset of diarrhea with greenish watery fecal material. Animals so affected have no appetite, are depressed, listless, and underweight. Dehydration with electrolyte imbalance is soon evidenced.

Diagnosis is made by microscopic examination of fresh feces for the presence of the trichomonad organism. It is thought by some that *T. equi* is a normal inhabitant of the caecum of the horse and that these protozoa flourish and increase in number only when some ill-defined bowel environment fosters their propagation. *T. equi*, then, is probably not the true cause of the profuse diarrhea, but is only the accomplice in the crime. The real causative agent is yet to be uncovered.

Treatment is quite successful in some cases by the oral administration of iodochlorhydroxyquin (Vioform). Recommended dosage is 20 grams daily for a thousand-pound horse, continued for one week. Intestinal protectives, such as kaolin, bentonite, and tannic acid, can be administered via the stomach tube as an adjunct to the drug.

Persistent and protracted cases will sometimes respond to the oral administration of yogurt or *Lactobacillus acidophilus* (acidophilus milk) purchased at your local grocery store. It can restore to the intestinal tract some of the beneficial bacteria lost through profuse diarrhea. Extensive oral antibiotic and antibacterial therapy for protracted periods of time might be equally responsible for reduced numbers of beneficial bacteria.

Another alternative treatment, although very old in origin, continues to be popular. Called *transfaunation*, it is a method whereby the feces of a healthy horse are transferred to the stomach of the ill horse. The colon contents are mixed thoroughly with warm water in a pail, then strained thoroughly through a porous, clean bag. The strained fluid is then administered to the sick animal through a stomach tube. Transfaunation is another way of replacing the vitally needed normal intestinal flora and other unidentified factors so necessary for healthy gastrointestinal function.

Constant or chronic diarrhea, no matter what the cause, when refractory to treatment, is most destructive to a horse's health and most frustrating to the attending veterinarian.

trypanosomiasis An infectious blood-borne disease caused by parasitic protozoa called trypanosomes.

Dourine, or equine syphilis, a naturally occurring venereal disease of horses and asses, is caused by the protozoan *Trypanosoma equiperdum*. It is transmitted during breeding and is characterized by inflammation and swelling of the genital organs, glandular enlargement of the testicles, and varying degrees of progressive hind leg and muscle paralysis.

Trypanosomiasis should be suspected when a discharge is noted from the genitals, combined with itchy, raised skin plaques and, of course, reduced fertility.

The diagnosis is confirmed in the laboratory from samples of exudates of drainage material.

Neoarsphenamine, suramin, or quinapyramine are effective drugs for treatment. If untreated, death can occur.

Fortunately, dourine has not been reported in the United States for many years. Veterinarians are constantly on the watch so that it will not reinvade.

For other diseases caused by trypanosomes, see the following chart, Equine Trypanosomiasis.

EQUINE TRYPANOSOMIASIS

Disease	Species	Vector	Natural Host	Clinical Signs	Diagnosis	Geographic Distribution
Dourine	*T. equiperdum*	Breeding (coitus)	Horse, ass	Edema of the genitalia; wheals	Trypanosomes in genital secretions (Laboratory-Complement-Fixation Test)	Cosmopolitan
Surra	*T. evansi*	Bites by horse flies (*Tabanidae* and *Stomoxys*)	Horse, mules, ass, buffalo, cattle, goats	Fever; anemia; urticaria; edematous swellings of legs and ventral abdomen	Isolation of trypanosomes in the blood	South America, Asia, Far East
Nagana	*T. brucei*	Bites by tsetse fly (*Glossina*)	Humans and all domestic and wild animals excepting goats	Fever; edema of lower abdomen; anemia; watery discharge from eyes and nose	Trypanosomes found in blood plasma	Africa
Murrina	*T. hippicum*	Bites by horse-flies and vampire bats	Horse, mule, ass, buffalo, cattle, goats	Anemia; fever; edematous swellings on ventral abdomen; watery discharge from eyes and nose	Trypanosomes found in blood plasma	Central America
Mal de Caderas	*T. equinum*	Bites by horse-flies and vampire bats	Horse, mule, ass, buffalo, cattle, goats	Anemia; fever; edematous swellings on ventral abdomen; watery discharge from eyes and nose	Trypansomes found in blood plasma	South America

ulcer   A hollow lesion on the surface of the skin or a mucous-membrane surface, caused by superficial disintegration and loss of skin continuity, often attended by suppuration (pus formation). A wound with a superficial loss of tissue from trauma is not primarily an ulcer, but it can develop into one if healing stops or infection ensues. Ulceration of the oral mucosa lining the horse's mouth is frequently encountered in veterinary practice. The cheeks, gums, and tongue tissue are especially vulnerable to sharp or overgrown tooth edges, ill-fitted bits, and heavy-handed handlers.

Treatment consists of local compression or application of tamed iodine once a day for three successive days, followed by a daily flushing of the oral cavity with a saturated salt solution for three days. *See:* VESICULAR STOMATITIS.

ulcer, corneal   The cornea of the eye is a thin, transparent membrane that covers the anterior (outer and front) curvature of the eyeball. Corneal inflammation (keratitis) and corneal ulceration are not infrequently found in horses.

The horse, by virtue of its large ocular globes, peculiar vision, and innately curious nature, is quite vulnerable to corneal injury and susceptible to subsequent infection.

Any sharp object, such as a tree branch, twig, thorn, or splinter, can contribute to corneal irritation or laceration. Shameful misuse of the whip sometimes injures the horse's eye.

If neglected, bacterial invasion will surely result in formation of an ulcer.

Symptoms are excessive tearing and blinking of acutely inflamed eyelids, usually forced closed by tissue swelling. All corneal lessions manifest an extremely painful eye condition, and affected horses are consistently difficult to examine. Sedation is indicated both for the patient's comfort and for expediting the diagnosis and treatment.

Ocular examination, although somewhat precarious, will reveal either a corneal laceration, puncture, or ulceration.

In any eye injury or ocular disease, the importance of dilating the pupil cannot be overemphasized. The pupil reacts instantly to inflammation with simultaneous constriction and closure of the iris. Although this is a vital protective action by the body, it is conducive to undesirable adhesion-formation and fixation of the pupil.

Treatment consists of typical instillation of a combination of antibiotics (chloramphenical, polymyxin B, genticin) and atropine sulfate four to eight times daily. Analgesics if needed, plus a protective head dressing or "hat," will suffice in most cases. The hat, made of gauze-covered cotton with two ear holes, is tied under the chin. It provides the sore eye comfort and protection from air currents, dust irritants, and sunlight. The hat can also serve as a moist pack for continuous cooling effect with medications.

A severe corneal ulcer requires hospitalization to properly treat and successfully salvage the eye and its vision. When severe injury occurs to the ocular globe, I always prefer, after surgery or treatment, to suture the eyelids closed. This forms a natural barrier to bacteria and irritants and provides a bonus in the form of the normal lubricating qualities of the conjunctival inner lining of the lids. This method has worked well. *See:* EYE.

undescended testicles   *See:* CRYPTORCHIDISM.

urinary stones   *See:* UROLITHIASIS.

urolithiasis (urinary calculi, bladder stones, urethral stones)   The equine suffers fewer urinary diseases than other species. Although the incidence of urolithiasis (stone formation) is low in horses, there are two kinds with which we have to reckon: urethral calculi found in the urethra, and vesical calculi seen in the urinary bladder.

Stones formed in the horse are frequently large and solitary. Although occasionally found throughout the urinary tract, calculi are most commonly found in the urinary bladder. These vesical calculi, varying from the size of a grain of sand to a large stone, affect adult horses of both sexes, although a higher incidence does exist in the gelding.

The mare, with her wide and short urethra, manages to pass a small calculus easier than does the male, which has a long, narrow urethral tract. In the gelding, a small calculus can pass out of the bladder with the urine, travel down the urethra, and become lodged, causing pain, discomfort, and difficulty during urination. In this case, the calculus can be dislodged and possibly passed to the outside by gentle and prudent use of a male urinary catheter.

If recognized early, corrective results may be achieved through frequent examinations, laboratory analysis indicating dietary changes, exercise, and therapeutic use of diuretics.

Large calculi, some reaching a diameter from 3 to 6 inches, cannot be passed and remain in the bladder. Unless such a stone is surgically removed, with time and a steady increase in size, the calculus will cause the animal's death.

Horses fed on hay, pasture grass, and food high in phosphorous content seem predisposed to calculi development. Chemical analysis reveals carbonate and mixed phosphate mineral content composing the stones.

Symptoms are dribbling of urine with a relaxed and semidropped penis, weakness with an ataxic gait, straining to urinate, intermittent fever, and frequent urination with small volumes escaping.

Urinalysis aids in the diagnosis. Rectal palpation usually reveals an oval hard mass located at the neck of the bladder. The urinary catheter will encounter blockage or resistance when introduced through the urethra.

The treatment is surgical removal. Postoperative attention includes dietary changes and occasional routine urinalysis and physical examination for detection of recurrence.

Prognosis is good.

urticaria (hives)   A skin manifestation of an allergic reaction in the horse's body. Lesions are characterized by round, steep-sided elevations on the horse's skin, as small as a nickel or as large as a quarter in size or circumference, with some coalescing of lesions into huge, flattened areas.

Horse people are seldom upset when a few lesions appear on the head and neck area in varying numbers and sizes; these usually appear quickly and disappear just as quickly.

Ingestion of hay or a pasture weed containing an antigenic agent is the most common cause of urticaria in the horse. Another possible cause is an allergic response to a specific drug (e.g., penicillin), or to the drug in combination with another, or to its route of administration.

If the allergic reaction continues or becomes severe, swellings can occlude the passage of air through the nasal cavity, and suddenly an emergency exists. In this event, the veterinarian may perform a "hurry up" tracheotomy to save the horse's life.

Most cases resolve themselves. Others require removal of close-by hay or roughage, and others are relieved by injections of sedatives and antihistamines. All courses of action should be directed by your veterinarian. *See:* ALLERGY, ANAPHYLAXIS, PULMONARY ALVEOLAR EMPHYSEMA.

vesicular stomatitis An infectious viral disease, communicable to humans, responsible for blisters, vesicles, and erosions on mucous membranes of the mouth (lips and tongue) and on the coronary bands and feet of the horse.

Although transmission of vesicular stomatitis is not thoroughly understood, it is believed by some authorities to be spread by biting insects (mosquitoes, stable flies, and horseflies) and by ingestion of food contaminated with saliva and excreta from these insects. Incidence of the disease is greatly increased in wet, low-lying areas during hot weather.

Vesicular stomatitis was first recognized in horses during World War I in Africa. Reported cases have ranged from Canada, Indiana, New Jersey, Mexico, and Central and South America.

The first symptom noticed is excessive salivation while the horse is eating; salivation can be so profuse that it literally drips into the grain. Then vesicle and blister formation develops on the lips and tongue tissue—all on the inside of the mouth. Shortly thereafter, appetite ceases abruptly from discomfort and mouth soreness.

Corresponding vesicles form on the sole of the foot, but more so on the coronary band tissue, which eventually becomes red and raw with bleeding.

Symptoms of the disease are diagnostic. Your veterinarian can confirm the diagnosis, however, by obtaining a skin-tissue sample and submitting it to the laboratory for identification of the virus.

Horse pox is the only known horse disease with lesions similar to those of vesicular stomatitis, but it has one distinguishing symptom: horse pox has a pus-containing lesion; vesicular stomatitis is devoid of pustules.

The course of the disease is from 12 to 18 days, principally creating inconvenience and inefficiency in growth or productivity, which usually translates into an economic loss, not a loss of life.

After the disease, during recuperation, a short-lived immunity develops, which, unfortunately, lasts only from four to six weeks.

Treatment consists basically of nursing care—comforting mouth washes—unless a secondary bacterial infection occurs. Then your veterinarian should be consulted.

Even in the presence of the disease, by keeping horses housed and free from biting insects and by feeding unexposed foods, the disease can be prevented and contained. Quarantine efforts combined with hygienic practices could not merely limit, but possibly even erase this disease.

Although the horse has been spared and is known to be resistant to the dreaded hoof-and-mouth disease seen in cattle, there is a striking similarity of the symptoms seen in vesicular stomatitis and in hoof-and-mouth disease.

At the time of writing, it was reported that 13 people, including several veterinarians, had recently contracted vesicular stomatitis. This disease is a public health problem and is classed as a reportable disease.

viral arteritis (infectious arteritis)   For many years, this acute infectious disease was confused with various types of influenza and even with some forms of conjunctivitis, or pinkeye. It is now known that a specific virus is responsible for this disease entity and its peculiar symptoms.

Symptoms are heavy mucous nasal discharge with inflammation of both the respiratory and gastrointestinal tracts. Fever with leucopenia (reduced number of white blood cells), conjunctivitis (swollen, red, and inflamed eyelids) with excessive tearing from the eyes and down the face, also are typical symptoms. The salient symptom of viral arteritis, however, is profound edema development in all four legs.

The virus of this dangerous disease attacks the arterial walls causing tissue degeneration and even necrosis (cell death) in severe cases, thereby compromising circulation. Swollen limbs are a direct result of circulatory inefficiency. Generalized weakening occurs as the disease runs its course of approximately 14 days, if uncomplicated by other (secondary) infection.

Good nursing care can influence the severity and length of illness. Pneumonia is a common sequel to viral arteritis. In that event, treatment is upgraded and the prognosis is downgraded.

Unfortunately, broodmares exposed to this virus notoriously abort. The virus is readily recovered in the fetal tissues, which aids diagnostic efforts.

Your veterinarian will make a differential diagnosis from various other respiratory diseases. If viral arteritis is determined, then absolute rest with antibiotic therapy is essential.

Prevalence of this disease is always greater on large farms with large numbers and concentrations of horses. Although a vaccine is not yet available commercially, quarantine measures, isolation of new members, and overall good husbandry can minimize or appreciably reduce this costly infection.

In my practice, I have seen a few cases of what I diagnosed as viral arteritis in horses. Careful, conscientious treatment with supportive fluids, isolation of the sick from the well, and supernursing efforts turned the tide and we suffered no losses or aftereffects. I was, however, dealing with a comparatively small number of horses. Equine viral arteritis has been a constant threat in Kentucky and Florida, where thousands of horses are housed, concentrated, and vanned frequently, especially during the short breeding season.

A recent outbreak of EVA caused closure of breeding sheds and general financial havoc. By late spring of 1985, Fort Dodge Laboratories developed a vaccine and made available this preventable drug to all breeding farms. Quarantines were lifted and the vaccine was welcomed with open arms by the devastated breeders.

A diagnostic blood test to identify carriers is available and the State of New York prohibits entry of breeding stock without a negative certificate. Control measures are inconvenient and expensive, but without them, disease and infections would run rampant!

viral rhinopneumonitis   *See:* RHINOPNEUMONITIS.

warts (cutaneous papillomatosis)   A wart is a small hard round excrescence on the skin. Warts are called papillomas because they originate from the papillae of the skin. Caused by a virus, warts that cover the mouth, nose, and lips of a horse are thought to differ from the warts found on other areas of the body.

Young horses, three years and under, are affected by warts, and once affected, they seem to establish an immunity. Older horses have immunity and escape subsequent reinfection even when placed amid young horses with "warty muzzles."

Transmission is through direct contact, nose to nose, and is also spread through contaminated feed tubs, water troughs, fences, and stalls.

Thorough scrubbing and disinfecting of these objects with strong solutions of pine oil, Lysol, or some viricidal preparation will kill the virus.

There are three methods of treatment for wart infection:

1. Topical application of castor oil, glacial acetic acid, olive oil, silver nitrate, or trichloroacetic acid

2. Electrocautery, possibly resulting in a small scar formation

3. Laboratory preparation of a tissue vaccine from wart material removed from the area

It is difficult to properly assess these treatments and their efficiency, since warts are notoriously known for their spontaneous remission!

wobbles (equine ataxis, inco-ordination) Wobbles is found as a sudden and alarming alteration of a horse's gait and body movement along with signs of inco-ordination. Symptoms are ataxia—an unsteady staggering, even swaggering, gait and a clumsy attitude.

Commonly found in young, fast-growing horses ranging from 16 to 24 months of age, and frequently affecting colts more often than fillies, wobbles is a fatal condition. The onset of symptoms in a colt prepared to begin training can be devastating to the owner, trainer, and veterinarian. This entity, with all of its abruptness, is actually an insidious condition that develops slowly and then appears without warning.

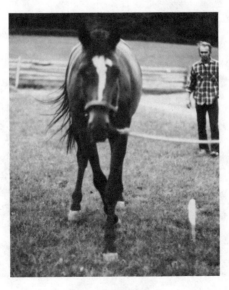

Ataxia (Wobbles)

wobbles continued

Currently we understand the cause of wobbles as compression of the spinal cord by the bony vertebral column. Lesions develop in the cervical (neck) area of the vertebral column and are usually found involving the third through the sixth cervical vertebrae.

The soft and sensitive spinal cord, full of nerve tracts, is infringed upon by the hard, bony vertebrae, which, under normal conditions, surround and protect the cord. For some unknown reason—either trauma, nutrition, or heredity—the vertebrae may shift physically, or the canal through which the cord passes may not be of sufficient size; in either case, compression of the cord results. Nerve fibers and tracts are literally pinched and compresssed with resultant inflammation of tissue and eventual necrosis (cell death). Innervation to the extremities, especially the hind limbs, is compromised and this results in degrees of ataxia and paresis. The word *wobbles* describes the clinical picture well. The hind legs swing outward in a characteristic staggering fashion.

To predict the course of the disease is easy, but to foresee the rate of progressive changes is difficult. Some animals are rapidly affected and become prostrate within days, whereas others may stagger around the paddock for several weeks before symptoms dictate euthanasia. The rate of deterioration depends upon the severity of spinal-cord compression.

Treatment has nothing to offer and nursing care with supportive therapy is usually unrewarding.

Intensive research with some experimental surgery is currently being conducted to reach an answer to this fatal entity that has taken a great toll in our horse population.

wound healing   *See:* GRANULATION TISSUE.

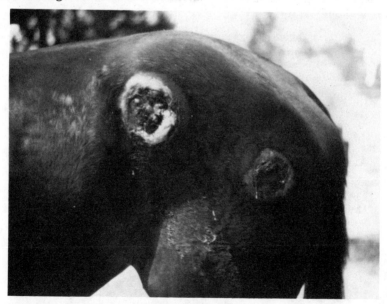

Bed Sores (Decubital Ulcers), a horse recovering from a protracted illness

LAMENESSES

anatomy   The science of the morphology (shape or structure) of living creatures. It has always interested me in my practice to observe how all the body parts, their proportions, and their relationships directly affect the quality of conformation in an individual animal.

I need hardly mention that a horse of excellent conformation is pleasing to the eye. More important, conformation bears directly on the horse's durability, its talent, and its capacity to remain serviceably sound. Conformation is not the only factor, however, that affects the horse's ability to perform successfully over a given period of time. Speed, stamina, and a good mental attitude are desirable traits exhibited by champion runners, and these traits, I believe, are inherited, not developed. Today we are assisted by computers in matching bloodlines to get a promising mix of complementary qualities in a foal. But no matter how ideal the mating may appear on paper, it is up to the purchaser to judge the results. This takes an educated eye and the advice of a veterinarian who has thoroughly scrutinized the prospect.

ankle   Fetlock or metacarpophalangeal joint. The ankle of the horse includes the joint where the cannon bone (metacarpus) articulates with the long pastern bone (first phalanx).

In the back of the ankle are the two all-important and unique sesamoid bones. These serve as a smoothly moving support over which the powerful flexor tendons pass on their way to the foot. The flexor tendons cover the front of the ankle.

The suspensory ligament, the major ligament of the lower leg of the horse, is a wide band positioned on the back of the cannon bone. It divides at the upper ankle level and sends a branch down on each side of the ankle.

Just above the ankle level the major nerves, arteries, and veins of the horse's limb converge into a complex protective fibrous sheath. This durable trunk continues down over the ankle into the lower pastern area, where the delicate vessels then enter the semirigid foot.

Superficially located on the inner and outer posterior border of each ankle, these vital structures of the lower leg are thus highly subject to physical trauma even though fully encompassed in a durable fibrous trunk.

The most common injury sustained by the nerves and vessels of the ankle occur when the horse's gait is altered for one of many possible reasons. Fatigue, poor footing, and the need for foot balancing or shoeing are a few examples, all usually founded in human abuse. As a result, one limb, usually the opposite extremity, may cross over and strike the other, causing injury. Or, the hind feet may bruise and even lacerate other limbs, especially during keen athletic competition. *See:* APPLE ANKLES, INTERFERING.

ankle continued

Conditions of pathology (or disease) of the ankle, in addition to gait trauma: osselet formation, intra-articular or joint fractures, sesamoid inflammation or fractures, osteoarthritis, strained ligaments or tendons, ankylosis.

ankylosis   Stiffening or fixation of a joint due to excessive use. This distressful entity is undoubtedly the result of abusive concussion or chronic infection in the ankle of long-standing duration. Ankylosis is found most often in the front ankles of Thoroughbred race horses and the hind ankles of Standardbreds. The condition invariably results from neglected osselets, untreated fractures, or concussive trauma.

Once soft tissue, cartilage, and bony changes in the ankle develop, and the irreversible process of ankylosis is initiated, treatment of any kind is futile.

Prevention is the only known treatment for ankylosis. *See:* OSSELETS, OSTEOARTHRITIS.

apple ankles   *See:* EPIPHYSITIS.

arthritis   There are many types of arthritis in humans stemming from many different causes. The single type of arthritis to which horses are prone is *osteoarthritis*. Although the condition is defined as simple inflammation of the joints, we veterinarians most often see it as an intense osteoarthritis in young horses in training. We know only too well that these cases are caused by physical trauma and concussion to underdeveloped and immature limbs and joints, a very different thing from the "old-age" osteoarthritis of the older horse that results from a lifetime of wear and tear on the joints.

Young race horses are especially susceptible to osteoarthritis because they are put into hard training before their skeletal systems have matured. A two-year-old's epiphyseal plates (growth lines) are not yet closed; its joints are not strong enough to withstand the stresses its trainers may impose in preparing it for competition. *See:* OSTEOARTHRITIS.

asymmetry   This term denotes an inequality in the size and shape of two or more corresponding parts, such as the massive gluteal (upper thigh and above-gaskin) muscles, shoulder muscles, or forearms.

"Sore" horses often show an asymmetric gait rather than a definitely lame stride. This uneven distribution of body weight is easier to hear (on a hard-surfaced lane) than to see. *See:* ATROPHY.

atrophy   Defined as a wasting of tissues, organs, or the entire body, muscular atrophy is a major clue to unsoundness.

To detect a difference in size between two identical muscle masses, stand well away from the horse when viewing it. Any change in the size or shape of a muscle is due to reduced use, disuse, or faulty (deficient) nerve innervation. If the matching muscle (which should be identical) is enlarged, it could be because it is compensating for the atrophying mate.

Often, the cause of muscle atrophy is a blow to the horse's body, occurring perhaps unnoticed in a van, stall, or starting gate. If nerve damage is sustained concurrent with trauma, inevitably there follows a paresis of the muscle area; even worse, a more generalized paralysis may ensue. In either case, the muscle's blood supply is compromised or diminished, resulting in muscle atrophy. Be suspicious of any animal exhibiting any degree of muscle or skeletal atrophy, especially when assessing its future usefulness or serviceability. *See:* ASYMMETRY.

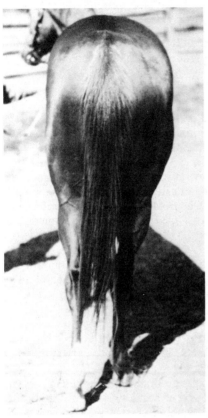

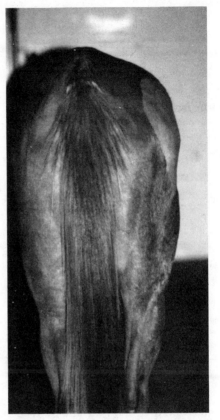

Symmetric Quarters, no indication of muscle atrophy

Asymmetric Quarters, indication of muscle atrophy from nerve injury or disuse

bog spavin *See:* SPAVIN.

bone spavin *See:* SPAVIN.

bowed tendon *See:* SUPERFICIAL FLEXOR TENDON, TENDONITIS.

breakover The area on the toe of the foot or its shoe from which the foot actually flexes and subsequently leaves the ground. Some elusive lamenesses, usually early in their development, create telltale breakover points on the bottom of the foot or shoe. These wear points develop as the horse attempts to compensate for its discomfort.

After watching the horse move on a shank, pick up the bare or shod foot and look for evidence of uneven wear. Consult with a veterinarian for a definitive diagnosis.

I have found that many gait alterations, regardless of cause, can be well managed, perhaps even permanently corrected, through the combined efforts of a skilled farrier and an equine practitioner. Many talented and deserving horses have had their useful lives greatly extended by conscientious caring professionals. *See:* FOOT.

broken down   A lay term for any competition horse that has suffered a severe injury during racing or training. Most often the term refers to "bowed tendons" or severely ruptured suspensory ligaments. Retirement from competition is usually mandatory with protracted treatment and rest. In some cases, euthanasia is indicated. *See:* TENDONITIS.

bucked shins   Inflammation of the tissue (periosteum) covering the front surface of the cannon bones.

Periostitis is the medical term used for this disorder. An acute attack requires cooling agents and rest; chronic "shins" require counterirritants (paints, blisters, or firing) and rest.

The condition originates from stress and strain, and from concussion to these areas caused by speed-related overextension of the forelegs. If soreness and inflammation persist, "firing" (q.v.) is indicated after a responsible person ascertains that the shins are cool to the touch. Before a horse can prudently be fired, it requires seven to ten days total rest for the average inflammation to subside.

Periostitis is so common in young race horses in the United States that some owners and trainers routinely accept such trauma as part of the training and racing careers of their horses. This need not be! There are few such cases in England, where racing is exclusively on grass and the maximum distance for two-year-olds is seven furlongs.

The answer to bucked shins does not lie with new medicines, fancy cures, or herbs. Rather, we should delay starting our two-year-olds until late in the year, better educate our trainers, improve track surfaces, and enforce stricter licensing. *See:* METATARSUS, PERIOSTITIS, TIMBER SHINS.

bursa   A small closed sac lined with synovial membrane and containing synovial fluid. Bursae are found throughout the body in areas subject to friction and provide a cushion for any bony area over which a tendon passes.

bursitis   Inflammation of a bursa, usually caused by physical exertion, fatigue, or overly strenuous exercise. Horses commonly suffer from bicipital bursitis (shoulder), trochanteric bursitis (hip), and navicular bursitis (foot).

Although this ailment develops quickly, it requires a lengthy period for recovery—if it *does* recover. Some acute bursitis cases, if treated promptly, subside in a relatively short period, but if the same area is repeatedly abused, the bursitis then becomes chronic, perhaps a crippling and permanent affliction.

Care of bursitis:

First aid before the veterinarian arrives:

1. Hose with cold water
2. Cold-water bandage where applicable
3. Alternate cold or cooling packs with heating pads
4. Manual massage with liquid braces of liniments

Veterinary care of bursitis:

1. Rest and the local application of cooling agents
2. Oral administration of 60-grain aspirin, three to four times daily, *or* a 1-gram tablet of phenylbutazone twice daily
3. Injections locally into the bursae under strict supervision by your veterinarian

BURSITIS

Types	Location	Stable Name	Common Causes
Supra-atlantal bursitis	Head: poll, between ears	Poll evil	Originates by a deep bruising of tissues, then bacterial invaders complicate.
Supraspinous bursitis	Withers	Fistulous withers	Originates by a deep bruising of tissues, then bacterial invaders complicate.
Spinous bursitis	Back: Top of thoracic vertebral spines (saddle area)	Bruised back	Trauma from ill-fitting saddle
Bicipital bursitis (intertubercularis)	Fore leg: point of shoulder		Trauma: colliding with stall doorway, posts, fence, starting gate
Olecranon bursitis	Fore leg: point of elbow	Shoe boil, capped elbow	Shoe of the same leg in contact with elbow when animal is down
Trapezius bursitis	Fore leg: shoulder area		Trauma; dirty hypodermic needles
Trochanteric bursitis	Fore leg: shoulder area	Whirl bone disease	Trauma: hind leg slipping backwards, jumping, loading on a ramp or from starting gate
Carpal bursitis	Knee	hygroma, capped knee	Trauma: blow to knee or self-inflicted by pawing at door, screen, and half door
Cunean tendon bursitis	Hind leg: front and inside hock	Hocky	Early spavin or arthritic changes
Achilles bursitis	Hind leg: point of hock	Capped hock	Kicking: self-inflicted in stall, trailer, or van
Podotrochleosis	All four feet: inside foot under the os pedis	Navicular	Abusive concussion, poor foot care, hereditary predisposition

bursitis continued

If the condition becomes chronic, continue to rest the animal, then apply counterirritants such as paints, internal or external blisters, or, as a last resort, firing.

Except for first-aid steps listed above, for all other treatment please consult your veterinarian.

Bursitis is a common horse ailment suffered by competition, pleasure, and draft horses. Since there are many bursae in the horse's body, inflammation can occur at any time in any of these little cushions. In fact, a large portion of my practice is concerned with such treatment.

Horse doctors use cortisone and its by-products with great care in order not to jeopardize the patient's future usefulness.

cadence A rhythmic sound useful for diagnostic purposes. To confirm lameness, it is not always necessary to *see* a horse when it is jogged on a hard or firm surface. It is enough to hear the cadence of the gait—whether symmetric or asymmetric—to determine whether the horse is sound or unsound.

capped elbow *See:* BURSITIS (CHART, PAGE 77).

capped hocks A bursitis over the point of the hock caused by kicking stalls, trailer walls, or anything solid. A soft swelling occurs initially which becomes firmer to the touch when chronic. Cooling agents, antiphlogistics, hosing with intermittent hot and cold water all help, but kicking is a vice and if the cause or environment is not changed, the same undesirable behavior will persist. In some cases the damage is so severe as to warrant destruction of the horse.

Change stalls, rearrange feeding tubs or feeding patterns; perhaps the habit can be broken. Early treatment can be helpful when a simple bursitis is evident, but once a chronically fibrosed hock results from repeated insults, treatment is worthless. I have never seen a case of capped hocks completely resorbed, regardless of treatment.

In chronic cases, mild iodine paints containing DMSO or DMSO and steroids can reduce the size somewhat simply by causing the superficial swelling to shrink, but the actual fibrous tissue will not disappear.

If any lameness is evident early, this subsides quickly and the capped hocks remain, not as an unsoundness, but as a cosmetic detraction or blemish. Capped hocks can greatly reduce a horse's value when it is offered for sale. *See:* BURSITIS (CHART, PAGE 77).

clubfoot A malformation in which the foot grows at an obtuse angle, with no appreciable toe growth but excessive heel growth. Long regarded as a foot problem, it is actually caused by a contraction of the deep digital flexor tendon, and is thought to be of congenital origin. Curable only by a recently developed surgical technique called *inferior check ligament desmotomy*.

The incidence of clubfoot development in young horses is increasing steadily, much to the concern of breeders.

The cure was impossible, the deformity ugly, and the lameness was lifelong. Many such cases were euthanized.

Today we have a miraculous surgery that produces a cure. *See:* DESMOTOMY.

contracted heels A condition in which the heels of the foot are narrower than normal, although the entire foot may be contracted. Contracted heels usually are found in the front feet and develop when there is a lack of or a reduced amount of

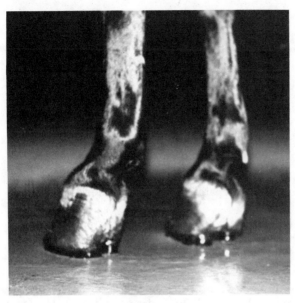

Contracted Heels

natural frog pressure. The cause usually is (1) a condition in the limb or foot that prevents the front from bearing normal support, or (2) incorrect balancing and dressing of the feet. Young animals are more sensitive to poor dressing than older ones.

It is my opinion that this condition in the heels is simply an extension and manifestation of contracted tendons that are affecting the entire limb, joints, and feet. Although external influences, both good and bad, bear somewhat on the degree of contraction, flexor tendon contraction, exerting its relentless tendon pull, is the true underlying etiologic factor.

Contracted heels invite unsoundnesses or predispose to the development of lameness. Any horse with this condition is a bad prospect for purchase. It is interesting to note that contracted heels often have a deep-seated thrush infection, usually quite refractory to treatment.

Contracted heels are seen often in horses whose feet have been allowed to grow long for show purposes—Saddlebreds, Walking Horses, and fancy driving horses. Who knows what other types will join them in the future. *See:* SHOEING.

corn *See:* FOOT.

cracked heels A lay term for a painful condition involving the heels of a competition horse. Two well-known causes are chemically treated track surfaces, and frequent baths (with heels left wet).

If all four heels are carefully dried after washing and are kept clean, dry, and protected (when necessary), such problems can be avoided. Enzyme and antibiotic preparations are excellent when applied to a heel and covered with a sterile dressing. Avoid contact with water, dirt, and air.

cracked heels continued

Dry heels well, then apply the following lotion:

Lead acetate	2 tablespoons
Zinc sulfate	2 tablespoons
Glycerine	1 pint

OR

Goulard's extract of lead	2 tablespoons
Olive oil	1 pint

Another excellent preparation for cracked heels or any dry irritated skin area:

Zinc oxide	10 ounces
Benzocaine powder	1 ounce
Cold cream	5 pounds

Do not confuse this condition with foot cracks. *See:* FOOT.

curb (*not* the bridle bit)   An inflammation and thickening of the plantar tarsal ligament, located on the back of the hind cannon bone just below the hock area. It can best be viewed by standing beside the horse and looking at the back of the leg, immediately below the hock. You will see a rounded (convex) swelling projecting backwards. Heat, swelling, and lameness can occur depending upon the degree of inflammation and the severity of the injury to the plantar tarsal ligament.

If the ligament is ruptured, a larger, warmer, and appreciably more painful swelling will persist as compared to a simple strained ligament. In either case, an antiphlogistic (anti-inflammatory agent) and cooling efforts, such as hosing, are in order. Rest, cooling agents (poultices), and perhaps even a mild paint may be prescribed by your veterinarian. With ideal treatment, curbs heal well, usually by fibrosis (a laying-down or interlacing of fibrous tissue by the body to heal and strengthen the area). With fibrosis, however, comes some degree of thickening or increased size. Once formed, curbs do not go away. The formation does not present a serious threat to unsoundness, just a cosmetic blemish.

Curbs may be blamed for soreness in a conformationally unsound leg, but I, for one, question the diagnosis. And although slipping, sliding, and physical abuse are all listed as reasons why curbs appear, I have yet to see a curb develop on a conformationally sound hind leg. Perhaps this condition properly belongs in the category of hereditarily or congenitally predisposed conditions.

Some foals are delivered with curbs on their hocks; some wait until later on in their youth to develop curbs on already crooked hind legs. Individuals with sickle hocks, cow hocks, and bandy legs are destined to develop curbs if they are not foaled with them already there.

deep digital flexor tendon   A tendon originating from three muscular heads located on the back surface of the radius (large bone above the knee) and ultimately attaching on the under surface of the os pedis (third phalanx, or coffin bone) of the foot. This flexor tendon, relatively small in circumference, very round in shape, and quite unimpressive in structure, is in my opinion the most important tendon in the horse's leg. It receives more stress and strain than any other part of the leg.

Recent research has revealed that when a bowed tendon occurs, the problem is not with the deep digital flexor tendon, but rather with its partner, the superficial flexor tendon. *See:* CLUBFOOT, SUPERFICIAL FLEXOR TENDON.

epiphysitis   An inflammation of the growth zone or plate in the long leg bones of young horses. It is first evidenced by an enlargement on the inside surface just above the knees. In normal youngsters, these plates will calcify and close at between 22 to 26 months of age. An open (immature) epiphyseal plate is very vulnerable to stress, strain, and undue exertion. An early, hard training schedule can easily jeopardize the animal's future soundness. Wise trainers will not start training a young horse until the veterinarian takes X-rays and approves the degree of closure of the growth line above the knees. This is a routine procedure in better-run barns.

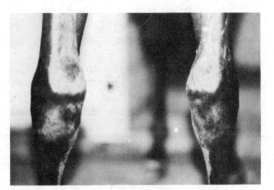

Epiphysitis, bilateral knees

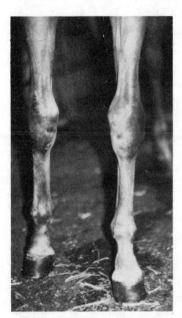

Epiphysitis, knees, growth line

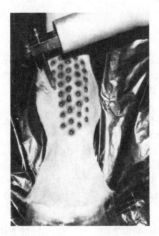

Firing Ankle on Racing Horse

epiphysitis continued

Nutritional epiphysitis can occur involving all four limbs; its signs are painful swellings above the knees and "apple ankles," a transitional condition of the ankles caused by overnutrition. If recognized early, the condition can be managed successfully with no veterinary treatment; only supervision is required. The regime consists of reducing grain by 50 percent, stopping all supplements, changing legume hay to timothy, and stall-resting the horse. These suggestions are mandatory for a successful outcome. The enlargements above the joints should slowly subside and "cool out" in approximately four to six weeks. For success, please abide by the rules!

Epiphysitis is another manifestation of an imbalance between nutritional intake and the rate of tissue and bone growth.

firing   The process of burning crevices or holes of various sizes and shapes into a horse's skin. It is most commonly used on the legs, although occasionally it finds application in other areas of the body.

In theory, firing is thought to be beneficial by stimulating an inflammatory reaction, bringing blood with all of its healing properties to the area. In fact, it is known to change a chronic condition to an acute situation, thus reactivating the healing process.

In my opinion, firing is sound in principal, and although I have fired horses for years and consider the process to have definite merit, it is interesting to note that the statistical success rate of firing continues to decline. Perhaps this controversial treatment has received its ominous reputation through misuse; perhaps it has erroneously been applied to normal tissue!

Unlike those who view firing as a cure-all, I see it as beneficial in a narrow spectrum of uses. They include:

1. Properly cooled-out bucked shins
2. Properly cooled-out splints or any other bony exostosis
3. Osselets
4. Sesamoiditis
5. Chronic arthritis
6. Bone spavin
7. Chronic curbs

Please note that all areas amenable to the firing process are of a bony or fibrous nature; these, I find, usually respond well to this old method of treatment. Soft-tissue lesions or injuries do not react well to firing and thus are contraindicated.

To prepare for firing, there are a few things you can perform in advance of the veterinarian's arrival:

1. Set up a clean, dry, well-lighted area in the barn.
2. Clear the barn of all excess personnel and pet animals.
3. Clean your horse and clip the affected area well and then scrub the entire leg with warm water and soap. Rinse well with clear water, and, above all, *dry* the leg well.

The veterinarian will probably sedate the horse mildly, scrub with alcohol, and quietly block the region to be fired with an appropriate local anesthetic (2 percent lidocaine hydrochloride). If the site is extensive and the horse requires in excess of 30 milliliters (cc), your veterinarian will add a minute amount of epinephrine to the local anesthetic. This very powerful drug acts to delay the rate of absorption of the local anesthetic and thus prevents a procaine reaction (sweating, shaking of the head, wide blinking eyes) commonly seen in horses that have received a large dose of local anesthetic for any reason.

The old-fashioned firing iron was a rod-shaped instrument, approximately 20 inches long, with a small point on one end and a cylinder in the handle to hold ether. "Ether irons" were difficult to keep at a consistent temperature and required many assistants. Today we have electric-powered firing irons that are efficient and reliable.

After firing, the veterinarian will cover all fire holes or crevices with a paste blister of choice, then cover with sterile gauze and dressing. A cradle is then applied and some additional tranquilizer is injected before the veterinarian departs. I find that a little consideration given the animal during the first 24 hours has rewards. There is no need for a horse to suffer unduly with our firing procedure today, no need for it to miss one oat.

The efficiency of firing depends upon the veterinarian's skill and technique, the type of paint or blister used after the firing, and the conscientiousness of the caretaker or groom in attendance.

foot The foot of the horse includes the hoof and its internal structures. The hoof is a thickened and cornified epidermis comprised of three layers—two relatively thin outer layers and a thick, tough inner layer that encases and protects the internal structures of the foot. The hoof is bloodless and nerveless; it derives its nutrition from the coronary band.

On the outside layer, just below the coronary band, is a narrow band of tissue called the periople, similar to the cuticle of the human nail. The periople produces a waxy material that migrates down over the hoof wall to help prevent drying out of hoof tissue. The innermost layer consists of tubules of hard keratin material that run longitudinally from the coronary band to the bearing surface; 25 percent of this layer is water held within the tubules.

Although the horny wall grows constantly, the rate of growth can vary dependent upon physical condition, nutrition, ground surface, and the care given to the feet. As a rule of thumb, foot tissue grows one-third of an inch per month; it requires approximately 12 months for the hoof tissue, growing from the coronary band, to renew itself completely.

Treatment and care of the feet is an integral part of daily care for every owner or caretaker. Feet should be picked out daily, with the aid of a hoof pick, before and after exercise. This daily examination shows up the presence of any foreign bodies (stones, glass, and nails), and allows you to check the condition of the shoes (to see if they are broken, shifted, or bent, or if there are any loose nails). This is the easiest way to prevent lameness.

For young and barefoot horses, regular dressing and balancing of the feet by a farrier to maintain proper angulation of toes and heels can alleviate the stresses placed on limbs at this early vulnerable age.

Foals should have the points of their toes rounded so that they "break over" at the center of the toe. If these points that grow naturally on all foals' feet are not regularly rounded with a rasp, the foal will tend to break either to the inside or

foot continued

the outside of the foot, directly affecting the stride and ultimately the angulation of its legs.

While unhealthy hoof tissue can occur because of poor diet, extremely dry, hard ground, or wet, deep mud, in my opinion it most likely originates from a congenital or hereditary predisposition.

Feed additives (dried brewer's yeast, vitamin and mineral supplements, gelatine) have been tried for promoting healthy growth, but with inconsistent findings. Although I cannot produce scientific documentation, I have had cases in my practice that responded dramatically to high doses of vitamin A over a period of eight to 12 weeks. I must admit that all these individuals had a history of questionable diet and care, giving unscientific credence to dietary deficiency as a cause.

Dry brittle feet, feet with cracks, or feet that refuse to grow a toe or heel can be visibly improved by daily use of Mollamentum, pine tar and lard mixtures, or Irish Reducine® poultices applied externally. These preparations are more effective if—besides covering the soles, frogs, walls, and coronary bands—they are massaged in manually 2 inches above and around the hoofline. New foot growth will thus be stimulated.

An old remedy for brittle feet is a mixture of 1 ounce of turpentine with 6 ounces of neatsfoot oil, applied once daily for two weeks.

If applied according to directions, a hot Irish Reducine poultice is, to my mind, superior to all other medications. Added effort and time are required, but the benefits far outweigh the inconvenience.

First, heat the can of Reducine and then spread the thick black contents generously over each foot—the sole and wall and up as high as 2 or 3 inches above the coronary band. Cover well with a light layer of cotton followed by two layers of aluminum foil. Then cover with two layers of feed sacking and tie well.

CAUTION: Do not allow air to enter, since this would cause blistering of the soft tissue. The use of the air-tight covering makes it unnecessary to grease the tender heel area with Vaseline, as is usual in the application of a counterirritant. Maintain the integrity of the covering by reapplying tape over the outside, and do not remove the covering for 14 days. The new growth that you will see and the improved texture of the foot will delight you.

Whenever you want a foot to grow, remember, bind it up well and keep it warm and protected from air!

When purchasing a horse for competition or pleasure, it is a good policy to scrutinize the shape and texture of all four feet and engage the services of your veterinarian to help you evaluate those all-important feet. A poor foot (or feet) can cause endless and immeasurable misery to both the horse and the owner, not to mention the farrier.

Lameness, shoeing and nailing problems, cracks, splits, and broken walls are all included in an unlimited grab bag of mostly unhappy surprises. A brittle-footed horse must show superior potential in every other respect to justify its purchase. Daily care is a chore you must anticipate! *See:* THRUSH.

foot bruise   A contusion usually deep in the underlying soft tissue of the foot. In order to classify as a bruise, the skin or hoof surface must be intact with no visible break.

A stone or any hard object contacting the foot with adequate force can transfer pressure through the outer semiprotective layers, causing capillary rupture. The result is a painful bruise to the horse's foot.

The sole of the foot is especially vulnerable to bruising, which occurs frequently when horses are subjected to rocky or hard-surfaced ground. Leathers or pads placed under the shoes can be used as a preventive measure.

A characteristic sore-footed gait and the horse's response to foot testers are signs that help to diagnose a bruised foot. Local fever or increased heat in the foot with arterial pulsation are inconsistent symptoms.

If extreme soreness exists, some people prefer to soak the horse's foot first and then apply a poultice of their choice.

A cup of Epsom salts (magnesium sulfate) with one-half cup of vinegar in one-half gallon of hot water makes a fine soaking solution, followed by poultices and rest. In addition, of course, there should be an update on the patient's tetanus vaccination history.

founder   *See:* HYPOTHYROIDISM, LAMINITIS.

iliac artery thrombosis (verminous arteritis)   Horses suffering with thrombosis (obstruction) of the iliac artery or aortic bifurcations usually show a transient unilateral hind leg lameness. Occlusion of this major hind leg artery can cause the horse to appear dramatically lame with virtually no lesions and no evidence of leg injury.

The condition is thought to result primarily from a parasitic invasion into the lumen of the large artery which has the effect of blocking the flow of vital oxygenerated blood to the entire hind leg. *Strongylus vulgaris* larva, the largest and most destructive bloodworm, is the main parasitic offender.

Symptoms are pain, elevated heart and respiratory rates, and profuse sweating all over the body except the affected limb, which is usually dry and cool to the touch. Often, the metatarsal pulse is imperceptible. All symptoms are exaggerated with exercise when the demand for blood to the extermities is greatly increased.

When a horse shows transient symptoms of hind leg lameness that increase with exercise, quickly check the temperature of the limb for evidence of digital pulse and for a prolonged venous refill time.

Rectal examination may reveal a disparity between the amplitude of the abdominal aortal branches and the two iliac branches. If an uneven supply of blood exists, this may account for the pain, coolness of limb, and reduced blood supply to the distal portions of the leg.

There is no known treatment for an occlusion of a main artery in the horse. Possibly in the future, surgeons will be able to repair the area with Teflon or some other prosthetic material.

Please worm your horse regularly and carry out all the recommended practices to break the parasite's reproductive cycle (hygienic care of the horse, environmental cleanliness, pasture rotation, chain dragging of pastures, avoidance of overgrazing, etc.).

inferior check ligament   Originating in back of and slightly below the knee in the fore leg, this ligament is incorporated into the deep digital flexor tendon and ends about midway down the back of the cannon bone.

The inferior check ligament occupies a similar location in the hind leg, originating just below the hock and ending midway down the back of the cannon bone.

The term *desmitis* means an inflammation of a ligament. When it occurs in a check ligament, desmitis results in lameness or intermittent lameness for a minimum of several months. Treatment calls for a protracted period of rest first and foremost, as well as cooling agents followed by paints, blisters, or firing. Prognosis is usually fair, but the results depend upon the severity of the injury and the inflammation at the time rest was instituted.

Most horsemen can recognize the swelling over the flexor tendon area just under and in back of the knee as a strained check ligament, but I would gamble that few could locate the affected structure. This ligament is concealed from sight, resting neatly inside the same sheath that protects the deep digital flexor tendon, and is palpable only by experienced hands.

A component of the "stay apparatus," the inferior check ligament provides an important means of correcting the "clubfoot syndrome" seen in foals and adults. *See:* CLUBFOOT, DESMOTOMY, STAY APPARATUS.

joint infection   An infection of the joint cavity and its contents. This entity is dreaded by horsemen and equine veterinarians. Accidental wounds, nonsterile injections, and careless handling are the usual causes.

When a disease-producing micro-organism gains entrance to a joint cavity in any area of the horse's body, the prognosis is automatically guarded and the "red alert" is activated. Once an infection is established in the synovial membranes, it seems to become walled off and insensitive to all conventional treatments. Routine medicines, antibiotics, and drugs prove ineffective, while the joint infection continues, usually unabated, to destroy joint tissues (intra-articular surfaces, synovial membranes, and bone tissue). Even adjacent tendons, tendon sheaths, and ligaments are affected, as their ability to function is impaired.

Symptoms are swelling, heat, and pain in and around the joint accompanied by a fever usually "spiking" over 105° Fahrenheit. A blood count reveals a high white cell count indicating a systemic infection, although it is difficult to treat systemically. Direct joint intervention is mandatory.

Treatment consists of an immediate aspiration of the joint fluid (arthrocentesis) for laboratory cultures, identification, and sensitivity tests. Simultaneously, it is urgent to flush the joint with sterile saline solution and to reinject a strong broad-spectrum antibiotic directly into the joint cavity, usually through the same needle used to obtain the laboratory sample of synovial fluid. Intravenous injections of the same antibiotic augment the joint treatment. With early and intensified efforts, some joints can be salvaged without permanent damage, but unfortunately only a small percentage of joints are restored to normal.

Most infected joints become enlarged, fibrosed, and ankylosed, losing all range of motion and ability to perform as in a normal horse. Many such individuals have only the role of reproduction to anticipate; a gelding has no future.

As a broodmare veterinarian, I have seen many race fillies sent to the stud much too early in their racing careers because of joint infection. Some have hobbled out of the van with an ankle or a knee swollen to the size of a large grapefruit. It is a sad commentary on the competence of their keepers.

joint inflammation *See:* ARTHRITIS, OSTEOARTHRITIS.

joint lesions Examples:

Foot   ringbone, navicular disease
Ankle   osselets, sesamoiditis, windpuffs, intra-articular fracture fragments
Knee   carpitis, hygroma, intra-articular fracture fragments
Hock   spavins, thoroughpin, intra-articular fracture fragments
Stifle   gonitis, intra-articular fracture fragments
Hip   coxitis

joint mice   A common term for any minute body, tiny fracture, or split-off piece of articular cartilaginous fragment found in the joint space. When these bodies become free and perhaps move around in the joint, they can cause great pain and even destroy some intra-articular cartilaginous surface if they are sizable and if considerable stress is exerted. Surgical removal is then indicated to prevent additional damage to joint structures and to relieve pain.

lameness   In the horse, lameness is manifested by an asymmetric or uneven gait. Undoubtedly, it is the most frequent problem besetting horse owners.

Lameness is readily apparent to an observant, sensitive person; you do not need great knowledge and experience of horses in order to detect it. When a horse is merely sore or *slightly* lame, however, then experience is helpful.

Whatever the cause of lameness, prompt attention can often minimize a problem that otherwise could develop into a lengthy and costly situation. Don't delay treatment.

Locating the precise site and cause of lameness is the job of the veterinarian. Drawing on years of experience as well as on diagnostic methods, the doctor can usually pinpoint the problem and promptly produce a definitive diagnosis, a precise prognosis, and a prescribed course of treatment.

Since 90 percent of all lameness occurs in the foot, you, as an owner, may prefer to apply first aid before calling for help or while waiting for the veterinarian to arrive.

First, feel for a pulse in the leg and for heat in the foot and adjacent coronary hand and pastern. If heat is detected, then remove the shoe, clean the entire sole and frog area, and subsequently apply a poultice to the entire foot area. This treatment reduces inflammation from such causes as a stone bruise, puncture, corn, loose or close nail, a lodged piece of gravel, or hidden abscess.

To counter heat, swelling, or pain in the horse's leg, you can safely hose, poultice, or apply wet dressings.

This first-aid approach could result in a sound horse again, but please do not embark on a home nursing project unless your horse has received regular Tetanus Toxoid boosters.

The use of a poultice is a great standby and its application can never do any harm. In my opinion, *when in doubt, poultice. See:* POULTICE.

lateral cartilages   A lateral cartilage is a specialized patch of cartilage located at the coronary band level on each side of the foot. These cartilages act as cushions

lateral cartilages continued

to absorb concussion to the foot when it strikes the ground surface. The foot and coronary area expands and contracts with each stride as weight is shifted onto and off the foot.

Normally, these structures are quite soft, pliable, and absorptive, typical of physiologically sound cartilage. However, when concussions are too great and/or too frequent, and when there is some contributing factor such as a questionable diet, marginal foot care and shoeing, or any other foot abuse, then ossification can occur. Hereditary predisposition is another factor in ossification of the lateral cartilages. This is the site of side-bone formation. *See:* OSSIFICATION OF LATERAL CARTILAGES.

metatarsus   The cannon bone of the hind leg, arranged similarly to the cannon bone (metacarpus) of the fore leg. The hind leg cannon bone, or third metatarsus, has corresponding splint bones located on the inside (medial) and outside (lateral); these are called metatarsus II and metatarsus IV, respectively.

The large metatarsal bone is not only 2 inches or so longer, but it is also notably stronger than that of the fore leg, due to the presence of a very thick and compact bony substance in the front of the bone and on the inside surface. Nature has fortified the weight and stress-bearing areas.

I have found that during exercise and competition, especially in timber races, fox hunting, and point-to-point events, the cannon bones of the hind legs receive great traumatic abuse from hitting the top rails at a high rate of speed. "Timber shins" develop after the race and are seen as a convex swelling on the entire front surface of the hind leg shin. The solid wooden fences leave their mark on these large, courageous jumpers.

Flat runners suffer a shin problem called bucked shins (periostitis) in the front legs. This is an inflammation of the periosteum on the third metacarpus, caused in this case by excessive speed rather than physical trauma. *See:* BUCKED SHINS.

myopathy   Any abnormal condition or disease of the muscular tissues. It occurs most frequently in the hind legs of rodeo horses, especially those used for sliding stops, but it can be sustained accidentally in any individual of any breed simply by simulating the same type of leg stress as that seen in Quarter Horse competition. Hind leg myopathy may subsequently develop if a horse gets a hind foot caught in the halter.

Caused by physical trauma to the semitendinosus, semimembranosus, and large biceps femoris muscles of the hind leg, an acute inflammatory condition develops initially which then becomes chronic. These large and important hind leg muscles are located above the hock, extending up to the hip and backwards on each side of the tail-head and dock area.

It is sometimes difficult to know exactly when the injury occurs, since lameness is not seen during the acute phase, only when healing begins. Adhesions causing lameness form between these muscle groups, and the developing adhesions create the lameness.

There is a characteristic hind leg gait which is almost diagnostic when viewed from the side and observed at a walk on hard surface footing. The peculiar hind leg gait is sometimes called "goose stepping." As the leg is advanced, the foot is suddenly pulled backwards 3 to 4 inches just before striking the ground surface. A sliding sound can be heard with each stride. As you stand behind the animal, a hard patch may be palpated in the muscle tissue halfway between the point of the hock and the ischium. Adhesions usually form between the semitendinosus muscle and the semimembranosus on the side closest to the tail, and also on the outer side of the leg between the semitendinosus and the biceps femoris.

Conservative treatment is ineffective. Surgical removal of the intermuscular adhesions is the preferred course of action. The success rate is very satisfactory, although I have experienced some delayed healing and excessive swelling where sutures have been difficult to keep in place. The end result, however, was gratifying.

navicular disease (podotrochleosis) Navicular is the name of a small but important bone in the horse's foot. Shaped like a shuttle, it is located just in back of and slightly under the main bone of the foot, the os pedis, or coffin bone. The navicular bone is coated with cartilage to serve as a cushion for the important deep digital flexor tendon to pass over before it attaches to the bottom of the os pedis. The navicular bone is notorious as the site of a common ailment that causes lameness in many horses, grief to the owners, and frustration to veterinarians.

Navicular lameness comes in two forms: The early incidence is usually seen as *navicular bursitis,* while the later-developing malady is called *navicular disease*.

Bursitis affects the bursal sac that lies nestled between the deep digital flexor tendon and the navicular bone. When inflammation occurs from trauma, pounding, and generalized abuse, inflammation develops. This will respond to rest, cooling agents (hosing, tubing, injections locally), and corrective shoeing.

With progression and time, however, the bursitis develops into navicular disease with chronic bone changes resembling arthritis. Not too much can be offered in the way of treatment for navicular disease, although corrective shoeing and injections into the bursa locally may cool the area and may sometimes mobilize any minute arthritic bony fragments that could be a contributing cause of pain. As a last resort, a posterior digital neurectomy may give some lasting relief.

Causes of navicular bursitis or disease are as numerous as the suggested remedies. Concussion, misuse, poor shoeing, contracted heels, and small feet are a few with which to reckon. My personal opinion is that predisposition for the development of navicular disease is inherited.

An early symptom of navicular disease is occasional lameness with a characteristic toe-catching gait; the outer part of the fore foot catches the ground and causes a bit of dust or dirt to fly up. This gait is almost diagnostic of navicular bursitis.

In spite of all efforts, this disease progresses slowly to the point of chronic lameness.

A clinical diagnosis should be determined with radiographs to confirm the diagnosis, but X-rays should not be the means of diagnosis. I have seen positive X-rays and a clinically sound horse.

There is no ideal treatment, but we do have methods available to relieve the horse's needs, if only in a temporary fashion. Treatment consists of corticosteroid

navicular disease continued

injections locally; as the disease progresses, a posterior digital neurectomy is indicated. *See:* NEURECTOMY.

These efforts, combined with a classical navicular-type shoe, can keep some exceptional horses in the mainstream of use or competition by remaining serviceably sound. Efforts should be made to achieve a 48-degree or greater angulation of the front feet. A navicular shoe comprises a wide web, rolled toe, and elevated branches. A 2- to 3-degree pad interposed between the shoe and foot will simplify the need for elevation.

In difficult cases I routinely inject a local anesthetic, 2 percent lidocaine, directly down into the navicular bursa to achieve a definitive diagnosis. In seven clinical cases over 25 years, I experienced a phenomenal response. In each case the horse became sound within minutes—the normal response to a local anesthetic—but, quite inexplicably and to my disbelief, each one remained categorically sound ever after. How to explain this? Was the foot sore from some cause other than navicular disease? Did the local injection of lidocaine swell the tissue and mobilize minute particles of calcium that were causing pain? It is impossible to say.

There is another treatment for chronic navicular to add to the already long list of medications. Although I would insist upon further research before using the drug, some veterinarians prescribe daily oral administration of heparin. Heparin is an old, reliable anticoagulant used for years to inhibit clotting and promote bleeding. Heparin's oral use has evoked great claims of success in the restoration of previously crippled horses; along with navicular it is reported to improve flow of blood through a foundered foot. Care must be taken to avoid any break in the skin or serious laceration, since hemorrhage without clotting is a true threat in the case of daily heparin use. *See:* HEPARIN.

Many fine show mares, loaded with talent, develop navicular disease and are immediately retired as broodmares to reproduce, most likely, handsome foals with the potential for early development of navicular disease. I see this most frequently in Quarter Horses, where the breeders want heavily muscled animals with tiny, malformed feet. If show judges stopped selecting huge-bodied individuals with mouse feet, they might discourage the breeders from this folly!

occult spavin   *See:* SPAVIN.

open knees   A lay term for enlarged knees exhibiting an irregular profile and questionable appearance. This open-knee condition is commonly found in large, well-fed horses under three years of age.

Diagnosis is quite easy based on the clinical appearances of the knees, although X-rays are essential for confirmation of the diagnosis. Specific X-ray views are necessary: The cone must be directed high on the knee to include the epiphyseal line located on the distal end of the radius.

Radiographic evidence of growth-line immaturity dictates the vital need for additional time for the horse to grow and mature.

Do not foolishly subject your young animal to the rigors of training and thereby risk the development of epiphysitis. Simply delay breaking and serious training until future X-rays reveal a sound, closed growth line. *See:* EPIPHYSITIS.

ossification of lateral cartilages (side bones)   The cause of ossification is not understood, although in the order of suspicion concussion ranks first, followed by conformation and hereditary factors. Side bones can be seen in all stages and degrees of development and can cause varying lamenesses with exercise.

In this condition bone cells are deposited into the cartilage, producing a change in texture from suppleness to rigidity and inflexibility in the inner part of the foot and in the coronary band. The transition is usually slow and gradual but very permanent.

Diagnosis is made by digital palpation on each side of the foot at the coronary band level to determine flexibility. Diagnosis must be confirmed by radiographs, however.

Side bones are seen more often in the fore feet and most often in horses over six years of age. Hunters, jumpers, and pleasure horses suffer with this malady; young race horses rarely are affected.

Treatment consists of rest with a variety of blisters over the coronary band area. I have had some success with an approach that calls for grooving the hoof wall directly over the lateral cartilage area, fitting on a bar shoe with beveled branches to spread the foot, and applying generous amounts of Irish Reducine daily. In some selected cases, the treatment has allowed the horse to continue working.

Side bones is a condition that—with the exception of severe cases—can be managed with careful supervision. *See:* LATERAL CARTILAGES.

osteoarthritis A form of arthritis affecting the bone surfaces in joints, with inflammation and erosion of the joint cartilage surfaces. Multiple bony changes and diverse calcium deposits result.

It is this author's opinion that trauma and physical abuse sustained in young, vulnerable race horses is the major cause of osteoarthritic lesions commonly seen today.

Osteoarthritis can affect almost every joint in the horse's body, not unlike the form of the disease seen in the human body. One major dissimilarity is the difference in ages at which this painful, deforming, and crippling condition occurs. It afflicts the very young competition horse and the older human being.

In the horse, osteoarthritis commonly manifests itself as navicular disease, ringbone, chronic osselets, carpitis (knee), or bone spavin (hock). Each and every one of these conditions is capable of curtailing a racing or athletic career. Some young castoffs continue on in less demanding roles such as pleasure hacks or hill toppers' mounts. Of course, of prime importance is the suitable disposition and level-headedness of the former race horse and its ability to adapt. *See:* HYALURONIC ACID.

Treatment of arthritis is basically palliative, not curative, so conscientious efforts should be made to prevent the permanent joint changes characteristic of osteoarthritis.

Some alert trainers and equine veterinarians insist upon X-raying the epiphyseal line at the distal end of the radius before placing a horse in training. *See:* EPIPHYSITIS.

Time is the most favorable factor, allowing for physical maturity and mental development which help the race horse to cope better with the multiple daily stresses of training, vanning, and racing.

Two-year-old horses in training often suffer inflammatory conditions. These *osteoarthritis continued*

can subside with rest and cooling efforts, or they can present persistent signs of osteoarthritis. The instant that pain, heat, swelling, or any limb or joint discomfort is detected in the youthful athlete, a judgment must be made as to whether the training schedule should be continued. The horse's competitive or useful future lies in the decision-maker's hands.

Treatment can consist of rest and cooling out the affected area. Then an evaluation, sometimes augmented with X-rays, dictates the preferred course of treatment: paint, blister, fire, or—among the newer techniques—ultrasound, laser, or cryogenics.

Once arthritis is established in a joint, treatment is directed toward relieving pain and increasing mobility. The drug hyaluronic acid (q.v.), released for use in the United States in 1984, was a major advance in joint therapy. Marketed under such names as Hylartin, Adequan, and Healon, it acts to promote regeneration of the articular cartilage.

Normal Foot and Pastern

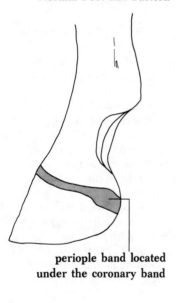

periople band located
under the coronary band

Sites of Leg and Hoof Conditions

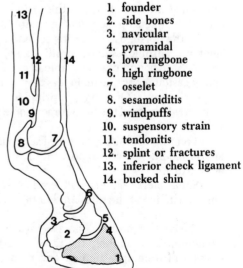

1. founder
2. side bones
3. navicular
4. pyramidal
5. low ringbone
6. high ringbone
7. osselet
8. sesamoiditis
9. windpuffs
10. suspensory strain
11. tendonitis
12. splint or fractures
13. inferior check ligament
14. bucked shin

Knee or Carpus

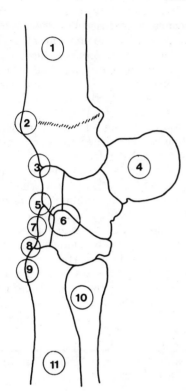

1. radius
2. epiphyseal growth line
3. upper joint
4. accessary carpal bone
5. lower joint
6. carpal bones (8)
7. slab fracture site/third carpal bone
8. fixed joint
9. tuberosity
10. splint bone
11. cannon bone

Also effective against pain are the prostaglandin inhibitors, which include that old standby, aspirin, and phenylbutazone. These drugs act to block the mediation of pain and are safe with minimal side effects. These less harmful drugs are used daily in race horses to help maintain a competition level.

osteochondritis dissecans (OCD) A partial or complete separation of a piece of articular (joint) cartilage and underlying bone. It occurs most often in young horses in the weight-bearing joints and produces lameness.

Radiographs are essential for diagnostic purposes. Poor blood supply to the joint surface and death of tissue with focal dimineralization occur, but the process is not fully understood.

The true cause of osteochondritis dissecans is not known, although hereditary predisposition and hypothyroidism have been suggested.

If the stress of exercise is stopped before the articular cartilage splits, the prognosis is somewhat better. Once the separation occurs, however, the joint will never be pain-free.

Many large, well-bred young horses have been destroyed as a result of OCD, most often diagnosed in the stifle joints. However, in recent years, with the use of the arthroscope and a technique called eburnation, some select cases of OCD have been treated successfully.

osselets   There are two types of osselets: green and true. Both types involve inflammation of the ankle joints. Osselets are found affecting both ankles on the front legs of race horses subjected to daily concussion caused by speed. Early training over poorly surfaced tracks can compound the amount of ankle concussion. Where there are other factors as well—breed predisposition, poor shoeing, poor nutrition—the horse will almost certainly develop sore ankles.

When green osselets appear, all activity must cease! The swelling and acute pain in the fore ankles is caused by the stress of speed which strains the fibrous joint capsule along with the extensor tendons in the leg.

Rest is foremost in treatment, augmented by hosing and poulticing with cooling agents (antiphlogistics). If the condition is severe, the veterinarian may suggest aspirin or Butazolidin tablets orally to combat inflammation.

X-rays taken at this time are customarily negative for any chronic bony changes, since green osselet formation is essentially an inflammatory reaction.

With green osselets, one month usually is required to properly cool the ankles and allow healing. If, however, all sound advice is breached and the horse is returned too soon to training, then the chance for further damage to the ankle is greatly increased and the development of chronic osselets is almost assured.

Chronic or true osselets are formed by a minute, continuous tearing away of the joint capsule from its bony attachments (cannon bone above and first phalanx below). This stimulates an inflammatory response of the bone covering. Deposition of fibrous tissue results in permanent disfigurement of the ankle. Osselets vary in size, resembling anything from an orange to a small grapefruit. Even the uninitiated can recognize this race horse entity.

Treatment, again, consists of cooling out any inflammation and then, discretion of your veterinarian, employing paints, blisters, or firing. Rest for a minimum of three months, if not longer, is mandatory.

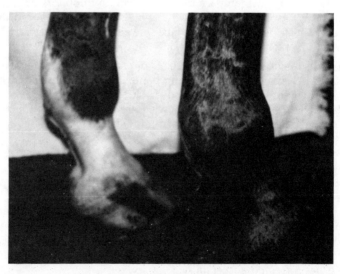

Osselets (Race Horse Ankles)

When I see osselets on any horse, I automatically know that I will find a tattoo under the upper lip, because this entity is synonymous with race horses. To carry this a bit further, I have never found osselets on any horse other than a race horse.

When complicated by other ailments, usually caused by continual abuse, osselets can quite easily progress, locking the joint irreversibly (anklylosis). With the inability to flex the ankles within a normal range of motion, the race horse is handicapped and thus represents a danger to itself, its jockey, and all other horses or people involved. *See:* FIRING.

pedal osteitis An inflammation of the bone of the foot, the os pedis, or coffin bone. Among the proposed causes are concussion, thin or tender soles, and poor dressing, balancing, and shoeing of the feet. I am of the opinion that this condition is of hereditary or congenital origin.

The numerous cases of pedal osteitis I have seen in my practice were all horses that had never been subjected to any form of hard work or use. X-rays of the feet, in all cases, showed a ragged and irregular border of the os pedis, with large areas of increased blood supply and a reduced amount of calcium.

Horses suffering with pedal osteitis can never live a normal useful life since they usually become sore after any light exertion. With rest they may become sound again, only to go lame with use.

periostitis *See:* BUCKED SHINS, METATARSUS.

peroneal paralysis (peroneal nerve) The peroneal nerve in the hind leg innervates the extensor muscles of the foot and the tibialis anterior muscle, the main muscle that flexes the hock. Degrees of peroneal nerve paresis are not uncommonly found in the equine; something as simple as slipping or falling can cause the condition. Other suspected causes are casting and/or tying legs for surgical procedures or during a general anesthetic where pressure exists between the body and the surface of the operating table.

It is symptomatic when the horse rests the hind limb with the anterior wall of the foot on the ground surface. The salient symptom, however, is the reduced ability to advance the limb during flight. The affected leg seems to trail behind with the front of the foot dragging as the limb is advanced, sometimes in a feeble fashion.

Prognosis and treatment depend upon the inciting cause of peroneal paralysis. If caused by restraint, the symptoms subside in 48 hours with local application of heat and massage. Anti-inflammatory injections seem to help in some cases, but I have seen cases of altered gait and function of unknown etiology that never improved.

podotrochleosis *See:* NAVICULAR DISEASE.

pyramidal disease A condition on the inside of the foot which causes lameness and progresses with a growth that results in malformation of the foot. Ultimately, the characteristic "buttress foot" develops, characterized by a noticeably concave, dish-like toe and a prominent bulge on the front of the coronary band.

The causative factor is thought to be strain or injury sustained to the common digital extensor tendon as it attaches to the pyramidal process located on the front of the os pedis (coffin bone). The adjacent periosteum (bone covering) becomes irritated, and inflammation occurs with subsequent deposition of new bone cells and numerous arthritic changes.

pyramidal disease continued

Symptoms are lameness with heat, pain, and swelling. The palpable heat is in the foot with localized swelling on the front part of the foot at the coronary band level. A full metacarpal pulse is usually present in the early stages and subsides somewhat as the condition becomes chronic. Pointing the foot during rest is characteristic of foot lameness.

Diagnosis can be confirmed by radiographs of the foot. Lateral views of both the foot and pastern area are especially revealing.

Attempts to inject corticosteroids locally, applications of blisters and paints, and even a low neurectomy performed to relieve pain, all receive failing grades in the way of treatment. Therapeutic shoes with rockers or rollers to help the foot move forward with less effort make little difference in the degree of lameness.

Pyramidal disease is most commonly found in the fore feet and is basically refractory to all treatment efforts. Its location is almost identical to that of ringbone formation, another futile condition with a poor prognosis. *See:* RINGBONE.

quittor   A common term for *lateral cartilage necrosis,* a purulent, inflamma-tory, and necrotic condition of the lateral cartilage in the foot. It is the result of a neglected puncture wound or laceration sustained in the pastern area.

Symptoms are swellings located over the lateral cartilage, low on the pastern area, or even on the associated side of the hoof wall.

Treatment is unsatisfactory. Surgical intervention to remove the infected lateral cartilage is the only known cure for this condition.

Prognosis is fair to good.

quarter cracks (toe cracks, heel cracks, sand cracks)   History shows that cracks in the foot wall have plagued the horse since the beginning of time, and nothing seems to have changed. Splits in hoof tissue continue to bedevil the modern owner and trainer. A simple foot crack can be so devastatingly painful that training and racing schedules must grind to a halt until the ominous little split is successfully repaired.

Old veterinary books contain large sections of written descriptions and multitudes of line drawings detailing foot cracks in all their various forms. Each text offers many types of treatment and countless shoe designs for corrective purposes. Even so, at this point in the battle of foot cracks, I would say that the cracks still hold a slight lead—although the "patch" treatment that has recently found favor appears to hold promise, in spite of misinformation and ignorance surrounding its use.

Although splits in foot walls seem to appear spontaneously, it is my contention that an underlying gradual weakening process exists that is aggravated by physiological forces of expansion and contraction in the foot during daily normal use. Add a slight amount of stress and the outside wall layer suddenly cracks open. Genes seem to be a factor too.

Standardbred horses and especially certain families within the breed are pestered with a high incidence of foot-crack maladies, regardless of intense efforts to improve the quality of training and handling.

Foot splits develop with greater frequency during speed than at slower gaits; cracks tend to appear subsequent to fast workouts and training sessions.

Assorted foot problems commonly occur in the wake of any foot change or recent shoeing. Dressing, rebalancing, and changing the angulation and/or the shoes, all seem to prompt pre-existing diminutive splits or cracks to become apparent. Shoes of different sizes, weights, and designs, with the angulation changes of the foot and pastern incorporated, can favorably affect the overall gait of the horse while at the same time directly contributing to the formation of splits and cracks in the hoof wall.

Cracks are designated by their location on or in the foot—that is, toe, quarter, or heel cracks. They are also classified as to origin: *Bearing-surface cracks* start at the bearing (ground) surface of the foot and extend up the foot wall; *coronary band cracks* originate at the coronary band level and extend down the foot wall. The former are decidedly easier to treat than the latter.

To discover and identify weakened areas in a so-called normal foot, scrutinize the coronary band and the distal bearing surface of the hoof wall before overt lesions develop. In horses prone to or suspected of hoof weaknesses, a weekly inspection of these areas using a magnifying device can uncover most hidden neophyte splits.

Immediate soreness as a result of a hoof crack is inconsistent, unless the crack is neglected and then soreness is a certainty! Untreated foot cracks split wider through stress and lack of support. If dirt, sand, or any form of contamination gains entry to the break in the foot enclosure ("sand cracks"), the chance of infection developing in the sensitive and soft underlying tissue is great.

In my opinion, successful treatment of any size or type of hoof defect entails two separate areas of concern: the hoof tissue and the metal shoe. The objective, simply stated, is to combine efficient foot-wall immobilization with an appropriately designed and applied shoe.

Basic treatment for all cracks consists primarily of securing the hoof wall to prevent movement during the normal expansion and contraction that occurs as body weight is alternately received and supported by the feet. Cleanse and precisely drill out all dead tissue on each side of the split or cracked area, being careful to remove no more hoof tissue than is necessary; do not inadvertently enlarge the existing defect. Then immobilize by applying your choice of wire, nails, staples, plastic, or any suitable material.

With a hoof rasp, remove a small section of hoof tissue at the bottom of the crack where it meets the shoe branch. Removing the support directly over the shoe helps reduce the expansion and contraction of the foot.

In the "patch" method of repair, rubberized patches are applied after the crack has been drilled out and filled with acrylic or methyl acrylate glue for adhesion and protection. The horse is able to compete or continue in training while healthy sound tissue slowly grows out. Although this may appear as an oversimplification of the principles of hoof repair, it is successful.

Hoof tissue grows from the coronary band level in a downward direction, in the same fashion as our finger nails. It grows at the agonizingly slow rate of about one-third of an inch per month, and thus constant surveillance and great patience are needed in the cure of a hoof defect.

Prevention of cracks and splits, when possible, has always been superior to any treatment yet devised. Coronary band injuries, poorly trimmed and neglected feet, and shoeing accidents are all too often part of the history of this problem.

quarter cracks continued

Try to avoid it with a program of daily foot care, cleanliness, and applications of foot dressings combined with a healthy diet to engender better foot texture and quality. *See:* FOOT.

ringbone   Osteoarthritis of the phalangeal joints (pastern joints). If the mere word *ringbone* doesn't strike fear in an owner's heart, the clinical finding of ringbone surely does depress this veterinarian. Although the list of medications is long, there is no treatment of any value for this crippling and career-limiting condition.

Soreness with constant lameness is the first and salient symptom of ringbone. Arthritic changes are found in one of two joint spaces. When diagnosed in the upper phalanx joint (between P_I and P_{II}), the entity is called *high ringbone;* when soreness is found in the lower phalanx joint (between P_{II} and P_{III}), it is then called *low ringbone*. High ringbone produces a clinically visible swelling situated on and around the pastern, in contrast to the equally painful low ringbone, located below the coronary band in the foot. Low ringbone requires radiographs (X-rays) to confirm its presence.

For want of a better clarification of causes, physical trauma has received the blame for ringbone. I am totally convinced that many other factors come into play, including hereditary predisposition, diet, and shoeing.

The formation of large bony exostoses (outgrowths) and arthritic changes in the joint are thought to result from severe injury to the interphalangeal joint surfaces. Nearby ligamentous and joint capsule injury also is sustained. Tearing away of surrounding ligaments incites the bone covering (periosteum) and soon periostitis develops as a result of tissue destruction. The painful process of osteoarthritis is under way.

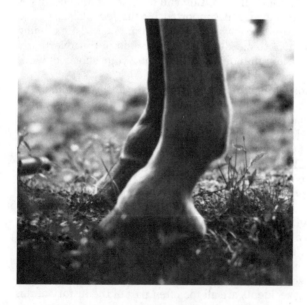

Bilateral High Ringbone Formation

True ringbone, as described above, includes both high and low osteoarthritis involving the joints of the pastern and foot. Some confusion exists about the terms "true" and "false" ringbones.

False ringbones are painful bony exostoses or periostitis on the surface of the pastern bones, but not near the joints. They also are caused by trauma, involving ligament and bone-surface injury rather than joint injury as seen in true ringbone. Lameness and soreness are present, but to a lesser degree. Many horses with false ringbone continue to provide varying degrees of service. Only your veterinarian with the aid of X-rays can offer a differential diagnosis and then a prognosis for soundness.

There is no known successful treatment for true ringbone. False ringbone produces the swelling above the coronary band and periostitis of the bone, but the area affected is between the joints on bone surface and *not* inside the joint space. False ringbone also can occur from subluxation of P_I and P_{II}, causing a swelling with a transient soreness. Treatment for false ringbone is rest and cooling agents. Contrary to the prognosis in true ringbone, the outlook is fair to good!

I have seen many ringbone cases in older retiree horses with no history of previous lameness. They suddenly develop a large swelling above the coronary band and go very lame. Some of these owners have added vitamins and minerals as dietary supplements in hopes of keeping the old pets healthy. Random and indiscriminate feeding of supplements to the very young and the aging gives me, as a veterinarian, cause for concern.

There is another form of so-called ringbone: *rachitic ringbone*. It is thought to be related to either a dietary deficiency or to some form of excessive nutritional condition. This may not be a true entity. Fibrous tissue enlargements are found on the pastern area of young horses; they resemble bony tissue when palpated but are negative when X-rayed. Your veterinarian can determine the deficiency or excess by studying the diet and running a blood chemistry.

Interestingly, these fibrous areas seem to respond to dietary changes and some subside almost as quickly as they appear.

sesamoid fractures There are two identical sesamoid bones (the proximal sesamoids) that sit as a pair in the back part of the horse's ankle. Being composed of cancellous bone, not considered true bone tissue, the sesamoids are thought to be originally a part of the suspensory apparatus which has, through evolution, ossified. With intimate attachment of the suspensory ligament branches on the sides and the back of the sesamoids, these small and durable bones serve as pulleys for the flexor tendons and fully qualify as working and supporting parts of the ankle.

Whether due to their function, their vulnerable position, or their cancellous nature, the proximal sesamoid bones receive a goodly share of injuries during competition or work. They are especially vulnerable to fracture during a race or any competition when muscle fatigue sets in from great exertion.

Depending on where fractures occur in the sesamoid bone, they are described as apical (top), basal (base), and multiple (body). Most of these fractures lend themselves well to surgical removal or some form of fixation. A lengthy, enforced postoperative period is necessary for rest and recovery.

sesamoid fractures continued

Prognosis is good when management is good. Untreated cases have a less favorable prognosis, since chronic sesamoiditis usually develops.

A horse suffering a fractured sesamoid during a race may or may not exhibit lameness during the first few post-race hours, but it will surely be lame by the following day. Radiographs are necessary to confirm the diagnosis and may aid in the direction of treatment, whether conservative or surgical.

sesamoiditis (proximal sesamoiditis)   An inflammatory process of the sesamoid bones and their adjacent ligaments. It is caused by stress, excessive strain, or physical trauma and can be either acute or chronic. In the acute form, it is quite painful to the touch with minimal soft swelling. In the chronic form, an enlarged and pointed area located over the sesamoid bone can easily be seen and is hard upon palpation.

Quite often fractures will occur simultaneous with injury to the soft tissue. If operable, all fracture fragments should be removed or immobilized surgically, thereby improving the recovery time, rate, and prognosis.

Conservative treatment consists of anti-inflammatory poultices and injectable drugs, with supportive casts if needed, but foremost and primarily, rest. Corrective shoes with elevated heels can be applied to relieve unnecessary pressure on the already sore attachments of the suspensory ligament branches on the sesamoid bones.

Prognosis depends upon the amount of damage originally sustained to the ligaments, bones, and soft tissue. But more important, the ultimate outcome depends upon the treatment. Early recognition and accurate diagnosis confirmed by local blocking and radiographs are the first necessary steps. Knowledgeable treatment and adequate rest will definitely minimize the amount of bone proliferation, arthritic response, and fibrosis of soft tissue that occurs during the healing process.

It has been my experience to find sesamoiditis on the inside surface of the sesamoid bone in 95 percent of cases. This hard knot is undoubtedly the result of repeated episodes of trauma and represents a source of chronic persistent lameness.

Although a horse with chronic sesamoiditis can function at a subdued level of activity for indeterminable lengths of time, intermittent lameness will assuredly be present with the everpresent threat of constant soreness. I have seen horses with sesamoiditis serve in a limited capacity, such as hacking for pleasure, but surely not as competition or working horses.

side bones   *See:* OSSIFICATION OF LATERAL CARTILAGES.

spavin   A term referring variously to bursitis, synovitis, and osteoarthritis occurring in the hock (tarsus) area. Bursitis is an inflammation of the bursa. Synovitis is an inflammation of the synovial lining of the joint capsule and the protective coverings of some tendon sheaths. Osteoarthritis is an inflammation of the bone at the joint surfaces.

There are four classifications of spavins:

1. Bone—osteoarthritic
2. Bog—bursitis and synovitis

3. Blood—combination of all the above
4. Occult—hidden, requiring X-rays for diagnosis.

Regardless of type, spavin development is thought to require a hereditary or congenital predisposition. Misuse, abuse, poor nutrition, and careless shoeing are all contributary causes, but I have yet to see a spavin develop on an anatomically sound hock or a structurally sound hind leg. It is my opinion that an unsound hock is always found on a fundamentally unsound hind leg. It is also my contention that the two are inseparable.

Poorly conformed hocks are destined to develop hock lesions (spavins, curbs, thoroughpins, etc.), and not necessarily work-related. Hind limb angulation (the angle formed by the large bones, the femur and tibia) basically serves to absorb concussion and thus reduces wear and tear on the body tissues and joint planes. A hind leg that is straight transfers greater stress to all joints and structures, ultimately inviting unsoundness of the hip, stifle, and hock. Obviously, the more the horse is made to work, the sooner the lesions will appear. However, just to be contrary, I will add that I have watched crooked-legged young horses over a period of time develop lesions of unsoundness while spending their lives at leisure in a pasture.

Avoid horses with conformationally crooked hind limbs or with any other leg deformity of congenital origin (bandy legs, cow hocks, sickle hocks).

Ideally, the leg should be straight when viewed from in front of or from behind the horse. Unfortunately, some judges prefer a hind limb to be straight also when viewed from the side, and insist upon pinning those individuals. Here is where the problem begins. Breeders continue to breed the winners and so we get more horses with hind leg trouble, or the potential for it.

A normally angled hind leg may be less pretty and less acceptable by conformation standards, but it is basically much sounder and less vulnerable to stress. To judge angulation, stand to one side of the horse and look at the large, long femur bone that lies between the hip joint and the stifle joint lower down. Then look still lower at the equally large tibial bone that lies between the stifle and the hock joint. The angle formed where these two bones meet at the level of the stifle joint determines the degree of straightness in the hind leg. This angulation can, in essence, determine the inherent soundness or unsoundness of both the stifle joint and the hock joint.

On the three types of spavins afflicting the hock, the bog spavin is by far the most common and the least harmful. Essentially it is a synovitis of the joint capsule which in turn produces a noticeable soft welling of synovial fluid on the front and inside of the hock.

When the joint becomes well distended with synovial fluid, quite often a smaller well-defined pouch can be seen on the outside of the hock. Careful examination will locate the swelling at the upper border of the joint ligaments and on a line level with the point of the hock.

Do not confuse a thoroughpin formation with this pouch of boggy hock. The two are in close proximity and have similar texture, but a boggy pouch is found lower than the normal location of the thoroughpin, closer to the hock joint, and it differs significantly upon palpation. A boggy swelling communicates with the swellings on the inside of the hock and nothing else does. *See:* THOROUGHPIN.

spavin continued

To ascertain a diagnosis, synovial fluid must be palpated. By placing one hand on the outside pouch and the other hand on the large swelling on the inside of the hock and simultaneously pressing, you can easily detect a fluctuation of fluid confirming the presence of a bog spavin.

In an older horse, bogs are caused by stress and strain and can be intermittently warm and painful. In young and growing horses, a bog formation usually is cool and insensitive to the touch, and lameness exists only if the swelling is sufficiently large to cause a mechanical interference during movement.

It is disturbing to see the increased incidence of bog spavins in exceptionally well-bred yearlings and young horses, especially in animals that are being fattened for sale or to achieve maximum growth for show purposes. Overfeeding of high-carbohydrate and high-protein feeds combined with reduced exercise has been associated with boggy hocks in young stock. These areas quickly subside when the rich diet is substituted for a normal horse regime. However, please do not confuse bog spavins with infected hocks. *See:* INFECTED JOINTS.

Classic bog spavin consists of a soft swelling of the hock, cool to the touch and painless. Although distressing to the owners, it does not singularly cause lameness. It is better to consult your veterinarian when confronted with a bog. Rest is always foremost.

If synovial fluid is excessive, your veterinarian may choose to aspirate the joint capsule to relieve local pressure. Aseptic and preoperative preparation to the area is essential to prevent entrance of a contaminant that might cause a crippling joint infection. This job should be left to the doctor! Avoid the use of steroids, since they produce undesirable effects two weeks after injection. I have found the use of intra-articular injections of hydroxyprogesterone after aspiration of joint fluid to be safe and quite therapeutic.

The hock joint does not lend itself well to any form of bandaging, and if bandaging is attempted for any purpose (sweating, painting, blistering), it will surely result in areas of undesirable pressure, especially on the Achilles tendon situated in the back and well above the hock area.

It is quite impossible to bandage a hock without creating pressure points. All types of spider bandages have been tried unsuccessfully, including an elastic tube-like bandage with a zipper. Someone, let us hope, will design a practical hock bandage in the future, probably using German springs to apply precise focal pressure points.

Bone spavin, or *jack spavin*, as it is commonly called, is a more serious type of spavin that has been known as a cause of lameness in horses for centuries. Most old veterinary books devote great space to treatments for "jacks." Bone spavin is a crippling form of osteoarthritis involving the intra-articular surfaces of the tarsal bones of the hock. Early in spavin development, a decalcification occurs followed by typical arthritic changes (periostitis, new bone formation, and calcium deposition in the form of an exostosis).

A bony spavin is a protuberance (palpated as a hard swelling) on the inside of the hock, and it can easily be seen. Stand in front of the shoulder by the fore leg and look backward and down on the inside surface of the hock for evidence of a small protrusion.

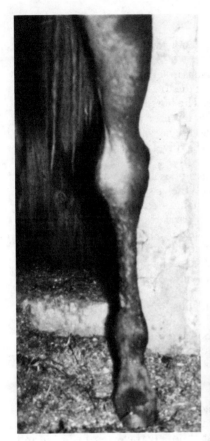

Bog Spavin, left hock

Bone Spavin (Jack), right hock

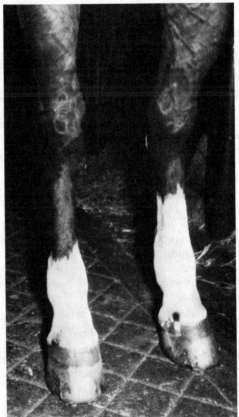

spavin continued

Be careful not to confuse an enlarged saphenous vein, where it traverses the front and inside of the hock, as a spavin.

Lameness is characteristic when the horse is first moved from the stall and is practically diagnostic when the animal hops on the toe, refusing to lower the foot and bear weight on the heel for several steps. The horse will then begin to warm out of the lameness, only to become sore again after a short rest period.

Another diagnostic method: Stand behind the horse and watch it walk away. With bone spavins, the horse customarily will travel wide-legged at the hock level.

Diagnosis can be confirmed by local anesthetics and by radiographs. Early osteoarthritic changes show decalcified areas on the tarsal bones; well-developed spavin cases reveal all degrees of arthritic changes and bony deposits.

A well-known "diagnostic" spavin test is carried out by an assistant who holds the animal's hind leg firmly in a fixed flexed position for some length of time. Suddenly the leg is dropped and the horse is moved off quickly at a jog and observed for signs of lameness. The value of this test has always eluded me, since all joints in the hind leg are flexed simultaneously. As far as I can see, this test proves nothing.

Conservative treatment consists of paints, blistering, and firing. Corrective dressing of the hind feet can be helpful by shortening the toe and elevating the heels. When shoeing, square the toe of the shoe and turn each branch into a high heel. The square toe directs the breakover point centrally, allowing for a straighter gait. The elevated heels provide a smoother stride with a quick and easier breakover.

Surgical treatment of bone spavin has virtually replaced all other corrective measures. A surgical procedure called *cunean tenotomy* has brought relief to many individuals, allowing them to continue to lead normal lives. Surgery consists of transecting the cunean tendon that obliquely traverses the inside and front of the hock. The cunean tendon exerts a restricting action on the hock which is freed by this routine procedure. A short postoperative period is advantageous, and moderate exercise is indicated to prevent formation of adhesions. "Cutting of the hocks" is a slang term for this surgery.

Blood spavin is an old and nonspecific term, and I am not certain that it describes a separate entity. Since the large saphenous vein courses over and near the tarsal joint, I can envision bruising or traumatization in specific situations. I have never diagnosed a blood spavin as such, however. Care must be taken not to confuse an enlarged vein with a spavin, especially in peculiarly shaped hocks. *See:* CUNEAN TENOTOMY.

splint   An exostosis or hard swelling that occurs on the splint bones, caused by a tearing of the interosseous ligament that binds the splint bone to the large cannon bone.

When the interosseous ligament is ruptured or torn away, the periosteum of the bone is irritated and a periostitis is initiated. New bone cells subsequently appear, forming an exostosis; this is called a *true* splint. Trauma is often the cause. Similar exostoses can be found elsewhere in the cannon bone area; the name used to identify the swelling—shin splint, knee splint, or cannon splint—indicates the location.

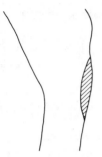 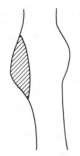 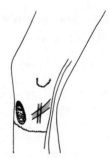

left hock,
curb formation
plantar ligament

left hock,
bog spavin
formation

medial left hock,
site of
cunean tenotomy

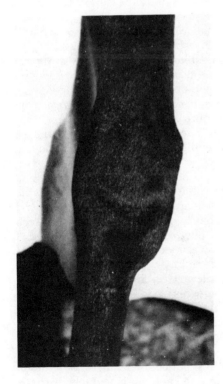

Splint, high on inside of right
fore leg near the knee, called
"high splint"

splint continued

Splints are common in young horses and frequently are found on the inside splint bone, since the horse's body weight is disproportionately borne on the inside of the legs.

Some causes of splint formations in young and old are overwork, stress, physical fatigue, and perhaps the breaking of horses before they are sufficiently grown.

Treatment consists of rest and cooling agents—hosing, poultices, wet bandages. At a later date, when all inflammation has subsided, then leg paints, blisters, or firing may be employed.

There are some cases where splints develop in the inside surface of the splint bones and impinge upon the suspensory ligament, thus causing a desmitis, an inflammation of a ligament. An acute lameness develops, although the cause is quite invisible. Exostoses that are not detectable to the eye are called *occult splints*.

The early stages in the formation of an occult splint, usually from five to seven days, are marked by a painful periostitis rather than a palpable exostosis. A neosplint site typically lacks heat, swelling, and detectable pulsation. Usually, the practitioner relies upon the use of a local anesthetic, lidocaine hydrochloride, injected into precise spots on the horse's limb to numb the area distal to the injection site. The injection that relieves the pain determines the exact seat of lameness.

It has been my experience, however, that occult splints do not respond well to local anesthetic infiltration, and that the results tend to be inaccurate and unreliable. I have learned a simple, dependable method of diagnosis. Merely flex the affected leg and methodically examine all borders of both splint bones by digital palpation. By holding the flexed leg in one hand and applying varying degrees of digital pressure with the other hand, one can recognize a true response to pain, one quite distinct from pure resistance to restraint.

Splints that persistently cause pressure on any soft tissue structure of the leg should be surgically removed, a technique similar to that used when removing splint-bone fracture fragments.

Veterinary practitioners are sometimes faced with an emergency situation when a valuable performance horse "pops a splint" and all measures to keep the horse on schedule are mandatory. The challenge is to relieve local pain and restore serviceability without allowing further injury to the star horse. In such uncomfortable circumstances, with no time allotted for a cooling-out period, I reach deep into my black bag and prepare a local injection of the sclerosing agent Osteum in equal parts and combined with Sarapin, a vegetable-oil base. After a surgical pre-op scrub, this is carefully infiltrated in and around the tender exostosis. This preparation reduces pain, increases blood supply, and stimulates a fibrosis between the splint and the cannon bone.

Another dependable drug, Hypodermin, a tamed iodine preparation, works in the same fashion. These two sclerosing drugs are safe measures and promote strength and healing in the splint areas.

For uninterrupted competition and no rest period, there is a major trade-off here, since the resultant exostosis will be large and perhaps inoperable, with the potential for producing pain at any time in the future.

In contrast, local steroid injections dramatically cool the tissues and reduce the swelling, sometimes allowing for a winning performance. The favorable cosmetic appearance is usually short-lived, however. Within two weeks' time, a typical steroid reaction occurs; a hot, proliferating exostosis, often much larger in size, reliably appears. Beward of promiscuous use of steroids.

In spite of the volumes that have been written on the splint and its many treatments, as veterinary practitioners we have few satisfactory answers for the distraught show-horse owner caught in the middle. Thus, the prognosis must be guarded!

splint bone fractures The splint bones are a pair of small bones of the horse's leg, located on either side and in back of the large cannon bone. The inside splint bone is called the second metacarpal bone in the fore leg and the second metatarsal bone in the hind leg. The outside splint bone is called the fourth metacarpal in the fore leg and the fourth metatarsal in the hind leg. The bone between the pair—the cannon bone—is called the third metacarpus in the foreleg and the third metatarsus in the hind leg.

The splint bones are nonsupporting and seem to serve no function except to protect and provide a channel two-thirds of the distance down the cannon bone for the suspensory ligament.

Splint bone fractures occur with greater frequency than is reported. Although the cause is insidious, most veterinarians and trainers agree that the chief offenders are physical blows, most often from the opposite foot, sustained during speed as the horse grows more fatigued.

Another well-known cause of fractured splint bones is the stretching of enlarged and thickened suspensory ligaments leading to displacement of the splint bones to the point of fracture during physical exertion. So when evaluating the soundness of a horse that has both a chronic desmitis and fractured splint bones, try to determine which came first, the chicken or the egg!

Diagnosis can be determined by digital palpation and confirmed by radiographs. To palpate, elevate the leg and, with all soft tissue relaxed, run your fingers along the inside and outside borders of the suspected splint bone. This method works quite well in uncovering all forms of splint bone aberrations, including malformed splint bones of congenital origin.

A fresh fracture with no displacement will cause only a transient soreness and a minute amount of local swelling and tenderness. The horse, with exercise, will again become sore. With tissue damage, an inflammation of the bone covering results and soon new bone cells are deposited (exostosis formation) at the fracture site. This serves to irritate the closely associated suspensory ligament and a desmitis occurs. With continued exercise, a palpable exostosis soon appears at the fracture site that consistently causes soreness after exercise. This hard, visible knot often is mistaken as a splint without the benefit of diagnostic X-rays. In most fractured splint bone cases, a period of rest, from a few days to a week, will produce a serviceably sound individual once again.

If soreness returns with exercise, surgical removal of the exostosis and the fractured distal end of the splint bone is indicated. This usually proves to be a very satisfactory method of correction.

stifle True stifle joint lameness, or gonitis, is an inflammation of the inner joint structure and is usually the result of physical trauma, stress, or strain caused by a

stifle continued

slipping-type injury. Deep joint injury is relatively uncommon in the average horse, but when it occurs, a poor prognosis for future usefulness is inevitable.

There is, however, a very frequently occurring stifle problem called "patellar fixation," which does not affect the joint proper but involves the closely located patellar bone and its three large surrounding ligaments.

The horse's patella, which is similar to the human kneecap, is loosely held into position over the stifle joint by these prominent ligaments that converge and attach on the tibial crest below.

As the hind leg flexes and extends during stride, focal areas of pain are produced when the one ligament, located on the inner surface of the stifle, inadvertently catches on or over the bony prominence on the femur. Intermittent catching or actual locking can occur during stride and result in panic by the patient and attendants. Thus, the name patellar fixation.

Less dramatic symptoms of this hind leg problem produce gait changes or alterations by the horse to prevent locking. The diagnostic audible sounds, ranging from a mere snapping to a loud popping, are indeed unmistakable. If neglected or ignored, toe dragging will gradually develop, followed by hind leg tenderness and eventual lameness.

A straight-angled hind leg is pleasant to a horseman's eye, but to the equine practitioner, it represents a headache. The straightness carries strong and persistent lameness potential for all individuals expected to work or perform.

Straight hind legs with obtuse-angled joints force the inner joint surfaces to meet and function at unnatural angles and positions. With any degree of work, stress and strain prevails inside of the joint. Show ring judges continue to pin straight hind legs—all with the potential for unsoundness. Although not nearly as pretty, the old-fashioned, acute-angled hind leg continues to remain a great deal sounder.

There is a distressing increase in the incidence of patellar fixation, especially in certain breeds. Breeders feverishly continue to mate straight-legged winners to other winners with straight hind limbs.

Fortunately, there is a surgical procedure to correct this inherited condition. It has answered many a horseman's prayer and has produced serviceable, trainable, sound, and comfortable horses that can perform and compete. *See:* MEDIAL PATELLAR DESMOTOMY.

stringhalt A sudden, spasmodic, high, jerking movement of one or both hind legs of the horse when it is first asked to move forward or backward. Although stringhalt has been reported in veterinary medical literature down the ages, the true cause, or even the mechanism of this perplexing hind leg malady is not yet known. Only one thing is constant in all the theories: that stringhalt is a neuromuscular aberration.

In some horses, the extreme superflexion of the hind limbs is almost violent, and for a split second the animal appears precariously off balance. Anyone or anything near the hind legs is in a hazard zone, especially when the horse is asked to move for the first time after a rest period. While the horse is standing still, the condition is not perceptible; only when it moves does the condition become evident. No wonder all insurance forms include in black print: "Did you watch the insured animal move outside of its stall?"

Interestingly, lameness is not associated with stringhalt. The exaggerated gait, controlled by involuntary movement, represents a mechanical interference with the ability to advance the limb in a normal stride. I have pondered how distressing this involuntary and uncontrollable jerking must be for a sensible and intelligent horse.

This unique gait is diagnostic in itself!

To this date, surgical correction is the only available treatment, and although it is not a cure, it does afford some comfort to the patient. A routine tenotomy of the lateral digital extensor tendon has the effect of reducing the animal's ability to flex the hind leg or legs, limiting height and range and thus inhibiting dramatic symptoms. Tenotomy surgery has been quite successful and the results have been satisfactory in a large percentage of cases. *See:* LATERAL DIGITAL EXTENSOR TENOTOMY.

superficial flexor tendon   One of two very important flexor tendons of the horse's leg. Both tendons are found on the posterior aspect of the leg, with the superficial flexor tendon covering the deeper-situated deep digital flexor tendon. This superficial tendon differs from its partner tendon in that it is much shorter, much wider, and thinner, and is specifically subject to tendonitis—which if not rested and protected will result in a "bowed tendon."

The superficial flexor tendon suffers degrees of tendonitis brought on by wear and tear. Minute, significant rupturing of fibrils occurs in focal areas, producing the pain, heat, and swelling known as tendonitis, the plague of the race horse.

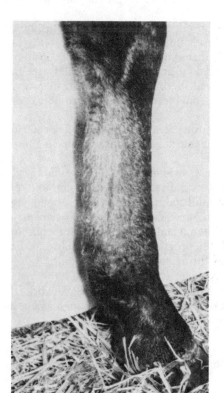

Tendonitis, precursor to a bowed tendon

superficial flexor tendon continued

I have observed, in post mortem examinations, that the deeper tendon, which runs on down to the horse's foot, is not involved in tendonitis entity, and I have been told of the same finding by another horse surgeon. *See:* TENDONITIS.

suspensory ligament   The largest ligament in the horse's leg, of primary importance as relates to soundness.

The suspensory ligament is a wide, thick band of ligamentous tissue snugly situated in back of the cannon bone with a splint bone on either side partially occluding the side borders of the ligament. Narrow edges of the suspensory ligament can easily be palpated two-thirds of the way down the cannon bone, as the ligamentous tissue emerges into full view from behind the splint bones. Originating from high under the knee, the suspensory ligament continues down the leg to divide just above the ankle level into two hardy branches. Each branch is semi-attached to the outside of its respective sesamoid bone as it passes down over the ankle and continues obliquely forward to become interlaced with the extensor tendon sheath, where it attaches to the first phalanx (pastern bone).

The main function of the suspensory ligament is to support the ankle and prevent hyperextension of the ankle joint. During excessive speed or exertion, the ankle is repeatedly subjected to great weight-bearing forces and, although split-second in duration, these could be very damaging without the support of the suspensory ligament.

Ligamentous strain, or desmitis, can occur from forceful slipping, sliding, stepping into holes, and abusive speed.

Any indication of desmitis is always an ominous sign to an astute horse person, since it calls into question the horse's future soundness and ability to compete with proficiency. This is not to say that a stricken horse cannot continue to perform, but rather that it most likely will do so at a much lower athletic level. Many horses with "suspensories" serve well in skillful hands even in racing circles, but the majority are forced to find suitable roles as pleasure horses or hunters or in various other capacities.

In Thoroughbreds, strains of the suspensory ligaments commonly occur in the fore legs during the gallop, whereas in Standardbred horses, the hind legs are the primary site of ligament strain.

Symptoms of desmitis are lameness, heat, swelling, and pain. Besides rest, cooling agents such as hosing and poulticing are indicated. When all symptoms of heat and inflammation have subsided, a mild iodine paint can be applied to stimulate circulation and tighen tissue. In some cases the veterinarian may advise blisters, sweats, and even firing. When ligament strains are sufficient to cause a slight dropping of the ankle level, the prognosis is questionable and the recovery period protracted. The animal's future usefulness is in doubt.

Rupture of the suspensory ligament is a very serious injury and if the main body of the ligament is involved, the horse may never resume normal work. If only one branch ruptures, the prognosis is somewhat better, although again, a lengthy recovery period is always necessary.

Symptoms are unmistakable when a suspensory ligament ruptures! The ankle drops almost to ground level, causing a horizontal and plateau-shaped pastern and a boxey-looking foot. As the ankle lowers almost to the ground, this

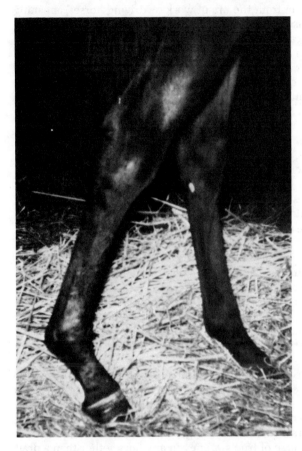

Ruptured Suspensory Ligament, right hind leg, subsequent coon foot development

startling change causes the entire upper limb to straighten and lengthen, losing normal angulation in all the leg joints. This reduction of joint angulation is seen chiefly when the hind leg is involved. Most noticeable when viewed from the side is the straight and strained appearance of the stifle and hock joints. It is interesting to stand behind the horse and note that the hip joint on the affected side is symmetrical with that of the opposite side. This confirms that the stifle and hock joints absorb the major role of compensation in this tragic limb alteration.

With repeated injuries or strains to the suspensory ligament, a horse will often develop a "coon-footed" appearance, in which the dorsal wall of the foot is steeper than the angulation of the pastern, and the ankle is somewhat lower than its counterpart on the other side.

There is no known satisfactory treatment for either chronic desmitis or rupture of the ligaments. Rest is the only course. Time will provide an abundance of fibrous tissue to strengthen the area, and eventually the horse will recover to the point of usefulness as a pleasure horse. It will not be a pretty-looking ankle and leg, but some horses are able to survive in a comfortable fashion and resume a quiet life.

sweeney An old horse term from the era of work or driving horses, meaning atrophy of the shoulder muscles caused by paralysis of the suprascapular nerve. The short but large suprascapular nerve branches out from the shoulder blade (scapula) and emerges from under and between the two muscles it innervates, the supraspinatus and subscapularis. With only skin covering the suprascapular nerve, it is virtually unprotected and is therefore extremely vulnerable to physical trauma in the shoulder area. Especially sensitive is the location where the nerve wraps around the lower part of the bony spine of the shoulder blade.

When injury to the nerve occurs, supraspinatus and subscapularis muscles shrink dramatically (atrophy), producing a hollow, flattened shoulder with unsightly bony projections. This is sweeney, recognizable by all.

Since these two muscles provide lateral or side support to the horse's shoulder, it is not unusual to see a horse with sweeney exhibit a momentary shoulder subluxation just as the body weight is shifted onto the affected limb. This gait defect, or "side movement" of the shoulder joint, can be detected by closely observing the horse's stride the instant the leg bears weight and is in a perpendicular position.

Lameness is inconsistent and varies with the degree of nerve paralysis and possible adjacent tissue damage. The presence of atrophy in the shoulder does not always mean loss of serviceability.

Diagnosis is never a problem, even for the neophyte. Simply walk to the head of the horse and look at both its shoulders. Compare the anatomical contour of each shoulder muscle mass for symmetry. Shrinking in size of a shoulder muscle creates an asymmetry of body form, and lopsidedness here should be quite obvious.

Years ago, it was quite common for heavy draft horses to suffer with sweeney of one or both shoulders. Wearing ill-fitted collars was the major abuse and cause of undue pressure on the suprascapular nerve. Other causes were kicks from fellow horses or self-inflicted blows sustained by running, bolting, or crowding through gates or stall doors and thus colliding with the posts.

I have never treated a case of true sweeney in any horse other than a draft breed. Although I have treated cases of mild shoulder atrophy in lighter horses—due to various causes—not one case was comparable to classic draft-horse sweeney.

Prognosis is always guarded, however. Treatment consists of hot and cold compresses applied over the affected shoulder during the acute stage together with oral administration and injections of anti-inflammatory drugs (phenylbutazone, aspirin, Banamine).

Later, when the muscles begin to shrink and innervation to the area has obviously been compromised, your veterinarian may suggest local injections of muscle irritants. Internal blisters are carefully injected under the skin to stimulate circulation to the affected area, and the irritated tissues respond with mild inflammatory symptoms. This is thought by some to promote healing by increasing the flow of fresh blood to the area. I can attest only that the associated swellings tend to mask or fill in some of the unsightly tissue deficits.

Although this treatment is not a cure, it consistently improves circulation and inconsistently produces cosmetic improvement. Depending upon the severity and extent of the injury, a lengthy series of internal blisters may be required to achieve some improvement or satisfactory function.

When administering an internal blister for any reason, it is not only important to aseptically prepare the proposed injection site, but also to massage the sites well after the injections are given. I would like to forewarn horse owners to expect some postinjection pain or some degree of discomfort immediately after the procedure. Be prepared either to sedate, tranquilize, or simply hand walk your friend for a short while to distract it from the possible burning or irritating sensation. The discomfort should be minimal and relatively transient.

Injectable counterirritants include:

1. Hypodermin, tamed iodine in a vegetable-oil base (most popular)
2. 2 percent silver nitrate
3. 5 percent aqueous solution of iodine (Lugol's Solution)
4. Equal parts turpentine and alcohol
5. Equal parts turpentine and chloroform

tendonitis (bowed tendon) An inflammation of tendon tissue. The term *tendonitis* denotes a poor prognosis for return to racing soundness.

Tendons connect muscle masses to bone tissue and endure varying degrees of stretching and accommodating, especially during the gallop. Initially the superficial digital flexor tendon sustains injury during speed primarily due to fatigue.

There are several causes of tendonitis. Physical trauma, poor shoeing, and abnormally long pasterns are some causes, but in my opinion the foremost etiologic factor is forced speed, usually greater than the horse is prepared to handle, with fatigue resulting.

Seldom ever does a horse bow during fox hunting, showing, or jumping, and innumerable bowed ex-race horses compete successfully in all these capacities. It is the speed factor encountered in racing that destroys compromised tendon tissue.

The superficial flexor tendon, located between the knee and the ankle, is the precise location of a classic bow. High and low bows occur in this area and are identified by their position on the back of the leg. Positioned deeper and closer to the suspensory ligament is the deep digital flexor tendon, which is seldom involved unless the injury is chronic and extensive and the entire leg is in danger of breaking down.

Symptoms of tendonitis commonly occur after a strenuous fast effort, usually soon after a race. Lameness, local soreness, heat, and swelling over the flexor tendons are typical signs of tendonitis. With this ominous finding all vigorous activities are cancelled and exercise is limited to hand walking. An anti-inflammatory treatment program is begun immediately. Icing and hosing, with cold-water bandages during the day and cooling astringent poultices applied overnight, are measures employed around the clock. The objective is to rapidly reduce all inflammatory changes in the tendon proper, and by so doing prevent or reduce adhesion formation. A tendon does not heal from within but relies on its covering, called the tendon sheath, which supplies the blood and fibroblasts that are responsible for healing. Adhesions that form between the sheath and the tendon tissue cause friction and discomfort.

For centuries, bowed tendons were subjected to all forms of irritants to promote healing, including blisters, paints, firing, and internal counterirritants. These agents caused more fibrous tissue to be laid down, with an abundance of

tendonitis continued

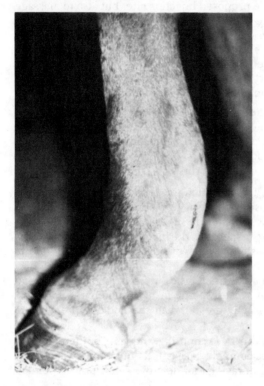

Bowed Tendon, "broken down"

adhesions resulting. The old rule was, the more fibrous tissue the better. Huge bows were commonplace and most were truly sore.

Today it is recognized that adhesions tend to interfere with the normal sliding motion of tendons, and thus irritating medicines have been discarded. A good rule to follow is this: Do not return a horse to exercise until strong digital pressure directly on the affected tendon area elicits no reaction.

Bowed tendons are synonymous with race horses. When a horse suffers a bout of tendonitis or bowed tendon, stop all training immediately. If through ignorance this animal is allowed to continue training, it will surely bow or break down completely. Be prepared to interrupt training for a minimum of one year and then re-evaluate the extent of healing before resuming work.

If a conformational predisposition exists, then arrange a career change for the horse before a weakened tendon brings about the animal's demise.

I have treated horses that had huge bowed tendons and nevertheless were used for jumping, hacking, steeplechasing, and point-to-point racing. They endured quite well the rigors of these endeavors. But if you were to subject any of these horses to a half-mile faster than a "two-minute lick" (sixty seconds), I guarantee that it would re-bow or break down. Speed *destroys* injured tendon tissue!

thoroughpin Synovial-fluid distension of the sheath of the deep digital flexor tendon of the hind leg as it passes through the hock area. This noticeable swelling can be seen both on the inside and outside of the leg and is found in the hollow tissue just in front of and at the level of the point of the hock.

A thoroughpin is located above the point where a boggy lateral pouch occurs, and although the two are similar to the touch and are closely associated, they can readily be distinguished and identified. With a thoroughpin, one well-defined fluid pouch is present; with a boggy spavin lateral pouch, the differentiating feature (as described under BOG SPAVIN) is the freely flowing fluid that communicates between the inside pouch and the outside pouch. A thoroughpin does not cause lameness and is considered to be much less serious than a bog spavin.

The cause of thoroughpin is simple or repeated strain, and the condition usually involves one leg.

Rest is the best treatment. Aspiration is indicated only if the swelling is very large or tense. Aspiration should be performed only by a veterinarian who is trained in aseptic procedures and who will remove just enough synovial fluid to make the animal comfortable. Aspirating stale fluid without reinjecting a drug will initiate formation of fresh fluid in the area and perhaps help the natural healing process. This method has worked quite well in my practice and has merit. Mild paints and blisters can be applied at a later date.

Once a thoroughpin has formed on a horse's hock, the telltale thickening in the deep digital flexor tendon will persist in spite of all methods of treatment.

Since most horses suffering thoroughpin formation surprisingly remain sound, the prognosis is good for serviceability, but only fair for cosmetic appearance.

Knowledgeable horse trainers are never upset by the appearance of a thoroughpin. I suppose they rationalize that things could be worse!

The Equine Foot

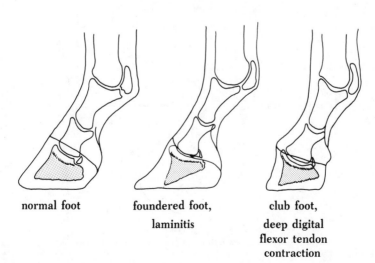

normal foot   foundered foot,   club foot,
                     laminitis   deep digital
                                             flexor tendon
                                             contraction

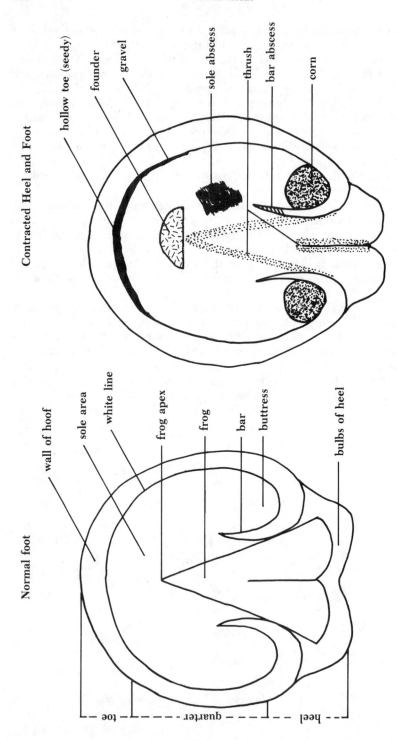

Contracted Heel and Foot

hollow toe (seedy)
founder
gravel
sole abscess
thrush
bar abscess
corn

Normal foot

wall of hoof
sole area
white line
frog apex
frog
bar
buttress
bulbs of heel

toe
quarter
heel

DIAGNOSTIC GUIDE
DIFFERENTIATION OF FOOT CONDITIONS

	Thrush	Gravel (Abcess)	Canker	Corn
Location	Frog	Sole, frog, or bars	Involves entire foot	Buttress only
Odor	Foul diagnostic odor	No odor	Offensive diagnostic odor	No odor
Sensitivity	Sore	Very sore	Sore	Sore; tender to hoof testers
Foot temperature	Higher only in severe cases	Warm to hot	Warm	Normal temperature
Pulsation	Only in severe cases	Strong pulsation	Present	No pulsation unless infected
Characteristics	Degeneration of tissue; cavities formed	Degeneration of tissue; pockets of infection form if untreated; discharges at coronary band	Foot tissue grows	Cavities filled with dried blood
Incidence	Commonly found in dirty or amateur barns	Associated with infrequent trimming; common during or after wet weather; result of punctures or foot bruises	Rare in light breeds; formerly common in hind feet of draft breeds	Found in fore feet of shod horses
Cause or etiology	Fungal (mycotic) plus bacterial invaders	Pus-forming bacteria	Causative agent unknown; dirty environment suspected	Poor shoeing

DIAGNOSTIC GUIDE
DIFFERENTIATION OF FOOT CONDITIONS

	Arthritic Changes	Contraction	Laminitis
Location	Navicular, side bones, ringbone	Contraction of the deep digital flexor tendon of the limb attached to the underneath area of the os pedis bone (malformed foot)	Sole area thins and opens at the frog apex
Odor	No odor	No odor	No odor
Sensitivity	No sensitivity to hoof testers	Sore	Very sore
Foot Temperature	Normal	Warm	Normal, warm, or hot
Pulsation	Inconsistent	Present	Strong pulsation
Characteristics	Osteoarthritic changes of bony tissue	Usually one foot contracted; symptoms simulate a foundered foot	Toe separation of tissue at white line with degeneration of sole at frog apex
Incidence	Common in young race horses and in older riding horses	Found with increasing frequency in foals and young horses	Common in fat ponies, fat horses, and in amateur barns
Cause or etiology	Concussion; use and abuse	Congenital origin	Poor husbandry; shock or stress; hereditary predisposition

COMMON FOOT PROBLEMS AND RECOMMENDED TREATMENT AND CORRECTIVE SHOEING

Common Name	Anatomic Location and Tissue Changes	Cause	Treatment	Remedial Shoeing
Canker	Excessive growth of abnormal tissue, entire sole, frog, and foot	Infection, dirty housing conditions	Dress away all excess tissue; pack well with formaldehyde solution	
Contracted foot (clubfoot)	Small foot circumference, short toe (slow growth), high heel (fast growth)	Congenital	Inferior check ligament desmotomy	Dress heels as low as possible; apply "tip" shores or shoes with feather-thin branches
Contracted heels	Very narrow heels, atrophied frog, entire foot narrow	Poor foot care, poor shoeing, infections in foot, thrush	Dress feet and balance; open heels well; apply Reducine around coronary bands, sole, and frog	Apply bar shoe, T-bar shoe, or chadwyck spring, beveled shoe branches to encourage the foot walls (heels and quarters) to expand
Coon foot	Steep foot angulation with a plateau angulation of the pastern	Ruptured suspensory ligament in leg causing the ankle to drop	Treat suspensory ligament; no specific foot treatment	
Corns	Bruised buttress area	Poorly designed, fitted, and applied shoes; shifted shoes or branches	Dress away all reddened and bruised areas; cauterize with medicine or a hot iron	Pack well with hoof packing and apply leathers with a bar shoe; avoid all sole or buttress pressure
Cracks: toe, wall, heel, quarter sole	Name indicates location	Poor diet, shoeing, or dressing; speed	Drill out all hoof tissue adjacent to the crack; treat with iodine or Reducine	Drill a horizontal groove above the crack and below, if possible; remove the foot tissue just below the crack and just above shoe

COMMON FOOT PROBLEMS AND TREATMENT Continued

Common Name	Anatomic Location and Tissue Changes	Cause	Treatment	Remedial Shoeing
Keratoma	Inner surface of horny wall	Tumor or unknown etiology	Surgical removal	
Laminitis	Sensitive and insensitive laminae of the foot	Excessive, deficient, or stagnated blood in the foot; separation of laminae with a ventral shift of os pedis	Acute: tube laxative anti-inflammatory drugs antihistamines methionine orally; pack feet in ice. Chronic: laxative, anti-inflammatory methionine, PBI$_2$ blood test for presence of hypothroidism	Dress heels down radically; shorten toes and remove all possible sole pressure; wide web-bar shoe for sole protection within heel area; roll toes for ease of breaking over
Navicular	Navicular bone found in back and under the P$_{II}$ and P$_{III}$ articulation	Bursitis develops followed by arthritic changes; hereditary predisposition or abusive use	Anti-inflammatory agents parental injections; oral preparations; local injections; posterior digital neurectomy	Press toes as short as possible, but do not touch heels; remove all sole pressure; pack sole with tar and oakum preparation; apply navicular shoe (thickened swedge branches, no heels); rolled toes with a 2°- or 3°-degree pad.
Pedal osteitis	Os pedis (coffin bone)	Decalcification of os pedis bone—hereditary or congenital	Anti-inflammatory agent after exercise	Keep well balanced; remove excess sole tissue; shoe often to maintain constant balance; hoof packing and pads to help protect sole area and reduce sole sensitivity

COMMON FOOT PROBLEMS AND TREATMENT Continued

Punctures or infections	All areas of the foot	Sharp objects; misdirected horseshoe nails	Remove foreign body and dead tissue; establish drainage; apply a poultice; tetanus booster; antibiotic therapy	Shoe is customarily removed and not reapplied until the horse is sound for at least several days.
Pyramidal (buttress foot)	Just under the coronary band in the front of the foot (front of os pedis)	Rupture of extensor tendon attachment to front of os pedis; strain, abuse, accident	Anti-inflammatory drugs; rest	Balance foot; apply shoe with elevated swedge heels; rolled toes
Quittor	Lateral cartilage	Infection and necrosis of lateral cartilage tissues; trauma; puncture	Surgical removal and cleansing of necrotic tissue; tetanus Toxoid antibiotic therapy	
Ringbone	High: P_I P_{II} Low: P_{II} and P_{III} articulation front of foot	Osteoarthritis, hereditary predisposition or abuse	No known treatment	Lower heels dramatically; apply smooth slipper-type shoe
Seedy toe (hollow toe)	Separation of sensitive and insensitive laminae	Results from chronic laminitis; infection established readily; hollow toe is portal of entry	Dress area and pack with Reducine or iodine solution pledgets	Trim feet well and keep balanced; shorten toes and lower heels; apply flat shoe with rolled toes
Sheared heels	Uneven heels	Abnormal heel growth with a tendency to contract under the foot; poor balancing; hereditary predisposition	Remove shoes and allow normal heel growth	Balance feet, especially heels, and apply a bar shoe with beveled branches for two or three shoeings

COMMON FOOT PROBLEMS
AND
RECOMMENDED TREATMENT AND CORRECTIVE SHOEING

Common Name	Anatomic Location and Tissue Changes	Cause	Treatment	Remedial Shoeing
Side bones	Lateral cartilages located on each side of the foot partially under the hoof	Ossification of lateral cartilages occurs with use and age	Groove hoof walls to relieve pressure and (by virtue of body weight) promote expansion of coronary band circumference of foot	Bar shoes; bevelled branches on shoes to cause walls to expand due to body weight
Sole bruise	Sole area	Sharp objects, stones, ground surface	Remove shoe; apply poultice	Protective plate for sole
Subsolar abscess (gravel)	Under the sole of the foot	Infection introduced through the sole causing abcessation with development of hollow cavities	Dress area open and establish drainage; pack with Lugol's Solution (aqueous iodine) and then apply poultice; tetanus booster; antibiotic therapy	Occasionally, if the condition is severe, a closed-in bar shoe with a removable plate can be designed to protect the sole
Thrush	Frog area, center sulci, lateral sulci, medial sulci	Fungal infection, filthy conditions, foot neglect	Dress areas free of excess tissue; allow air to enter; avoid water; cleanse with alcohol and cotton; treat with strong tincture of iodine and pack with cotton pledgets to keep clean and dry	
Shoe boil	Elbow area (olecranon bursa)	While down resting, horse allows heel of front shoe to press on the elbow of the same leg, creating a bursitis	Use of shoe boil boot, adequate bedding, surgical correction	Design shoe with shorter branches and no heels
Fracture of os pedis (coffin bone)	Os pedis (P_{III})	Trauma, uneven surfaces	Rest, compression ortho-screws, posterior digital neurectomy	Bar shoe with medial and lateral clips

thrush The universal term for a commonly known foot infection affecting the frog area of the foot.

Thrush is caused by an infectious organism called *Spherophorus necrophorus* in combination with a suspected but unidentified fungus; it can quickly establish a deep and degenerating foot infection. *S. necrophorus* prefers a lack of oxygen to propagate itself, so undressed feet with areas of overgrowth and deep tissue grooves are ideal habitats for this foot infection that results in semipermanent foot damage.

Thrush customarily attacks the lateral, medial, and center sulci of the frog. Sulci are the deep foot ridges bordering the frog on both sides and in its middle section. Poorly trimmed, neglected feet exposed to a wet and dirty environment are typical candidates for the development of thrush infection.

Early in the disease, it limits its ravages to the borders of the apical-shaped frog of the foot. If uninterrupted by treatment, it will progressively deepen and destroy the sole and frog tissue.

Timely recognition and prompt treatment can minimize typical tissue damage—the clefts, crevices, and ugly void spaces that persist even after healing as evidence of a thrush infection.

Thrush invades foot tissues forming cavities, the distinct opposite of another, less prevalent, foot infection, canker. The former destroys tissue, whereas the latter produces an excess of undesirable and unhealthy tissue. Both have a repugnant smell.

Prevention is always the best treatment. Provide a clean stall and good hygiene in a pollution-free environment. A regular schedule of trimming and shoeing affords a built-in inspection time. Most farriers will volunteer information as to the health of the sometimes hidden surfaces of the foot. At shoeing time ask your farrier to look for evidence of early thrush. Remember, thrush organisms dislike air, so if your horse wears leathers or pads, be certain to take a critical peek each time the shoes are changed.

It has been documented that a stall used by a "thrushy" horse presents a hazard to any new occupant. The causative agent can survive in clay or dirt floors for an unknown length of time. It is advisable in this case to remove the clay or dirt surface and soak the underlying layer with a Lysol solution. As daily maintenance, clean the stall, rake all corners, allow air to enter, dust a light coating of hydrated lime and then reset with fresh bedding. Pick all feet and inspect them for moist areas and odor.

When I am presented with a horse that has a thrush infection, I lay more stress on the preparation of the infected areas than on the treatment itself.

The first step in treatment is to engage a farrier to dress the foot and then trim away all excess ragged overgrowth of horny tissue. This permits needed air to enter and exposes the tissues to oxygen. The farrier should disinfect his tools after use.

Cleansing is the next step. Avoid the use of water by all means, since moisture only serves to propagate the condition. Arm yourself with plastic gloves and a generous amount of alcohol (70% isopropyl or rubbing alcohol) and disposable cotton. Clean and dry all accessible areas. Continue the cleaning process until the white cotton swab returns white after probing into the crevices. Protect your hands and clothing, because the offensive odor can be overcoming

thrush continued

and it tends to linger stubbornly. A horseshoe nail is an excellent tool for reaching down into some of the minute cavities and distant infected grooves. To repeat: Unless there is a conscientious advance cleansing and preparation of the foot, all treatment is negated!

Routine treatment after cleansing consists of applying one of many drying agents: iodine in its various forms (tincture, solutions, crystals), formaldehyde, turpentine, Methylene Blue, Clorox, Lysol, Koppertox, or other. Regardless of which drug is used, I strongly recommend that it be applied with an eyedropper. In my experience, the horse invariably moves or jerks away at the critical seconds during instillation of the drug. These solutions are caustic, and most will burn normal tissue, therefore spillage is to be avoided. The highly sensitive and tender heel area is especially vulnerable to skin burns.

An eyedropper holds the required amount of solution, permits accurate delivery, and reduces wasteful spillage. Alcohol-soaked cotton swabs can quickly neutralize any accidental spreading of the irritant preparation onto normal tissue and thus prevent your having another problem to treat.

Finally, roll cotton impregnated with the medicine into cigarette-shaped pledgets and introduce into the crevices, firmly pushing down to secure them in place. Although these pledgets prevent air from entering, they serve well to hold the drug against the infected areas and they simultaneously protect against moisture, dirt, and contaminants.

Ideally, normal care of a horse's feet can prevent thrush infection, and most astute horse people consider the presence of the infection to reflect unfavorably upon the horse's environment and the standards of its owners or keepers. Yet I have seen horses develop thrush infections in spite of the finest treatment combined with the best husbandry. These horses continue to evidence some degree of the infection throughout their lives. Hereditary predisposition to this foot condition has been mentioned in some literature.

timber shins   *See:* BUCKED SHINS, METATARSUS.

BREEDING: THE BROODMARE

abortion Expulsion of an embryo or fetus, complete or incomplete, alive or dead, before it is capable of maintaining life outside the uterus.

The causes of abortion in the broodmare are numerous:

1. Weak anatomical reproductive system
2. A high incidence of early embryonic death, often undetected
3. Imbalances within the hormonal system
4. The presence or sudden invasion of the mare's body by infectious disease, either (in order of prevalence) viral, bacterial, fungal (mycotic), or protozoal in origin
5. Physical, psychological, or environmental trauma
6. Genetically malformed or incomplete conceptus (fetus)

The broodmare is notorious for her inefficiency in being able to maintain pregnancy. Her ability to conceive is highly sophisticated, but her capacity to maintain a fertilized egg is far from efficient at best.

The mare's uterus is anatomically primitive, her placentation is unstable, and her cervical closure is extraordinarily fragile. She tends toward hormonal imbalance, which makes the safety of the long gestation period (11 months) even more critical.

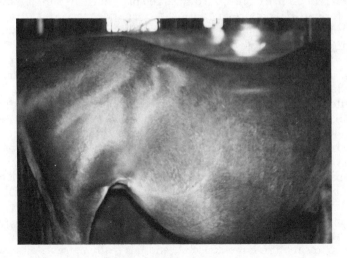

Pregnant Mare, imminent

125

abortion continued

The evolutionary process has not treated the broodmare kindly. Compared to other breeds of livestock, mares possess a reproductive system that is more complex and far less dependable than that of *any* other known species.

acidosis A metabolic disorder accompanied by an excess of acids throughout the body tissues. This condition is most often seen in broodmares approaching term, the end of their gestational period. Acidosis has been referred to as "pregnancy disease."

Affected individuals usually are lethargic, exhibiting inappetance and dullness, and swellings appear as edema on the ventral abdomen and most often on the lower leg. Edema can be identified by the telltale finger indentation left in the swelling after fingertip pressure and release.

A dietary change in the way of enticement (sweet feed, carrots, and the like), coupled with forced exercise, will improve the mare's attitude and appetite in most cases. Then hope for an early or on-time delivery. Injections of sodium lactate and sodium bicarbonate can, in some cases, be helpful.

A large percentage of imminent mares suffer degrees of depression, inappetance, lethargy, and edematous swellings. Such a mare may not be truly ill, but a conscientious owner will keep close watch over her condition.

True acidosis, characterized by intense symptoms, requires immediate veterinary attention.

afterbirth mass *See:* AMORPHUS GLOBOSUS, HIPPOMANES.

agalactia The absence of milk in the mare's mammary glands soon after parturition (delivery). Failure to lactate can be caused by many things: hormonal imbalance, more often seen in the maiden mare; poor nutrition or parasitism during gestation; retained placenta or parts thereof; psychological upset; and on and on *ad infinitum*.

Your veterinarian should be called. Undoubtedly he or she will sedate the mare, then request to examine the discharged placenta to be sure it is complete. If your veterinarian is not present during the mare's delivery, be sure to save the precious placenta. It should be stored in an absolutely safe place and closed container for prompt professional examination.

It is not uncommon to find that a portion of the placenta has been retained inside of the mare. Your veterinarian will start treatment immediately. Meanwhile, you can apply well-rung-out hot towels to the mare's udder every ten minutes. If milk fails to appear, your veterinarian may, with discretion, administer a minute dose of oxytocin or reserpine.

Oxytocin is used routinely in all other species, but it does present a risk for the broodmare, especially the older mare. Oxytocin is beneficial because it stimulates milk production and flow and increases smooth-muscle activity. But, at the same time, it increases blood pressure and has been associated with postpartum hemorrhage of the large vessels within the uterine walls. Obviously, an old mare that has endured many pregnancies possesses what might be termed a "worn out" uterus; oxytocin surely increases the risk in such cases.

Most mares respond by producing milk following the drug administration, but some mares require hours to lactate and this really presents a threat to the newborn foal. It must receive its mother's precious colostrum (first milk) soon, for it needs the nutrients, the laxative properties, and the vital antibodies of the colostrum.

If all efforts fail, you can turn to a milking mare (if you can find one), or a colostrum bank, or a commercially prepared synthetic formula (colostrum substitute).

Listen to your veterinarian's advice. You must realize that your foal's life is at stake! See: COLOSTRUM.

amnion   Part of the placenta, the smooth, grayish-white sac that envelopes the fetus during gestation. The foal remains within it during the passage through the birth canal. If the newborn is healthy and vigorous, its fore feet will break through the rugged amniotic membrane when it is about three-quarters of the way into the world. Weak foals can be delivered into the bedding still entirely enveloped in the sac and can perish if parturition is unattended and no one opens the sac.

An astute attendant will routinely open the amniotic sac and deflect the ends at about the time when both fore legs appear. The exposed legs facilitate the application of mild, considerate, and rhythmic traction by the attendant.

amniotic fluid   Fluid within the amnion in which the embryo is bathed and which it continuously swallows during the entire gestation period. See: HYDROPS AMNION.

amorphus globosus   An arrested abnormal conceptus, or a failure of a would-be twin pregnancy. Amorphus globosus is a rounded tissue mass possessing its own umbilical cord attached to the placental tissue. Fortunately, its growth and development are arrested early in gestation, preventing interference with a normally developing fetus through competition for nutrients and space in the uterus. The broodmare owner can be startled at finding the spherical dark ball in the placental layers. It does therefore justify an explanation.

The amorphus globosus is the curious result of an additional ovulation with subsequent fertilization occurring concurrently with the fertilization of the normal full-term foal. It is ordinarily found as a large ball, 3 to 6 inches in diameter, hidden in the layers of the placenta. When it is cut open, a thin layer of cartilage is encountered and the remaining fluid escapes: otherwise, it is a mass of unidentifiable tissue.

I have examined placentas that had as many as six amorphus globosus masses attached, quite obviously the result of a superovulation—not a normal happening in the mare, unless under the influence of hormones indiscriminately used. It is a wonder how a normal fetus can grow and can be successfully delivered after sharing the placental functions and housing with these round masses that represent potential twins or even a litter!

A passing thought to bear in mind when viewing such an expelled mass in the placental tissues: Be thankful that it did not continue to grow into an abnormal pregnancy and directly cause the abortion of the normal and supposedly healthy foal. Ninety-five percent of all twin pregnancies abort. See: TWIN PREGNANCY.

artificial insemination   Defined as the deposit of a stallion's semen by artificial means through the vagina and cervical canal directly into the body of the mare's uterus. This technique has medical advantages, for it precludes the worry over

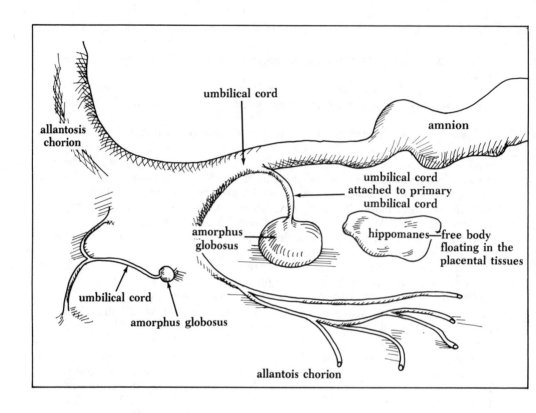

Afterbirth Membranes
(or Placental Tissue)

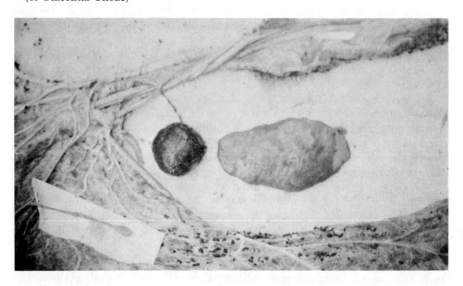

This demonstrates potential triplets, unknown in the equine, although a single normal birth occurred.

nature's way, with all the built-in weak links and amazing inefficiencies of natural breeding.

With today's enormous economic investments in the world market for bloodstock, there is great demand for improvement in breeding success. The food-animal industry has pioneered in artificial insemination (AI) and in techniques for the freezing and storage of semen and its beneficial applications. The research has established a foundation of knowledge upon which the horse-breeding world can draw.

Research concerning equine AI, and particularly the use of frozen semen, is developing in spite of "specie specific" problems. Horse semen seems to be more fragile than that of bovine or porcine males. It does not lend itself easily to handling, environmental threats, extenders, additions, or freezing procedures.

Even though a number of horse-breed registries (e.g., Morgan, Standardbred) have permitted the practice and registration of the products of AI, the Jockey Club, which regulates the Thoroughbred breed, firmly resists this procedure. Perhaps this is the main reason why research is stagnant for the time being.

It is also acknowledged that in spite of advances in the quality of animal production through the use of AI techniques, the horse world is reluctant to accept the practice because the net effect would be to make redundant many of the people and services that generate money in the horse industry.

Without doubt, artificial insemination provides certain benefits:

1. Allows control of hygienic standards for both mare and stallion
2. Permits control and screening of quantity and quality of semen
3. Makes possible early recognition, identification, and treatment of genital disease in stallion and mare
4. Allows insemination at the optimum time
5. Helps eliminate the danger of breeding-shed accidents and the risk of contagion for a lactating mare with foal at foot
6. Avoids the high cost of transport and boarding
7. Allows breeding "the best to the best," regardless of the geographical location of the stallion and mare

With all this to be said for AI, what can be said against it?

Primarily, from the evolutionary view, there is a danger that breeders would turn only to those relatively few genetically superior stallions and eschew lesser horses. The long-term effect of such concentrated lineage cannot be predicted. It could prove deleterious to the breed.

From the industry point of view, the need for breeding farms and stallion stations would be radically reduced, as would the businesses concerned with the vanning, boarding, and handling of broodmares and their sucklings.

For the same reasons that it refuses the legalization of AI, the Jockey Club continues to deny and stand firm against such practices as embryo transfer, superovulation in superior mares, use of surrogate mothers, and use of frozen semen that can be mailed anywhere in the world.

Imagine watching 12 horses leave the starting gate—all by the same sire!

artificial vagina The condom, or artificial vagina, is routinely used for semen analysis and evaluation. It is constructed of a rubber tube enveloped within a warm-water jacket (the temperature control is critical) that simulates the temperature and pressure of the mare's vagina.

artificial vagina continued

Several types of artificial vaginas are available commercially. Each has its own individual design and adaptations, and each promises success, but only if it is used by a skilled technician on a properly prepared stallion will a suitable *total* ejaculate be obtained. Most horses are reluctant to accept this routine for the collection of semen. Some resent it and absolutely refuse to co-operate.

A stallion's semen should be evaluated at the time of his sale, at the time of his retirement to stud, or at any time when fertility efficiency is in question. When there is a need for semen collection in condition suitable for gross and microscopic analysis, the artificial vagina is by far the best technique.

I would not advise amateurs to attempt the collection of stallion semen. Leave this job to the experienced! However, the following suggestions, though far from complete, may be helpful:

1. *All* personnel should be clean, equipped with hard hats, and prepared for animal restraint.

2. The artificial vagina should be absolutely clean and the temperature under perfect control.

3. It is necessary to provide a mare in season. Any small and experienced, usually older, mare that will tolerate the horse and his possible antics is suitable.

4. Both animals should be scrubbed clean.

5. Use the mare as a teaser until the horse has an erection, then allow the horse to mount the mare. With a clean hand deftly direct his penis to the side and into the artificial vagina. This appliance should be held in position by strong, "horsewise" assistants. They must wear hard hats.

6. Careful handling of the ejaculate is essential, because stallion semen is notoriously sensitive to jarring, temperature changes, and environmental insults such as wind and sunlight. The method of handling depends upon the use intended for the semen.

bagging up   A lay term to describe the enlargement of mammary tissue when the end of gestation approaches and parturition is close.

breaking water   The first sign of the second stage of labor during parturition, when the foal passes from the uterus, through the pelvic canal, and into the outside world. Moments before delivery begins with a great release of water—usually several gallons in volume—from the placental sac that envelops the fetus during gestation. The fluid eases passage of the foal by lubricating the reproductive tract. *See:* AMNIOTIC SAC.

breech delivery   Abnormal presentation of a foal at parturition. The hindquarters appear first, the opposite of a normal presentation. The hind feet, then the hocks, and finally the trunk appear, followed by the neck and head, with fore legs last. Most breech deliveries, although startling, are relatively smooth and work out satisfactorily.

Danger does exist if any delay in the birth process occurs. Most mares normally takes a "breather," if for only 30 to 40 seconds, in midstream of delivery. If this natural pause occurs while the umbilical cord is vulnerably positioned over the maternal bony pelvis, then entrapment can easily develop, impairing vital oxygen transport through the cord to the fetus.

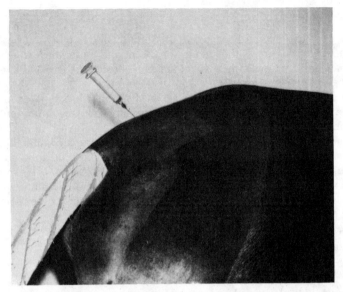

Epidural Anesthesia, site of injection used in all gynecologic procedures

CAUTION: As a matter of routine, be sure to monitor carefully and supervise your foal for the first few hours and days until you are sure it is absolutely normal.

Caslick's operation *See under:* SURGERY.

cesarean *See under:* SURGERY.

dystocia A difficult birth. Before our modern inhalation anesthetics, when a mare suffered a dystocia, the veterinarian's only choice was the use of chemical hypnotics followed by an embryotomy or fetotomy. These terms are synonymous and mean the removal of a lodged or twisted fetus, dead or alive, from the distressed mare's reproductive tract. Ideally, a simple dystocia will respond to correction and a timely repositioning of the fetus, resulting in a delivery through the combined efforts of the mare and the veterinary obstetrician.

Because 90 percent of all dystocias are caused by contracted foals, usually already dead from arrested normal development at the time of parturition, our major concern is then the broodmare. All energy must be turned toward caring for the mare, preserving her life, and saving her reproductive tract for future pregnancies. Cutting the fetal mass into smaller sections while it is still within the mare requires skill, knowledge, determination, and a great deal of strength and dexterity by the attending veterinary obstetrician. This surgical technique requires a special set of instruments designed for the intricate, detailed, and sometimes lengthy procedure. Reducing the circumference of the fetal mass allows for a much smoother delivery through the mare's cervix and vaginal vault, while providing protection and relief to the unfortunate mare.

Regardless of veterinary advances, I still see problems facing the broodmare in an isolated country barn who may encounter problems during parturition.

dystocia continued

Birth in the equine inevitably occurs in the middle of the night, and by the time the attendant recognizes the need for help and summons the sleeping veterinarian, the precious minutes that may well decide the fate of the mare and her foal have been lost forever!

After 20 years of correcting dystocias in distraught broodmares under the most adverse conditions, I must impart my dream for all heavy, imminent mares. It is that broodmare owners will someday have the option of admitting their nearly due mare to a fully staffed equine maternity ward comparable to our facilities for human beings. There all mares would be monitored around the clock by equine obstetricians and surgeons. The only losses suffered by mares and owners would be those that were absolutely unpreventable. Equine maternity wards are the answer to the midnight crisis, when help cannot come soon enough to save the savable. *See:* CESAREAN.

eclampsia *See under:* COMMON DISEASES.

fetal anasarca *See:* HYDROPS AMNION.

foaling *See:* LABOR.

gestation (pregnancy, fetation) That period from conception to parturition, approximately 340 days in the mare.

hippomanes A brown, free-floating mass found in the placental tissues. The uninitiated owner is likely to be startled at the sight of this amorphous mass, with its liver-like consistency and irregular shape, ranging in size from 4 to 6 inches long, 3 to 4 inches wide, and 1 to 1½ inches thick.

The function of this mass in the placental tissues remains unexplained. Basically it is fibrinous in nature, with no clearly defined cellular structure. The hippomanes is thought by some scientists to be associated with progesterone production and thus with maintenance of pregnancy.

hydrops amnion A condition of broodmares in which an excessive amount of amniotic fluid accumulates *in utero* during gestation. The resident foal is believed to be the cause. A normal fetus constantly swallows amniotic fluid and apparently keeps pace with production, whereas in hydrops amnion cases, the faulty foal seems unable to swallow adequate amounts, or perhaps none at all, and suffers anasarca, an accumulation of fluid in the tissues.

This relentless fluid build-up also causes increasing intrauterine pressure, creating undue stretching of the mare's uterus and abdomen, and presenting a clinical picture of a mare carrying a litter of foals! The mare usually aborts at around five to eight months of gestation, and because of inability to contract and expel the fetus (uterine inertia), veterinary assistance is needed to aid in diagnosis and delivery. Twenty to 30 gallons of tepid amniotic fluid releases quickly, drenching the veterinary obstetrician, and the slightly swollen, bluish, and lifeless foal then emerges.

It is ill-advised to breed the mare back to the same stallion, since this condition is thought to be of hereditary or congenital origin.

labor The process of expulsion of a fetus from the uterus at the normal termination of pregnancy. This definition describes the second stage of labor or actual parturition as seen in the broodmare.

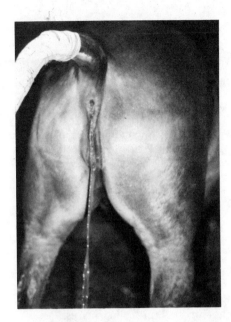

**Breaking Water, signals the be-
ginning of stage 2 in the delivery
process**

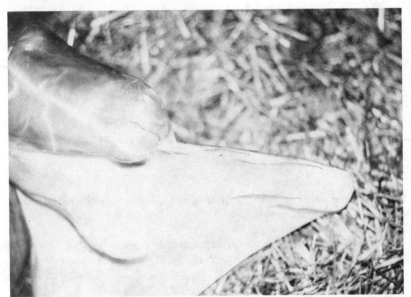

Appearance of Amnionitic-Covered Forefeet and Head of Foal

There are three stages of labor in the mare:

Stage 1. Internal or invisible preparations for parturition, ending in the "breaking of the water"

labor continued

Stage 2. Parturition, or the birth of the foal

Stage 3. Passage of the placental membranes (afterbirth), involution of the uterus, repair, and, with it, return of the reproductive tract to a normal healthy state

See: BREAKING WATER, DYSTOCIA.

lacerations, bruises, and hematomas It is not uncommon, especially in maiden mares, to see shortly after foaling evidences of lacerations, bruises, and hematomas. They can be found just inside the vulvar lips on the walls of the vestibule entering the vagina. Quite swollen and inflamed, the appearance is worse than the state. Normally no specific treatment is required, and within a few days the areas will be healing well. The regenerative power of genital tissue, compared to that of other body tissue, never ceases to amaze me.

leptospirosis *See under:* COMMON DISEASES.

mastitis *See:* UDDER.

middle uterine artery Rupture of this uterine-wall artery is common in mares that have produced several foals. Rupture can occur prior to delivery, but most often hemorrhages occur after parturition. Leakage or total rupture of this vessel is the major cause of fatal postpartum hemorrhage in foaling mares.

The worn-out arterial wall is thought to weaken gradually from the constant strain and stretching experienced with each pregnancy, and it is especially vulnerable to the large fetal weights that accrue during the latter days of gestation.

By virtue of its location, nestled deep in between the uterine muscle layers, this major artery is quite inaccessible for treatment of any kind, and thus continues to bleed unabated. Desperate efforts to encourage coagulation by means of injectable coagulants usually are in vain.

If time will allow for proper cross-matching, I have found that whole-blood transfusions buy time and have, in two isolated cases, saved the broodmare's life. The owners of these mares were informed to never breed back. Retire them, *please!*

milk *See:* COLOSTRUM, ORPHAN FOAL.

obturator nerve paralysis The obturator nerve is found in the pelvis and hind limb area where it innervates four large muscles: the obturator externus, pectineus, adductor, and gracilis.

This nerve is responsible for holding the limb close to the body (adduction). When its function is impaired—either by trauma, infection, bone calluses, or tumors—the limb diagnostically migrates laterally, that is, outward from the body.

Gradually developing symptoms of questionable hind leg stability (e.g., slipping to the side and away from the body) that worsen over a period of days to several weeks, progressing to reduced ability to control position or even bear body weight, indicate paresis of the obturator nerve caused by either an irritated old fracture site, calcified hematomas, or an active, growing tumor in the pelvic area.

When similar symptoms appear immediately after a mare delivers a foal, the diagnosis then would suggest a bruise or injury which the obturator nerve sustained from foal pressure during a protracted or very strenuous delivery. Some predisposed mares suffer varying degrees of paresis with each pregnancy, although outward appearances give no sign of anything amiss.

Many times I have watched a mare deliver a foal and then discovered that she was unable to rise. The frantic expression in the mare's face is not easily forgotten. As soon as a diagnosis is made, the newborn is hurried to safety with someone specifically assigned to remain with the foal. Distraught and sweat-covered, the mare usually benefits from some sedation while a crew attempts to set up a sling. Using heavy bales, a temporary straight stall is then constructed to give needed support to the heavy matron.

The outcome of this desperate and unannounced situation depends heavily upon the veterinary treatment, but more so upon the number of dedicated people who are willing to stay with the mare and foal around the clock.

Most mares regain innervation, or a functional obturator nerve, within 24 to 48 hours. This can be a long, long period, especially when you are faced with a high-strung, well-bred mare, constantly screaming and searching for her new foal.

With sheer physical strength provided by sufficient volunteers, the foal can be cradled and guided to the swaying mare and permitted to nurse regularly. Maintenance of the all-important mother-baby link is vital to prevent rejection by the dam.

Time usually rewards those waiting, and when the mare seems steady, the baby foal may be returned and the wall of bales removed.

I have known certain mares to have a history of repeatedly suffering degrees of paresis after each foaling. These mares deserve special consideration, and some thought should be directed to the question of breeding a mare that is known to have this deplorable nerve problem.

When you see your first obturator nerve paralysis, it is not the end of the earth—it only looks that way!

ovariectomy   The surgical removal of both ovaries, also called *spaying*. A filly or mare is then comparable to a gelding, with the exception that in the female the evidence of the surgery is hidden. It is easy to determine the absence of testicles in the horse, but who can tell by observation that the ovaries are missing in the mare? Only the gynecologists.

Indications for an ovariectomy are ovarian tumor, cyst, or any abnormal ovarian condition. Ovariectomy is not indicated in the mare as a means of preventing pregnancy, as in other species, but with some mares it is thought to improve disposition or behavioral pattern.

An ovariectomy can be performed in two ways: through a flank incision, or through the vaginal canal. With the second method, there is no scar or incision line as evidence that the surgery was performed.

The practice of ovary removal has gained popularity in recent years as a way of producing an even temperament in a filly or mare in the hopes of producing a more consistent performance. Other reasons for its acceptance are the ease of the surgery, the minimal postoperative problems, and the short recovery period.

Unfortunately, this otherwise sound procedure has inadvertently created

ovariectomy continued

an ethical problem. Traditionally, good race mares are purchased for reproductive purposes. When these mares are subsequently examined and found to have an incomplete reproductive tract, thoughts of litigation occur. There have been many such incidents, and I, as an equine practitioner, expect to see many more before some rule is adopted to protect the innocent purchaser.

parturition   *See:* LABOR.

persistent hymen   The hymen is a thin membranous curtain occluding the external vaginal orifice in the maiden mare. A persistent hymen is usually thicker than normal in texture and cannot be ruptured by the stallion; breaking it requires surgical intervention.

On efficiently run breeding farms, maiden mares are routinely examined prior to cover for any departure from the norm. I have found not only persistent hymens, but fragmented, divided, and holey membranes that presented the potential for mechanical problems, pain, inflammation, and subsequent infection for both the stallion and the broodmare.

placenta   A mare's placenta is comprised of two main layers, the *allanatois chorion,* a heavy outer layer attached to the uterine lining, and the *amnion,* the inner layer that envelops the foal.

The placenta is simple and diffuse, insecure in its attachment, and hormonally unstable. From an evolutionary point of view, it could be called antiquated. Placentation is directly responsible for the provision of nutrients, exchange of all gases, and removal of waste materials. It is literally the lifeline of the foal.

Abortion can result from uterine infections. Invading micro-organisms usually attack the site where the placenta attaches to the endometrium of the uterus. Infection here causes separation of the membranes, which results in reduced placental functions. Either a weak, sick foal survives, or abortion occurs.

During normal parturition, the foal, encased in its protective slippery amniotic sac, penetrates through the allantois chorion layer and proceeds to enter the outside world. The foal is delivered *in advance* of the placenta and *within* its amniotic sac.

Following parturition, the average healthy mare expels the placental membranes. When she regains her feet immediately postpartum, the membranes are very much in evidence, hanging through the lips of the vulva. Nearest the vulva is the allantois chorion—heavy, gray, white-veined, turned inside out by the direct pull of the attached umbilical cord. Lower down, most likely trailing in the straw, is the glistening, slippery amnion.

An angry red area on the surface of the now inside-out placenta is no cause for alarm. This is the part of the placenta most intimately attached to the uterine surface during pregnancy, where all gas and nutrient interchanges occur.

The placental membranes, or "afterbirth" should be expelled naturally by the mare at any time up to 45 minutes after delivery. If a mare has not passed the afterbirth within two hours after delivery, it is considered to be "retained," indicating a pathologic disorder. In this event it is essential to summon your veterinarian, who will examine and properly treat your mare to promote physiologic release of the attached afterbirth. Placement of intrauterine capsules

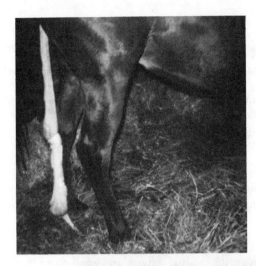

Retained Placenta, ready to be re-tied or elevated

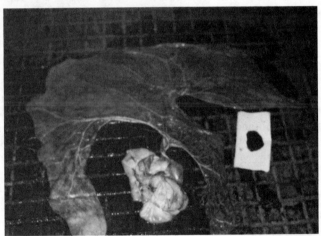

Normal, Healthy and Complete Placenta

or boluses containing antibiotics, urea, or sulfonamides is the first line of defense. (A retained placenta usually indicates an intrauterine infection.)

Manual traction to aid in the expulsion of a mare's afterbirth is strongly opposed by equine authorities because it will certainly result in untold damage to the endometrium, directly affecting future fertility.

When the membranes have passed, they should be placed in a tightly covered container to protect them from curious dogs and cats until a professional inspection can be conducted. The veterinarian will carefully spread the placenta out on the ground to determine its completeness and consistency. Size, weight, and color will be checked, and from these an overall impression of health or disease can be determined.

placenta continued

Incomplete passage or retention of a fragmented part of the afterbirth can cause septicemia and laminitis in the postpartum broodmare. If examination of the placenta shows that some fragment is missing, the veterinarian will administer intrauterine medication to promote physiologic release.

The placenta is eloquent evidence of the genital health of the mare and her chances of regaining fertility. It is an invaluable indicator not only of the immediate postpartum needs of the mare, but also of any unusual needs of the newborn foal. The whole complex story is there and can be interpreted swiftly by an experienced eye.

pneumovagina (windsucking)   The voluntary inspiration of atmospheric air through the vulvar lips into the vagina, causing a ballooning effect. Contaminated air is the primary cause of simple irritation, inflammation, and finally infection.

A predisposing condition to pneumovagina is the conformation of the mare's dock and the angulation of the vulvar plane. Mares built with the tendency to inspire air or to drop manure near the vulvar edges are candidates for pneumovagina and subsequent reproductive-tract infection. These individuals will be subfertile unless a Caslick's operation is performed.

It has been reported that with each pregnancy a mare loses a bit of tissue tone in her perineal area, so a multipara mare may, after a few pregnancies, require a Caslick's to prevent pneumovagina. *See:* CASLICK'S OPERATION.

Windsucking is a vice usually acquired when the animal is young and idle, during prolonged estrus cycles, or by suggestion while in the company of other mares in season.

postpartum problems in broodmares   *See:* ECLAMPSIA; LACERATIONS, BRUISES, AND HEMATOMAS OF THE REPRODUCTIVE TRACT AS A RESULT OF PARTURITION; OBTURATOR NERVE PARALYSIS; MASTITIS; INTERNAL HEMORRHAGE; RUPTURE OF MIDDLE UTERINE ARTERY; RETAINED PLACENTA; RECTO-VAGINAL FISTULA; RECTAL PROLAPSE; UTERINE PROLAPSE; UTERINE RUPTURE.

pregnancy examination   This is always a period of anxiety and anticipation for those involved with the breeding process—the owners, who have both an emotional and financial stake in the outcome, and, of course, the veterinarian, who may have followed the mare through her cycles and cover. Early pregnancy diagnosis provides an invaluable service to commercial breeding farms and is a skill that can facilitate the efficiency of the farm.

Manual or rectal examination is the most accurate and satisfactory method available, and results in an on-the-spot diagnosis. It does, however, require a skilled and gentle equine veterinarian.

Proper restraint is a prerequisite for a pregnancy examination. A stock is preferred but is not essential. Equally effective is a plywood board placed across the stall door to serve as a protective barrier between the examiner and the mare. The board should be wide enough to overlap the sides of the stall door so that it cannot fall in on the mare. It should be tied to the sides of the stall door (holes cut near the top are convenient for carrying it and for looping ropes through). The correct height for the board—as I have discovered from experience—is 42 inches. This height is critical for the safety of the veterinarian. A higher board could result in a fractured arm if the nervous mare slips or throws herself down

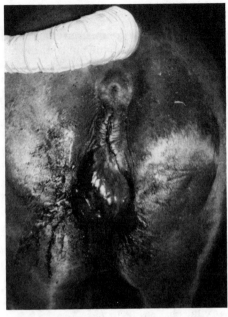

Vaginal Tumor, discovered after foaling

while the examiner is reaching inside her bony pelvis. A slightly lower board could allow kicking feet to clear the barrier.

The practitioner waits until the mare's hocks are pressing against the board and then, wearing sterile, disposable, polyethelene, shoulder-length sleeves, proceeds with the examination. A practiced equine veterinarian should be able to determine pregnancy accurately as early as the 18th day from the last cover.

If a question arises, due either to a difficult mare or an inexperienced operator, and if the manual examination is unsatisfactory, three laboratory tests for determining pregnancy are available:

1. *Friedman Test*—From day 45 through day 100 of pregnancy, a blood sample can be drawn from the mare to determine the amount of gonadotropic hormone present. This test is 99 percent accurate. The only time I have found false results with this blood test was when the sample was taken at the wrong period in gestation; human error was the problem.

2. *Mare Immunological Pregnancy Test (MIP)*—Taken between day 45 and day 130 of pregnancy, this blood test, a hemagglutination-inhibition test, is based on the presence of serum gonadotropins (PMSG). This immunologic test is considered very accurate.

3. *Cuboni Test*—After 120 days into gestation, the mare's urine can be tested for estrone contents. This urine test produces 90 percent accurate results.

prepubic tendon rupture The prepubic tendon attaches the abdominal muscles (rectus abdominis) to the pubis (pelvis) and helps to serve as the main abdominal support.

In any broodmare heavy in foal, especially one with many previous pregnancies, the pubic tendon attachment holding the weighty mass can quite

prepubic tendon rupture continued

easily rupture or tear away. Slipping, sliding, physical trauma, or a fall could cause partial or complete release of tendon attachment from the pubis, throwing all weight onto the remaining abdominal muscles.

Symptoms are unmistakable. The abdominal contour suddenly becomes lowered almost to hock level, with the udder positioned just in front of the hind legs. This condition is a problem at parturition. In the absence of muscular function and prowess, the fetus may not be positioned correctly for eventual delivery, and dystocia may result.

For the safety of the mare and foal, when a prepubic tendon rupture is diagnosed, it may be wise for all concerned to plan a cesarean section and thereby avoid complications or costly mistakes. Discuss this with your veterinarian. *See:* CESAREAN.

rectal prolapse   External displacement of the anal tissue; the consequence of excessive straining, usually during a difficult and lengthy delivery, or in response to some other painful stimulus.

Treatment is as for any prolapse in the perineal region: sedating the animal, injecting anesthesia after careful preparation of the epidural site, meticulous cleansing of the exposed "inside-out" tissue, and manual replacement. As a final step, a purse-string suture is customarily placed around the perimeter of the anal ring to maintain stability and yet allow vital passage of feces.

Diet should consist of limited hay and soft bran mashes daily for a few weeks.

Prognosis is fair to good.

pyometra   An accumulation of pus in the uterine cavity. Any severe case of endometritis or metritis, treated or untreated, can conceivably develop into pyometra.

During rectal palpation a uterus containing pus can closely simulate early pregnancy. Consequently, this dangerous infection has been erroneously diagnosed.

If the infection goes unrecognized and untreated, mares suffering with pyometra can become critically ill, run high fevers, and develop blood poisoning. To add further misery, founder will assuredly become an additional complication for the sick mare. Even death has occurred in neglected cases.

Prompt treatment is imperative, requiring vigorous uterine flushing, antibiotic therapy, and antihistamines, along with daily attentive care.

I have never known a mare to reproduce once she has developed pyometra, no matter how thorough or efficient the treatment.

rectovaginal fistula   This is one of the destructive consequences that can occur in the broodmare during an unattended delivery. Unless properly managed, it can threaten the mare's reproductive future. Although 95 percent of all broodmares foal successfully, the remaining 5 percent do not, and the fistula is one of the complications that keep equine practitioners humble.

Rectovaginal fistulas occur when an emerging foal's foot (directed upward) penetrates the dorsal wall (roof) of the vagina and continues on through the rectal floor above, thus creating a rent or hole. In some cases, the foot does not retract, but continues as the delivery progresses to tear backwards through the rectal area, ripping away all perineal tissue. When the anal sphincter and vulvar tissues are destroyed, this results in the formation of a cloaca, a common opening between the rectum and the vagina.

Occasionally during delivery of the foal, the broodmare sustains not only lacerations and tearing, but deep bruising as well. For this reason, immediate surgical repair is contraindicated and should not be considered. Devitalized tissue will not heal! Corrective procedures must be deferred for a minimum of 14 days to permit time for regeneration of damaged tissue.

The repair requires a series of reconstructive surgeries to rebuild a functional solid-tissue membrane between the vagina and rectum. Any minute leakage of feces or rectal contaminants into the vagina establishes an infection that causes not only infertility, but the eventual destruction of the mare's reproductive tract and capability. A good patient and a determined surgeon are essential to a happy outcome.

Rebuild the anatomical fault as soundly as nature allows. Culture, treat, and clean up the mare's reproductive tract as soon as possible. With good luck your mare may reproduce again.

tetany in the mare   *See:* ECLAMPSIA.

twin pregnancy   It is well documented that broodmares can easily conceive a twin pregnancy but are notoriously unsuccessful in supporting the duo. Abortion results in 90 percent of the cases, occurring at almost any time—from before the fetus reaches detectable size to commonly around the eighth month of gestation.

In my opinion, almost all such failures, especially those late in pregnancy, are nutritionally caused. The mare's uterus and its placentation are poorly equipped for maintaining twin pregnancy, since both fetuses develop simultaneously and require double the nutritional supply. Moreover, the equine fetus doubles its weight during the last two months of gestation, and in a twin pregnancy the demands for room and nutrition are far too great for the average mare. The weaker of the two fetuses is the first to be affected, with death usually following. The dead twin creates a "foreign body" reaction in the mare, causing abortion of both foals.

It always saddens me to see the stronger, apparently normal foal aborted along with the weaker individual. Unlike some other species, a mare lacks the ability to wall off a dead fetus and consequently aborts immediately. If the fetus is contracted or cannot be expelled rapidly, the broodmare becomes violently ill.

I have seen a few twin foals carried to term and born alive. On these rare occasions, the mother was always a large and roomy mare. Regardless of the sex, one twin always seemed a little larger in size, strength, and vigor. All these survivors, in my experience, had tender, loving, round-the-clock care that assured equal amounts of milk—supplementary milk is needed—and plenty of attention. *See:* BOTTLE FEEDING, COLOSTRUM.

udder   Common name for the mammary gland. This gland is responsible for the production of colostrum for the newborn and for continued lactation for nourishment of the foal or suckling.

The udder is of no great interest in the riding or pet mare—except, of course, for a teat inflammation caused by dirt or trauma, which can be treated locally and routinely with antibiotic-cortisone mammary ointment.

The broodmare presents a different set of circumstances. The health of the *udder continued*

broodmare's mammary gland is imperative to the young foal for many reasons. To the newborn, the mammary gland means survival with a direct effect on its immediate and future health. The nutritious and laxative properties of the milk are important in the transfer of preformed antibodies for immunity. The udder represents the singular source of immune protection for the newborn foal.

Often an udder will be hard, hot, caked, and sore immediately after foaling. A sore udder, especially in a maiden mare, can cause the mare to reject the foal or, worse yet, to become hostile and injure the foal as it approaches her to nurse.

An alert attendant can avert this tragedy by giving the mammary gland immediate attention, applying hot towels, "wrung dry," locally. This serves to soften and cleanse the udder and actually aids the "let down" and flow of the first milk (colostrum). Mother and child may then become friends.

Later on, during the period of heavy lactation, trouble can reappear in the udder. Bacteria can enter, especially if skin of the teat is bruised or has a pinpoint laceration. This can lead to an inflammatory process called *mastitis*. Seek your veterinarian's advice. Milk out the area of infection locally, then instill an intramammary ointment (e.g., bacitracin, neomycin, prednisolone). If the mastitis is severe, perhaps antiobiotic injections will be needed to fortify the mare's system. Body-temperature readings are an important guide in cases of udder infection.

The possibility of mastitis is always imminent during and shortly after weaning time on the farm. Experienced broodmare management can virtually preclude mammary gland complication and its various problems and treatments.

A painful case of mastitis that is allowed to develop in a pregnant mare can adversely affect her health, producing high fever, poor appetite, and other symptoms. Mastitis is a condition of neglect and is strictly inexcusable. Though well-developed cases are commonly seen in amateur operations, they are not to be found on knowledgeable breeding farms.

An old tried and proven system at weaning time suggests that all mares separated from their foals be given a hay-and-water diet, with no concentrates, for a seven-day period. Provide each mare considerable freedom to move around—open shed, open stall door with adjacent paddock. An essential visual check on all udders carried out twice daily by conscientious attendants can uncover early changes, relieve excess pressure, and prevent illness. As important as it is to remove a few streams of milk for relief of pain and pressure in the udder, it is equally important to limit the amount released. With each stream of milk the body is signaled to produce more milk. Therefore, milk out only a stream or two. With this old system, 90 percent of weaning-related mastitis cases are prevented.

Call your veterinarian if a hot, swollen, congested, and painful udder develops. Proper, prompt treatment can shorten the duration, minimize scar-tissue formation, and preserve sound mammary tissue for the future foal.

uterine prolapse External displacement of the uterus, resulting from a dystocia, a very difficult or protracted delivery. It is a desperate, life-threatening situation for the matron, and a very frightening one for the owner.

Quickly summon the veterinarian. The mare will be sedated (I.V. or I.M.) and prepped immediately for an epidural anesthetic (comparable to the "spinal" used in human medicine) to numb the entire perineal region and prevent undue resistance and straining. The veterinarian must be astute in regulating the dosage so that pain is relieved and the mare does not lose her footing; to achieve replacement of the organ, the animal ideally should be standing. Profuse flushing with copious amounts of sterile saline solution can aid in cleansing the "inside-out" uterus. A generous application of sugar reduces the swelling somewhat, and facilitates manual replacement.

The prognosis is guarded to poor. Broodmares, unlike other species, poorly tolerate this injury and usually develop an infection or septicemia.

uterine rupture   A tear in the wall of the uterus, admitting the intestines into the uterine space. This is a very grave finding. It can result from excessive straining; undue fetal weight or prolonged pressure over the mare's bony pelvis; a large fetus in a worn-out uterus as seen in multapara mares; a contracted foal causing a strenuous, lengthy delivery, or a poorly performed embryotomy (cutting a contracted fetus for removal from the mare's reproductive tract).

My mother owned a precious broodmare that had not only distinguished herself at the races, but had produced three beautiful foals. Although two weeks overdue, very pendulous and slightly edgy, she was still eating and acting healthily. Because of the delay in foaling, everyone felt a little tense, so her dates were checked and found to be accurate; she was then three weeks overdue! That evening, however, she went down in the straw and began forceful, active labor. We watched anxiously but quietly, and after several powerful contractions, there was no evidence of the amniotic sac. I scrubbed quickly in the prepared antiseptic pail and slipped my hand into the vagina with full expectations of palpating a foot. No foot was there and my heart sank as my hand felt and grasped intestines. I knew this meant a ruptured uterus and certain death for the mare. Further examinations revealed a hopelessly contracted foal inside of the uterus—totally locked and lifeless. Mother and I agreed to put the mare to sleep immediately.

uterus   Intrauterine conditions that affect the health and functional ability of the mare's uterus:

Endometritis—Infection of the lining of the uterus or the endometrium.
Metritis—Infection of the uterus.
Pyometra—Pus or purulent material collected in the uterus.
Retained placenta—Attached placental tissues with delayed release from the endometrium of the uterus.

See: UTERINE PROLAPSE, UTERINE RUPTURE.

windsucking   *See:* PNEUMOVAGINA.

PEDIATRICS

acidemia An acid condition of the blood brought about by metabolic changes. Metabolic acidemia occurs in newborn foals already sick with a systemic infection. Symptoms can vary; those commonly found are weakness, convulsions, respiratory distress, and degrees of diarrhea. Although acidemia is a secondary development of a primary infectious disease, usually a septicemia (blood poisoning), the importance of prompt recognition and treatment cannot be overemphasized.

An accurate diagnosis can identify the cause, then both conditions can be treated simultaneously.

Specific treatment for acidemia consists of 5 percent sodium bicarbonate solution intravenously, which can be repeated at two- to three-hour intervals, concurrent with specific treatment for the existing septicemia.

actinobacillus equuli (Shigella equuli) A deadly micro-organism that affects newborn foals. It produces a lethal septicemia (blood poisoning) in the young, who are referred to as "sleeper," "wanderer," or "dummy" foals.

If the foal is infected *in utero,* it may be aborted or delivered dead. If it manages to arrive alive it is likely to be weak, semicomatose, and unable to stand.

If the diseased foal is strong enough to stand, it will persistently circle the outer edges of the stall, usually in one direction only, "nursing" ceaselessly on the stall walls, feed tubs, buckets, or anything it can reach on its rounds—except its mother! Affected foals appear almost to resist their mothers. When exhausted, they stand as though in a deep stupor, seemingly unable to lie down, hence the term "dummy."

Other symptoms are subnormal temperature, severe dehydration, prominent bluish white nictitating membranes (the third eyelid), and a fetid, yellowish, distressing diarrhea (one can smell the diagnosis when entering the stall).

Some years ago, 90 percent of these foals were lost. With the advent of broad-spectrum drugs, combined with supportive therapy, most of them now survive and show no apparent aftereffects.

Your veterinarian will undoubtedly recommend the treatment accepted as standard today:

1. Feedings of colostrum and Milk of Magnesia by means of a stomach tube, sutured in position; a plug is inserted in the open end of the tube when not in use to prevent air and contaminants from entering.

2. Oral administration of chloramphenical (1 gram three times daily) and chloromycetin I.V. (2 grams, three times daily).

144

3. The administration of fluids and electrolytes is supportive and an essential addition to the treatment.

adenoviral infection A fatal viral disease of purebred Arabian foals; reported in England, Australia, and in parts of the United States. Symptoms are nasal and ocular discharge, depression, unthriftiness (thin or in poor flesh), with developing pneumonia and intermittent fever. A diagnostic blood study will reveal a shocking reduction of lymphocytes (a type of white blood cell). A differential white cell count can alert and guide the attending veterinarian.

We have begun to hear reports of adenoviral infections in horses other than those of the Arabian breed. Although symptoms are identical, all the animals affected have been identified as immunodeficient. (The veterinary profession has observed a profound increase in the prevalence of immunodeficient individuals—or perhaps it is the diagnostic skills that have increased.)

ascariasis A parasitic infestation that can be life-threatening in foals if untreated. Ascarids are roundworms commonly found as intestinal parasites but they overtly invade all organs of the body, especially the tissues of the lungs.

Affected foals manifest respiratory symptoms, including coughing and nasal discharge, along with potbellies and general unthriftiness. Neglected foals often develop pneumonia, requiring emergency measures.

Foals constantly reinfest themselves with ascarids, so regular repeated worming is imperative. Have your veterinarian set up a strict worming schedule and follow it religiously. *See:* WORMING.

atresia Congenital absence or pathologic closure of a normal opening, passage, or cavity. It is very rare for a foal to be born with an incomplete colon (in which case it must be euthanized) or incomplete vaginal passage (such a foal can easily live a normal life, but can never reproduce). Although surgical correction has been attempted, the results have been totally unsuccessful to date, in both colonic and vaginal atresia.

babysitter A quiet animal whose personality and presence is used for the purpose of settling or calming young, insecure animals, especially at weaning or any time when schedules or surroundings are abruptly changed.

A complacent gelding or preferably an old, fat, even foundered pony will serve well as a stabilizing companion. Mildly lame animals are ideal because they are less active. Donkeys, goats, or even chickens are sometimes used for this role.

barker foal *See:* CONVULSIVE SYNDROME OF THE NEWBORN.

bottle-feeding A lifesaving procedure used when needed to care for a weak newborn or a sick older foal. The colostrum that is vital to the neonate, as well as the nutritious milk needed by the sick foal, can easily be fed by a bottle.

A standard human infant's nursing bottle with the nipple holes slightly enlarged serves a young foal perfectly. Nutrition is thus made easily accessible to the foal, and the feedings can be served on time and at frequent intervals.

Some old-time horsemen are reluctant to feed a weak foal by bottle, believing erroneously that such a foal will ultimately reject its mother, or vice versa, once it is strong enough to nurse naturally from the udder.

Nothing can be further from the truth! Feed your sick or weak foal, provide the precious nutrition it needs, and I guarantee that when the foal is strong

bottle-feeding continued

enough, it will nurse naturally on its own, as nature intended. Without receiving this simple assistance, many foals have needlessly been lost. *See:* COLOSTRUM, ORPHAN FOAL.

cleft palate   A fissure in the hard and/or soft palate that together form the roof of the mouth; a malformation of the palate of congenital or hereditary origin in the form of either a split, crack, or crevice opening.

In the human this defect is usually accompanied by a harelip. The only symptom seen in the newborn foal with a cleft palate is milk flowing out of both nasal cavities as the frustrated foal attempts to nurse. This symptom is diagnostic! The afflicted foal's vigor and nutritional level depend on whether it can swallow more than it loses out of its nasal cavity. Lowered nutrition and nasal irritation result in pharyngitis, laryngitis, and even pneumonia if allowed to go untreated.

Surgical intervention, called a *palatosynthesis*, is the only alternative, but at the present time this procedure needs further refining and study. As you might suspect, the prognosis is guarded to poor.

colostrum   A thin but sweet milky fluid secreted by the mammary gland a few days or hours before parturition (delivery); it is the mare's "first milk," essential to the foal's health because it contains and thus transmits vital preformed passive antibodies to the foal. It exists only for a limited period of time, about 48 to 60 hours after parturition.

Colostrum is highly nutritious, contains an essential laxative substance vital to the foal's gastrointestinal health, and is the *only* source of antibodies available to the completely unprotected newborn.

Some mares leak unusual amounts of precious colostrum into the bedding when delivery is delayed for any physiologic or pathologic reason.

Other domestic species (bovine, caprine, feline, canine) have a built-in system, superior to that of the mare, whereby the fetus receives an antibody supply from the mother *during* gestation, regularly dispatched on time. These newborns arrive into the outside world with adequate protection against infectious agents and stress conditions. Foals are "second-class citizens" in that they are provided with no natural immunity for the outside environment during fetal development; thus handicapped, they endure parturition, umbilical detachment, traumatic struggles to stand, and the ultimate insult, the search for the inconveniently placed, partially hidden udder. Once it is found and nursing is achieved, all can sigh in relief!

A newborn foal fails to receive preformed protective antibodies in the following circumstances:

1. Death of the mother at or immediately after foaling
2. Agalactic (dry) udder, no milk available
3. Incompatibility of milk and foal (isoerythrolysis)
4. Total rejection of foal by mother
5. Faulty immune system in the mother with delinquent development of antibodies in the udder
6. Faulty absorption of maternal antibodies through the foal's duodenum

A newborn without colostrum or, for that matter, without milk, is not uncommon in the horse world, *but it is an urgent situation*. There are a number of ways to meet the emergency:

1. Many large breeding farms have established their own frozen colostrum banks for just this emergency.

2. There are agencies that provide "milk mares," usually crossbred, placid, docile mares with milk aplenty, all available for a fee. Best, of course, is a milk mare that has just foaled, since she has colostrum in her udder.

3. Today we are fortunate in having commercial colostrum substitutes, such as Foal-Lac®, made by Borden. These preparations provide all nutritional requirements in abundance for the neonatal foal. These do not supply antibodies, however.

Orphan or rejected foals not receiving normal colostrum should be routinely injected with antibiotics for seven to ten days to protect against infection. Veterinary observation should detect those individuals who require some additional protection, usually in the form of a serum transfusion literally loaded with antibodies.

In my experience, when a foal is fed the milk substitute conscientiously and according to directions, and when there is veterinary supervision with provision of needed antibiotics and serum transfusions, it can grow into a better-developed and visibly superior individual compared to mare-fed foals in the same environment. It is important to continuously provide a free-choice milk substitute and later make available milk pellets mixed with grain at all times.

At the risk of being labeled a traitor to motherhood, I am inclined to suggest weaning all foals very early, perhaps at eight weeks, and providing a good diet in lieu of the mare's milk, which has no nutritional value after three months. This method would provide additional benefit in freeing the perhaps re-bred mare from her burdensome foal. *See:* AGALACTIA, ORPHAN FOAL.

NUTRITIONAL PROPERTIES OF MILK

	Protein	Fat (Percent)	Fiber	Lactose	Ash
Mare's milk (colostrum stage)	19.6	14.2	0	53.4	3.6
Foal-Lac	20.2	14.4	0.2	52.6	7.2
Cow's milk	23.8	41.6	0	42.5	5.04

constipation *See:* RETAINED MECONIUM.

convulsive syndrome of the newborn The popular term for this condition—barker foal—derives from the unmistakable sounds made by the affected foal shortly after its delivery; the newborn usually falls on its side in the bedding and is unable to rise. Most of these foals convulse and "bark" endlessly until exhausted.

The cause of this condition in unknown. According to one theory, deprivation of oxygen to the brain prior to or during delivery causes these convulsive seizures in the newborn. The oxygen deprivation may be caused by:

1. Premature separation of the placental membranes before delivery
2. Delayed delivery

convulsive syndrome continued

    3. Pressure on the umbilicus by the mare's bony pelvis
    4. A breech presentation
    5. Untrained human intervention and cutting the cord too early.

    To care for such a foal is complex and calls for round-the-clock supervision: light tranquilization and sedation, stomach-tube feedings every half hour (tube affixed by a ligation suture), electrolyte replacement (dextrose, saline), IV.

    The owner or caretaker will be helped by the support techniques just listed, but the situation remains grim. Unless there is day-and-night nursing care, the barker foal's frequent and unexpected convulsive seizures will result in head smashing, uncontrolled muscle contractions, and self-inflicted wounds. Perhaps some such foals have been saved, but I have never been fortunate enough to witness a recovery.

diarrhea (scours)   An abnormally frequent discharge of watery fecal matter from the bowel.

    Mechanical, inflammatory, or infectious agents are causes of this symptom of illness. It is the first sign of trouble in foals, but it often proves to have some mechanical cause, such as parasitism or copraphagy (eating manure), or is associated with the mare's foal heat, or first heat following delivery.

    Because the causes are many, it is essential to establish proper treatment, since the affected ones dehydrate rapidly and can die before the problem is recognized and treated. While waiting for your veterinarian to appear, you will find that foals respond well to intestinal astringents and antidiarrhetics such as: acacia, activated charcoal, albumin tannate, bismuth, catechu, kaolin, Kao-pectate®, Milk of Magnesia®, opium, paregoric, and tannic acid.

    Diarrhea is often a first sign of systemic disease. A temperature check and a blood count can alert you to the early signs of foal septicemia (blood poisoning). *See:* FOAL HEAT SCOURS, PAREGORIC, SEPTICEMIAS.

foal diseases   *See:* SEPTICEMIAS.

foal-heat scours   An expected diarrhea that occurs in the newborn foal from the sixth day to as late as the twelfth day of its life. It is caused by the nursing foal's inadvertent ingestion of secretions from the mare's vulva that flow or drip down over the mammary gland. This exudate is more profuse during the so-called foal heat, when the mare's body is cleansing itself after her recent delivery. This discharge is full of micro-organisms and debris that can easily cause a gastrointestinal upset in the foal.

    Foal-heat scours is accepted by everyone as a normal happening, unless the diarrhea continues beyond the heat period of the mare and the foal is so severely affected as to cause it to weaken. Diarrhea can create a fluid and electrolyte imbalance *more quickly than any other known condition,* and dangerous dehydration follows shortly. During this period a septicemia could take advantage and rapidly develop in your foal while it is temporarily weakened by diarrhea. A watchful eye, some kaolin-paregoric oral mixture, and regular temperature and visual check-ups are all that is normally required.

    I have found that a few injections of penicillin combined with dihydrostreptomycin I.M. help the weaker foals through these occasionally stressful days and help to prevent other illnesses.

Be sure to wash the foal's tail and adjacent areas with white soap and warm water, then grease well with Vaseline to avoid scalding and subsequent loss of hair.

isoerythrolysis   *See:* NEONATAL ISOERYTHROLYSIS.

joint ill   *See:* SEPTICEMIAS.

leaky navel   *See:* PERVIOUS URACHUS.

navel ill   *See:* SEPTICEMIAS.

neonatal infections   *See:* SEPTICEMIAS.

neonatal isoerythrolysis   A highly fatal hemolytic (destruction of red blood cells) anemia of newborn foals that ingest poisoned colostrum from their mother's mammary glands. It is caused by isoimmunization by the mare during gestation that is directed against the red blood cells of her own foal! (The prefix *iso-* means "within itself.")

This strange twist in nature occurs when the broodmare is bred to a stallion with any blood type incompatible with the mare's blood type. If the fetus inherits its dam's blood type, all is well. If it inherits its sire's blood type, the fetus is automatically foreign to its own mother, and as a result the foal's red blood cells trigger the dam to begin the formation of antibodies in her own blood serum specifically designed to destroy her foal's red blood cells.

Fortunately, *no* harm is done during gestation, since no transplacental exchange exists in the mare (contrary to the process in humans and other species), and, excluding other problems, a normal healthy foal is delivered. All is fine until the foal nurses and ingests the colostrum (the first milk, teeming with natural—but in this case "hostile"—antibodies). These antibodies are capable of

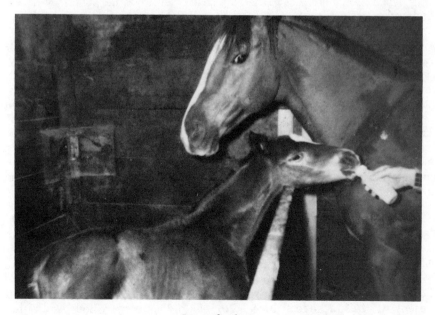

Isoerythrolysis

neonatal isoerythrolysis continued

destroying the newborn's red blood cells, producing a severe anemia in a very short time. If the condition is unrecognized and unchecked by emergency treatment, death can ensue.

This potentially tragic entity in the foal is analogous to the Rh factor in human disease. Although similar in many ways, it differs greatly by its quiescent and insidious development during gestation only to explode with the first few swallows by the foal immediately postpartum.

If the foal is allowed to continue drinking the "poisoned milk" produced by its mother, it will suddenly weaken and sink down in the bedding, unwilling or unable to rise. With a rapid respiration and heart rate, pale or yellow oral mucosa (gums), and a subnormal temperature, it will rapidly deteriorate and, unless treated, will die in from one to three days. Yellow (jaundiced or icteric) membranes indicate the destruction and death of red blood cells and their hemoglobin contents.

Blood tests at this time will reveal a profound anemia; sometimes the vital volume will lower to a startling 50 percent of normal (3–5 million per cubic millimeter; normal is 10–12 million per cubic millimeter).

Blood transfusions are lifesaving if promptly and properly carried out. Detailed care in determining compatibility for transfusion is essential in this urgent situation; although it is time-consuming, it must be performed without error or it can in itself cause death. Never transfuse from the dam since she is the cause of the problem and her serum is loaded with antibodies lethal to the foal. Select several possible donors and cross-match each until you or the laboratory can confirm compatibility.

Once a broodmare has carried a foal that sensitizes her, she may have a tendency to maintain a future blood titer of antibodies.

To prevent isoimmunization, check blood compatibilities prior to booking your mare. All that is needed is to take a blood sample from the prospective stallion and one from your mare, and then submit them to a reliable laboratory.

If you suspect that a mare may be carrying a foal of incompatible blood type, and if she exhibits jaundiced membranes, depression, edematous swellings, although all are nonspecific symptoms, you should draw blood serum from the mare any time after the eighth month of gestation and request a sample from the stallion for agglutination tests. If a positive titer is present in your mare, then the veterinarian will probably administer supportive therapy and will suggest a monthly blood sample to monitor the progressive degree of antibody formation through the remaining period of gestation. Feel fortunate to be alerted of an impending problem, since it allows you and your veterinarian to forestall the event.

Preparation is the key to success in cases of isoimmunization in the mare. The following is a suggested procedure in either diagnosed or suspected cases:

When the foal emerges, capture a drop of blood from the ruptured cord on a glass microscope slide. Then promptly mix a drop of the mare's milk with the foal's blood, stir lightly, and observe for "clumping" of erythrocytes on the slide—either grossly evident or seen under the microscope. If agglutination is present, MUZZLE the foal. Proceed to milk the mare every hour, and rather than discard this precious colostrum, store and freeze it for use in other foals. It is *not* toxic to other foals, only to its own.

The neonatal foal should be fed via baby bottles with colostrum from other mares, or with a commercial milk substitute (include antibiotics, laxatives, etc.). Some people prefer to use a "nurse mare." Although it is a splendid and admirable thought, critical acceptance by the mare and the question of timing for the needy foal probably will make its use impractical.

The foal's blood sample and a sample of colostrum should be sent immediately to the laboratory for a baseline value, then a repeat of each sample should be sent every 24 hours until all incompatibility is gone (all antibodies disappeared from the milk). When the laboratory sends the word, then mother and baby may be put together again.

As a rule, this is a round-the-clock endurance test for a minimum of three days. It is imperative for the mare and foal to be in sight of each other so that rejection will not transpire when they are placed together again. It is also vital to keep milking the mare on a frequent and regular schedule so that not only will the milk be released, but lactation will be undisturbed and her mammary gland will continue to function.

I have supervised several of these isoimmunization cases and have been fortunate in that all mares and foals survived. When I realize the vast and detailed knowledge earned and recorded by our forefathers in medicine, I feel a prevailing debt of gratitude. My appreciation becomes stronger when I see a healthy viable foal standing and nursing that otherwise would surely have perished through ignorance!

orphan foal Foals can find themselves without a mother for milk, comfort, and protection under numerous causes and conditions, but there is one sure thing, it is always abrupt!

Broodmares frequently die during delivery or shortly after parturition, leaving the orphan foal to fend for itself. Foals rejected by a "nasty" mother experience the ultimate insult, perhaps leaving a lasting psychological scar. A rejected foal is, in essence, an orphan!

In any case, the foal is suddenly alone and the job of feeding around the clock and providing safe exercise and companionship must fall upon its hardy and devoted human friends. We all know that young thrive well on milk from the same specie, so a "milk mare" is the ideal alternative—if you can overcome the logistics of timing, transportation, availability, and the costs of a nurse mare. Usually, however, although the nurse mare is lactating, she does not have the vital colostrum (first milk). It still must be provided!

Years ago, it was necessary to mix a milk formula of cow's milk, Karo syrup, lime water, and laxative.* The orphan foals who lived on this concoction suffered nutritionally, usually developed intractable diarrhea, and ultimately were stunted. It was quite easy to pick an orphan foal from a group of young horses by its pathetic undersize.

---

*This is the old-fashioned formula: 1 quart whole cow's milk, 2 tablespoons cream, 2 tablespoons lime water, 1 tablespoon corn syrup, 2 tablespoons Milk of Magnesia; feed several ounces of this mixture every half hour.

orphan foal continued

Today, when a mother and/or her milk are unavailable, most large farms have a frozen colostrum bank to meet the emergency. This provides the foal with the vital antibodies and natural laxative properties of the first milk. (In lieu of frozen colostrum, the human colostral substitute, Similac, can be used, together with antibiotic therapy.) This is second best as no protective antibodies are provided. For maintenance, the foal is given a synthetic milk substitute, usually Foal-Lac. The powder is formulated specifically for foals, and when mixed according to directions, it makes a superior nutritional fluid food for the neonate. It is best fed via a baby bottle every half hour round the clock.

At three days of age, in addition to the fluid food, a feed tub should be placed low enough to be easily accessible to the foal; it should be filled with equal parts of Mother's Oats and Foal-Lac pellets. It is my experience that foals raised on this schedule thrive better than their stable mates raised in the conventional fashion.

In the case of an orphan foal that has been denied colostrum, I give daily injections of antibiotics for the first week of life to afford some protection against infection. I also maintain vigilance on the condition of the navel cord stump, and ensure that a small amount of Milk of Magnesia is added to the diet daily for about three weeks. A serum transfusion, easily administered and loaded with protective antibodies, should be a serious consideration in any and all unfortunate foals that for any reason miss the all-important colostral meal.

The benefits that accrue from daily critical glances at any newborn during the precarious and sometimes turbulent neonatal period cannot be overrated. I call this watchful period the "third eye." *See:* COLOSTRUM.

pervious urachus Leaky navel, a rather common condition found in the newborn foal. During gestation, a ureter-like structure in the umbilical cord is attached to the fetal urinary bladder and excretes urine into the placental tissues. Upon birth, this structure customarily dries up and closes when the umbilical cord ruptures and recoils. Occasionally, it fails to close, remaining patent, and

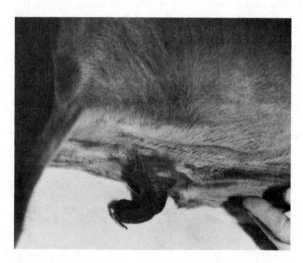

Foal's Navel Stump

leaks urine when the foal urinates. Although thought by some to be unimportant, I view a patent urachus as a potential for infection, since the umbilical stump is constantly wet and dirty from the leaking urine.

Treatment consists of daily inspection for drying and shrinking in size together with cauterization with either strong iodine tincture or silver nitrate.

As a practicing veterinarian, I have learned to associate previous urachus with foals suffering from systemic infections. Because of this knowledge, I always view this condition as a warning, and respond by giving the foal a complete physical, including a complete blood count. *See:* SEPTICEMIAS.

renal abscess in foals Renal abscesses occur often in foals that have a septicemia (blood infection). *Actinobacillus equuli (Shigella equuli)* is the causative pathogen of kidney abscesses in the foal. Streptococcal infections also locate in foals' kidney tissue. *See:* SEPTICEMIAS.

retained meconium A form of constipation seen in the newborn foal. Meconium is dark, sticky fecal matter that accumulates in the foal's intestine during fetal life and development. Normal meconium usually is defecated shortly after birth and is helped along by a laxative principal in the mother's colostrum. Sometimes the meconium is of the wrong consistency, lacking sufficient moisture to allow it to move along normally in the intestines. As a result, the foal comes into the world with a stubborn and painful constipation, which it shows by straining, discomfort, and tail switching as early as two hours after arrival.

Although a routine enema will evacuate the rectum, promote intestinal movement, and probably produce some fecal material, it cannot reach the colon or higher, where the meconium is normally retained. Passage of feces does not preclude serious constipation in the foal at a later hour.

Electrolytes intravenously can prevent dehydration and promote intestinal movement. Laxatives, analgesics, enemas, and warmth applied to the abdomen are all helpful, but it requires a tireless and loyal crew for a round-the-clock surveillance to protect the rolling foal from self-injury.

If treatment fails to produce a comfortable foal or a passage of feces within 24 hours, surgical intervention then becomes a serious consideration. Surgical removal of hard meconium from the upper colon is by now a standard procedure when indicated in newborn foals.

It is thought by some people that a less than ideal diet and improper exercise of the broodmare during gestation have a significant bearing on the number of foals born with retained meconium. *See:* SEPTICEMIAS.

ruptured urinary bladder in foals A condition not uncommonly found in the newborn, thought to be caused from either excessive compression of the abdomen of the foal in the bony pelvic cavity during delivery, or from extreme tension applied on the umbilical cord after birth. With a leaky urinary bladder, the urine escapes into the abdominal cavity.

After delivery, the neonatal foal will *appear* normal for the first 24 to 48 hours. I contend that an astute attendant, one who is truly interested, will notice that micturation (urination) is scanty and sense the hidden presence of a problem. The size of the tear or rent can vary greatly, thus symptoms range from very slight to overt.

The exact cause of bladder rupture is not known, but with abdominal *ruptured urinary bladder in foals continued*

retention of urine the symptoms are classic. Periodic straining, abdominal distention, slight temperature elevation, and dullness with a "panting" respiration are characteristic of a ruptured bladder. Depression then develops, mucous membranes become white, and the foal ceases nursing! This is now a "red alert." Call your veterinarian!

If untreated, vision will be affected and convulsions may develop from the retained urine and its toxicity.

Your veterinarian will, after a thorough examination, aseptically prep the foal's abdomen and perform an abdominal tap (paracentesis). If free urine is retrieved in the syringe from the abdominal cavity, then emergency surgery for repair of a ruptured urinary bladder is indicated. During the paracentesis, an effort should be made not only to diagnose, but also to remove as much accumulated urine as possible. This helps provide a "better risk" patient to the surgeon.

Early recognition with prompt diagnosis greatly enhances the foal's chances for a complete recovery after successful surgical repair.

septicemias   Systemic diseases caused by bacterial invasion of the circulatory system. They occur commonly in young foals and can affect all parts of the foal's body.

The micro-organisms or their toxins may enter the bloodstream *in utero* and result in the abortion of a dead fetus. In spite of the infection, in some cases embryonic growth and fetal development continue in an infected uterus and placental membranes, and a sick foal is born. Some of these foals are saved by prompt recognition and treatment of the acute form of infection.

A healthy foal can be born and then acquire a systemic infection in three known ways: micro-organisms may enter through the open navel stump, through the mouth (ingested), or through the nostrils (inhaled).

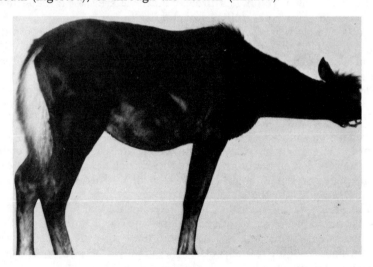

Septicemic Foal, typical unthrifty appearance

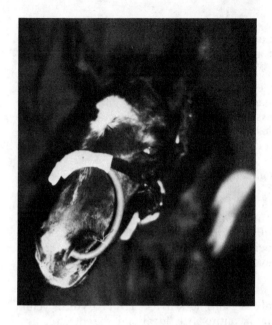

Septicemic Foal, naso-gastric tube sutured into place for feeding purposes

SEPTICEMIAS IN NEWBORN FOALS

Causative Agent	Symptoms
Streptococcus	*Navel Ill, Joint Ill:* Hot, swollen, painful joints Infected navel, leaky navel Lameness, unthrifty Temperature elevation
Escherichia coli	*Loss of equilibrium* Neck periodically drawn to the side Temperature elevation Depression
Actinobacillus equuli (Shigella equuli)	*Dummy, Sleeper, Wanderer Foals:* Disorientation Poor nurser Abnormal temperature Scours/diarrhea/leaky navel Depression
Corynebacterium equi	Temperature elevation Constipation Pneumonia Good nurser Fat condition

Known Offenders:
  Pseudomonas aeruginosa
  Salmonella typhimurium
  Salmonella abortus equi

Thanks to modern antibiotics, conscientious supportive measures, and the attentions of alert veterinarians, many septicemic newborns are surviving today that would have succumbed but a few years ago.

shaker foal syndrome   A group of symptoms, not as yet an identifiable disease; seen in foals one to six months of age. Most affected foals exhibit a sudden onset of weariness and inability to nurse, as all muscles of the body and limbs tremble uncontrollably. Trembling progressively worsens into total body shaking and the foal soon becomes recumbent despite even heroic supportive measures. No specific treatment is administered, as the etiologic agent has not yet been identified.

One foal can be striken among many in a barn, thus the cause is believed to be infectious and not contagious.

This foal syndrome has been highly fatal.

There is hope on the horizon, however. Researchers have released data indicating that *Clostridium botulinum,* the causative micro-organism of the dreaded disease botulism, has been associated with the shaker foal syndrome.

Thus, a new treatment has evolved: Magnesium sulfate (Epsom salts) as a laxative is indicated to clear the bowels of ingested toxic material. Oxygen therapy or source is essential since death occurs by respiratory paralysis.

Potassium penicillin is the only safe antibiotic to use. Avoid oxytetracycline and amino glycosides. *C. botulinum* antitoxin is ideal and sought after as a possible miracle cure if available—the cost is almost prohibitive. *See:* BOTULISM.

tympany of the guttural pouches   *See:* GUTTURAL POUCHES.

Tyzzer's disease   An acute and highly fatal liver disease of young foals, usually observed during the first month of life. Caused by *Bacillus piliformis,* it is thought to be spread by ingestion and perhaps carried by rodents who also may serve as a reservoir for the infection.

There are at present no known control measures and no treatment available since the course of the disease is so rapid and so lethal; the disease is actually diagnosed at autopsy.

SURGERY

arthroscopic surgery   A method of joint surgery in which an arthroscope, a fiberoptic viewing device, usually 4 millimeters in width, is introduced into the joint space for surgery diagnostic purposes. If indicated, surgical instruments can be slipped through another tiny incision a short space away under the continual guidance of the arthroscope. The surgeon, viewing the inner surface through the scope, is able to remove small fracture fragments, trim and shave areas of pathology, and centrally flush and clean the joint.

There are many advantages to this method over the former open-joint approach—the two small puncture incisions, the atraumatic nature of the surgery, the reduced chance of infection, and the short recovery period, to name a few.

The greatest advantage, from a trainer's standpoint, is that the average case can resume training in about one month, as opposed to the ten-month compulsory postoperative rest period with conventional joint surgery.

Great skill and experience with the use of the arthroscope has a direct bearing on the success rate of arthroscopic surgery.

cesarean section   The surgical extraction of the fetus by way of an incision, made successively through the abdominal wall, the uterine wall, and the placental layers enveloping the term fetus. This surgery is performed in lieu of a natural delivery when the safety of the mother and child is in question. (The name of the method derives from Julius Caesar, who is said to have been delivered by "C section.")

Until a few years ago, a cesarean section was rarely attempted in equine surgery, largely because the prognosis was uncertain, and because the people concerned, being unsure, waited until it was too late before they elected a surgical delivery.

When a natural delivery is precluded for any of various reasons and surgery is decided upon, time is of paramount importance. Quite dissimilar to the prognosis for human and other species, the success or failure of all deliveries in the mare, whether normal or by other means, depends totally upon *prompt* recognition, diagnosis, and action. This responsibility rests heavily and squarely on the shoulders of the attending veterinarians. The reason for the urgency has to do with the peculiar and unique placental arrangement in the mare. The placenta's attachment to the inner lining of the uterus is unstable and easily vulnerable. When it is affected, the vigor, oxygen, and nutrients available to the fetus are diminished. Not a minute can be wasted in making decisions and initiating action.

157

cesarean section continued

To clarify my point: If I receive two simultaneous urgent calls, one for a mare ready to deliver and the other about a cow approaching parturition, I answer the horse call as fast as my car will travel. I then return home, have a snack, put on warm dry socks, and go out again to answer the cow call. The fundamental difference here is in the type and innate efficiency of the cow's placenta, which secures and protects the fetus not only through gestation, but also during the period of labor.

The need for "C" sections occurs most often in maiden mares or very old mares. In all age groups, the major cause of cesarean surgeries is contraction of the equine fetus *in utero*. Dystocia, a difficult or impossible delivery, is inevitable, with the degree of difficulty depending upon the severity of contraction and the size of the affected fetus. When you are fortunate enough to witness the delivery of a normal healthy foal through a normal mare's bony pelvis and reproductive tract, look closely and observe that there is little or no room for error. Everything just fits!

Contraction is just what the word describes. In contrast to the freely movable and adjustable limbs of the normal fetus, handy for delivery purposes, a contracted foal's flexor muscles pull the limbs and body into a distorted position and lock the entire body into a rigid, fixed position, presenting a solid mass. The veterinary obstetrician is unable to manually straighten the limbs, neck, or body for passage through the mare's narrow pelvic canal to the outside world.

There are degrees of contraction. Some foals come into the world appearing almost normal with a slightly perceptible tendon and muscle overpull; some have a single contracted limb, while others suffer the ultimate degree of contraction and are dead in the uterus before labor begins in the mare. These most severely affected fetuses resemble a twisted solid mass of bony tissue, and almost certainly require manual sectioning (embryotomy or fetotomy) for removal in pieces. This can be performed in the barn, not requiring the surgical environment of a hospital. In this instance, loss of the foal is absolute as it is sectioned for careful, gentle removal from the mare. The mare's life is saved, although at a risk to her reproductive canal. I should also add that this procedure demands herculean effort and presents a hazard to all attending personnel, especially if the mare is a well-bred, high-spirited animal.

It is possible for a skilled practitioner to diagnose rectally a contracted foal prior to the onset of labor symptoms, if afforded the opportunity.

The cause of contraction is unknown. Several researchers have established a correlation between the coexistence of scoliosis of the spinal cord of the foal and limb contraction. Others suggest that "supernutrition," the overfeeding of protein and vitamin supplements during gestation, has been associated with a large number of contracted foals. In one season I personally experienced seven contracted foals in a group of forty mares. When all fancy additive feeds were deleted and replaced by a good old-fashioned nutritious diet, all foals the next year were quite normal. My rule is that I have never seen a contracted fetus or foal in a poor man's barn!

Other causes of dystocia are worn-out uterine tone, hormonal imbalances, a ruptured uterus, malformed fetus, and (rarely) an abnormal bony pelvis due to old fractures.

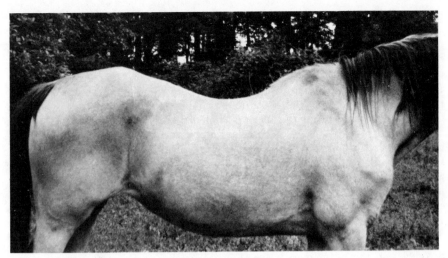

Lordosis (Swayback)

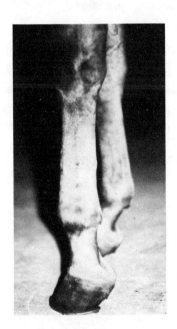

Nutritional Contraction, 18 months

Encouraged by the increasing number of horse hospitals, better methods of transportation, and greater knowledge among horse people, cesarean surgery has become an integral part of veterinary medicine today. Much credit for success must be given to the safer and smoother general anesthetics that have been developed, which allow for precious operating time and proper positioning

cesarean section continued

of the patient. A C-section, in my opinion, is the superior approach for all involved—the fetus, the mare, the surgeon, and all loyal helpers. This method offers both mother and offspring a chance to live. *See:* DYSTOCIA.

Caslick's operation A surgical procedure performed on mares to prevent pneumovagina ("windsucking" air into the vagina). Named after its developer, a Caslick consists of suturing the upper portion of the vulvar lips into apposition. In a few weeks the vulvar edges become sealed by skin growth and the sutures can be removed. Although not mandatory, removal of sutures can preclude irritation from accumulated fecal material and serve as a courtesy to the mare. The effect of a Caslick is to prevent inspiration of contaminated air and fecal material, thereby inhibiting irritation and the secondary inflammations that are usually followed by infection. The operation thereby enhances and preserves fertility.

Clues indicating the need for perineal suturing:

1. Reduced vulvar tissue tone due either to nutritional causes or to multiple deliveries in the older mare

2. Anatomical shape of perineal region (dock, tail, and anus) that predisposes to pneumovagina, found even in some maiden mares

The ideal time for a Caslick is:

1. After an infected mare has been properly treated and is starting a period of rest

2. Immediately after a well-timed cover and ovulation

3. At the time of pregnancy determination

Record on the upcoming spring schedule a date for opening the expecting matron roughly one week in anticipation of foaling. Open a mare a few days prior to cover by a stallion. This time period allows the initial skin-edge soreness to subside and can prevent unnecessary discomfort for the mare—perhaps even avert a breeding shed accident.

To open a mare for any reason:

1. Apply a tail bandage

2. Scrub perineal area and dry well

3. Instill a local anesthetic

4. Open with sterile scissors

5. Apply antiseptic powder to raw vulvar edges.

I recommend Caslick surgery as a prudent and sound practice in broodmare care. By some trick of evolution, the design of those structures that are so important for reproduction—the mare's tailbone, dock, anus, and vulvar angle—is not very efficient. Many older broodmares, and even some maidens, benefit from a Caslick.

castration The surgical removal of the testicles in a colt or the ovaries in a mare (*see:* OVARIECTOMY). Castration is carried out for various reasons and is unquestionably the most common surgical procedure performed on horses.

Intractability, aggressiveness, and unpredictability are a few good reasons to consider castration in the normal healthy stallion. Other reasons have to do with the animal's genetic potential. Individuals with poor conformation, medical conditions (testicular malfunction, inguinal and scrotal hernias, tendon contraction, clubfoot, etc.), or lack of talent and willingness to achieve should not be left entire to perpetuate themselves.

Basic rules for castration procedure:

1. Avoid dirty and dusty areas
2. Avoid poor ventilation
3. Avoid high temperatures and humidity
4. Control insects (flies)
5. Reduce grain intake by 50 percent for three days postoperative and incorporate a bran mash
6. Provide adequate exercise under restraint

It is especially important to have the patient's abode prepared in advance of castration and free from all dust, dirt, and debris.

Surgery can be carried out while the horse is either standing, cast on its side, or cast up on its back. The veterinary surgeon will make the judgment, taking into account the horse's size, age, disposition, and general normalcy of the reproductive tract (not necessarily in that order of importance).

The drugs used for sedation and for anesthetic purposes will vary with the method of castration employed and with the number of assistants and their experience and capability.

In some breeds of horses standing castration can be routine, with the assistance of experienced personnel. In contrast, small ponies, donkeys, and green or unbroken horses should always be cast in recumbency and secured to protect the safety of all.

Follow the advice of your veterinarian by all means and ask questions if in doubt as to postoperative care and attention. Your veterinarian will administer antibiotics, a tetanus booster, and probably some additional sedation to quiet and maintain the patient's comfort for the first few hours postsurgery. Now is the time to keep a vigilance for postcastration hemorrhaging. An occasional drip of blood from the incision area is acceptable for the first few hours, but if at any time the drip increases in frequency or if the drip rate forms a stream, then an emergency exists! The blood must be stopped before a large volume of blood is lost, or the animal can become dangerously ill or perhaps die.

Good nursing care greatly enhances the recovery time by minimizing any and all "postcastration blues."

First of all, do not touch or allow anyone to touch the operative site with *anything*. It is my contention that the majority of postcastration complications are people-related. Well-meaning people insist upon cleansing the area and actually introduce contamination, whereupon infection develops. Do not permit hands—no matter how clean—cotton, or any other object to contact the areas after surgery. This form of treatment is outmoded and unnecessary. In fact, it can be harmful!

Quietly hand walk the new gelding for 15 minutes daily for the first three days following surgery.

On the fourth postoperative day, begin twice daily to hose the area with water, preferably before and after the scheduled daily hand walking. Quietly *castration continued*

walk your horse to the water faucet and patiently ease a gentle stream of tepid water up under his inguinal area. Most horses will readily accept this, so continue for about 15 minutes to hose the entire region thoroughly, including the two surgical incisions hidden within the scrotal tissue. Repeat the hosing after exercise. Continue this regime for about one week. By using the water treatment you avoid direct manual contact and the transfer of contaminants. Healing can progress uninterrupted.

Since I adopted this method, my cases of inguinal, prepuce, and sheath swelling, as well as other minor complications have practically ceased to exist! No swelling, no soreness, and *no infection!*

The question of when to reinstitute serious exercise is crucial. It varies somewhat with the individual horse. Judgment is required, so don't hesitate to ask your veterinarian for advice.

Before leaving this subject, I want to emphasize my point by recalling the following incident:

One night about 11:30 P.M., early in my practice, I received an emergency call from the owners of the adjacent horse farm. They were hysterical about a recently gelded young horse that was hemorrhaging. I rushed over to their farm and found both major testicular arteries streaming blood. The stall and the horse were red with it. After injecting a sedative and quietly applying a twitch to his lip, I managed to clear away some blood with cotton and antiseptic water, finally isolating the exposed arteries. I placed sterile surgical hemostats strategically on each bleeder and the escaping blood ceased and all was quiet! Everyone in the barn sighed with relief. The horse would live!

I learned a special lesson that night which I have never forgotten these many years, and which I always try to communicate to others. Six colts had been operated on the previous Sunday morning by a very competent, experienced veterinary surgeon; 36 hours later, one gelding was hemorrhaging! Vigilance in postoperative care is an essential element in any surgery!

If the groom had decided to retire at eleven as usual without a late-evening check, this young horse would have bled to death before dawn.

cryogenics   A branch of science that deals with the phenomenon of extreme cold, especially its therapeutic applications.

Extreme cold was used in the treatment of cancer as early as 1845 and although reports of successful cures or remissions were scanty, they were encouraging. It was not until the 1970s that cryosurgery gained a respectable place in the fields of both the human and veterinary medicine. A new technique applied to an old method has opened a horizon of new and exciting applications.

The *double-freeze method* of killing cells has proved amazingly beneficial in the treatment of nonhealing skin wounds and tumors. In this procedure of killing cells, liquid nitrogen, in either spray or probe form, is applied to a growth and rapidly frozen to $-25°$ Celsius, then the frozen tissue is allowed to thaw slowly. The lesion then is promptly refrozen to $-25°$ Celsius for the second time, then thawed again. The objectionable odor created by the dead tissue after freezing is the only disadvantage I have noticed in treating large skin masses. After a week or ten days, as skin sloughs off, a pink area begins to appear underneath the dead tissue. The worst is now over, healing is in evidence!

With the development of accurate methods of monitoring the temperature of the skin surrounding the lesion, the success rate of cryogenics in both human and veterinary medicine has been greatly enhanced. Some authorities believe that cryogenics will, in the near future, become the treatment of choice for all equine skin growths, in preference to other techniques such as surgical excision, radiotherapy, electrosurgery, chemotherapy, or autogenous vaccines.

Four prime examples in horses where cryogenic surgery has been tried successfully are: squamous cell carcinoma, equine sarcoid, equine habronema, and excessive granuloma formation.

cunean tenotomy A surgical procedure for the relief of early bony spavin formation. Cunean tenectomy, also called Peters spavin operation, is the transection of the tendon of the tibialis anterior muscle as it obliquely crosses the front and inside of the hock.

The transection removes the ever-constant irritating movement of the overlying tendon when there are periosteal and osteoarthritic changes in the tarsal bones. Besides bringing relief from pain, the procedure increases the freedom of the hock during flight of stride.

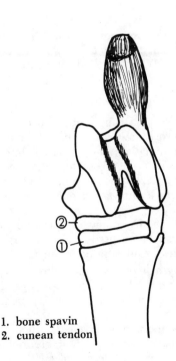

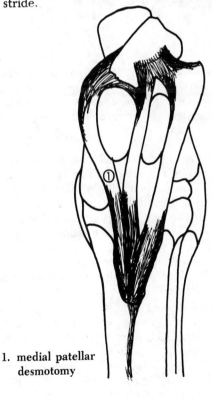

1. bone spavin
2. cunean tendon

1. medial patellar
   desmotomy

Left Hock

Left Stifle

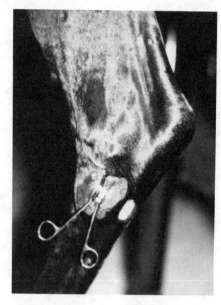

Cunean Tenotomy, right hock inside surface

electrocautery A technique to cauterize bleeding tissue or to reduce beds of excessive granulation tissue by local application of a specifically designed instrument heated to a red-hot temperature. When applied, it destroys, coagulates, and reduces unwanted tissues.

CAUTION: This instrument is safe only in a veterinarian's hands.

Lacking a veterinarian and an electrified cautery instrument, the procedure can be performed by a skilled farrier using an iron of his own fashioning. It should have a small, spoon-like point to fit the area of granulation. The farrier will bury the tip in the red-hot coals and when it is cherry red he will press it for four or five seconds against the granulating tissue, causing a sizzling sound and a burning smell. This should leave a flat area, usually with no unwanted bubbly proud flesh.

Either method is acceptable, although it seems somewhat barbaric to perform or watch unless you are aware that granulation tissue lacks all nerve function and that the entire operation is painless. Only the odor remains!

electrosurgery The use of energy created by a high-frequency alternating current to make incisions in tissue. Used for removal of tumors, warts, and pimples. Electrosurgery is excellent for making the initial skin incision. It is neat and virtually bloodless.

Other advantages are: precise control of the incision; no tissue destruction or sloughing; little scar tissue; no bone damage; usually heals with first intention.

Although I use electrosurgery frequently in my practice (e.g., coagulation of blood vessels, hemostasis, and puncturing to create scar tissue for contraction purposes), I for one do not expect it will replace the scalpel in surgery.

herniorrhaphy   Term used for surgical correction of hernias. Hernias are classified by anatomical location—umbilical, inguinal, scrotal, and abdominal.

There are two standard methods for repairing hernias: the *closed* and *open* methods.

Closed hernia repair employs external aids—clamps, plugs, tapes, etc.—and relies upon tissue reaction for healing, with the excess tissue sloughing away.

Open hernia repair involves surgical reduction of the sac contents and closure of the opposed tissues with appropriate and precise sutures.

I consider the various contraptions used in closed repair to be hazardous, archaic, and primarily life-threatening for the animal. If the primitive device fails to remain securely in place until adequate healing occurs, a circulatory compromise or infection can develop with possible escape of abdominal contents. This is lethal.

Proper surgical correction is the only sound and safe way to perform herniorrhaphy. *See:* HERNIA.

inferior check ligament desmotomy   A surgical procedure performed to relieve contraction of the deep digital flexor tendon and prevent the malformation of foot growth and shape known as "clubfoot."

Some foals arrive in the world with contraction and are unable to walk as a result of the intense pull exerted by the deep digital flexor tendon. The feet of these foals appear perfectly normal, while the legs are pulled into a flexed attitude. If there is immediate surgical correction, the animal can live a normal life with no residual evidence. This is the ideal age for correction.

Clubfeet also can develop at a later age from a lesser degree of tendon pull and secondary abnormal foot growth.

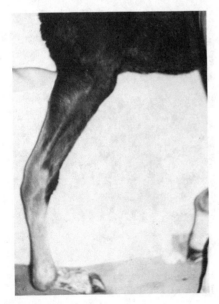

Contraction in Newborn Club Foot, caused by deep digital flexor tendon contraction (3–5 months)

inferior check ligament desmotomy continued

A desomotomy (transection of a ligament) in effect lengthens the tendon without interfering with the tendon tissue. The inferior check ligament, just below the knee, encompasses and lightly supports the deep digital tendon. By transecting the ligament, the tendon is released and lengthened by several centimeters. The added length allows the os pedis inside the foot to rest flat on the inside on the sole where it belongs, and the heel of the foot to rest comfortably on the ground.

This is a very successful surgery offering a total cure for clubfooted individuals and also those with various degrees of contraction and associated lameness. Prognosis is fair to splendid, and postoperative care is minimal.

Immediately postoperative, the foot should receive proper balancing and lowering of the heel. This is essential during the first six weeks after surgery.

Normal exercise can begin one month after surgery. *See:* CLUBFOOT.

lateral digital extensor tenotomy A surgery to relieve the symptoms of "stringhalt" affecting the hind leg. The procedure consists of removing a portion of the lateral digital extensor tendon as it crosses over the outside surface of the hock joint.

Two half-inch incisions are made through the skin, one above and one below the hock. The tendon, located directly underneath the incisions, is then freed by blunt dissection and transected. Usually, a 7-inch length of tendon tissue is removed. Each incision is closed with two sutures and healing is swift and efficient.

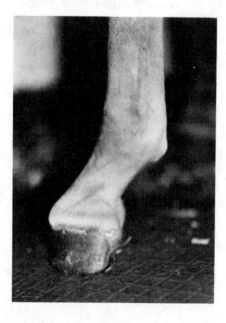

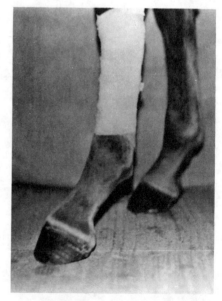

Club Foot, pre-op

Club Foot, 5 days post-op, inferior check ligament desmotomy

Prognosis is good for a functional recovery.

Postoperative, the gait is improved and closely resembles a normal stride. The patient is more comfortable, too. *See:* STRINGHALT.

medial patellar desmotomy This is a surgical procedure designed to relieve undue restriction and locking caused by the medial patellar ligament in an obtuse-angled stifle joint.

It is a simple surgical operation that can be performed on a standing horse which is under adequate local anesthetic. Ample skill is necessary to deftly locate, isolate, and then precisely transect the wide medial patellar ligament. Then, one small mattress suture is required to close the small incision, centrally located over the stifle area. No incisional scar is detectable.

If the original diagnosis is correct, the prognosis is good to excellent!

neurectomy (nerving) Excision of a nerve segment. My concept of neurectomy, as applied to veterinary medicine, is the transection of a nerve fiber to reduce sensitivity distal to the operative site. The primary purpose of this surgery is to relieve pain.

Many abuses of this procedure have occurred, motivated by the desire to win purses or prizes, with no consideration given to the welfare of the horse. For this reason, the terms *neurectomy* and *nerving* have earned a shady reputation over the years, and in some cases even today, the label is justified.

All neurectomies are performed for one purpose, to relieve pain. The location of the incision on the horse's leg decides the prudence or imprudence of the operation. Any neurectomy, partial or complete, performed above the ankle level is considered by conscionable horse people to be nothing short of criminal. There are some exceptions—although few—to this cardinal rule: broodmares, stallions, pet horses that are never ridden or driven, and retirees are candidates when relief of pain is the sole desired end, and supervision of the area is carried out on a daily basis.

What happens to the area deprived of innervation?

With reduced sensation to a tissue area, the integrity of cells and vessels depreciates, and although the functions remain, they are less efficient than in normal tissue. The numbed area is vulnerable, by virtue of inhibited sensitivity, to undetected skin breaks and punctures. It is also susceptible to the threat of an insidious developing infection.

Selected cases can benefit from this operation. In competent hands, a carefully considered neurectomy (usually a posterior digital neurectomy, heels only) can be performed with impunity. For success, however, we must have a consenting and informed owner, one who will maintain vigilance over the condition of the horse's feet and soles (no thrush, no infections, and no foreign bodies), and especially watch for "close nails" and other careless shoeing incidences. For total understanding, an owner must be apprised of the potential for neuroma formation and its relatively easy removal.

When an animal loses its ability to perform or carry out the task for which it was purchased, in most cases, it becomes a burden for the owner to support; the horse's future automatically dims and becomes uncertain. At this time the horse needs a champion, an advocate, someone who will help it stay healthy, serviceably sound, and usable. This is how I see my job as an equine practitioner. I have performed hundreds of neurectomies and credit the procedure with

neurectomy continued

restoring the animals to a useful, comfortable existence in the majority of cases. Especially in cases of the common arthritic ailment of navicular disease, the heel neurectomy has given many older horses additional years of pain-free life. *See:* NEUROMA.

neuroma A bulb-like swelling that forms on the end of a nerve branch after a neurectomy. A neuroma can vary in growth rate and size from minute to that of a small lima bean. The degree of tenderness can range from insensitive to extremely distressing. Most neuromas are painful, especially when touched or palpated, and their development under the skin is associated with the return of lameness. Some horses with prior neurectomies become hypersensitive and quite lame when the neuroma begins to grow.

In routine neurectomies (there are about ten different techniques at present), an owner can expect neuroma formation from as early as three months postoperative to as long as three years, depending upon the horse's innate ability to regenerate tissue. Certain breeds of horses are notorious neuroma formers.

Your veterinarian can best diagnose and determine whether the neuroma is in fact the cause of lameness and arrange for surgical removal if necessary.

After the first neuroma removal, it has been my experience that the future rate of formation is greatly slowed in all breeds and individuals, and even slower the second time around.

Prevention of neuromas has plagued the surgeon, both human and veterinary, for centuries. A satisfactory answer has not come, in spite of the innumerable methods employed to inhibit the open nerve fiber from reacting to transection.

The chance of neuromal formation should always be a consideration in deciding whether or not to perform a neurectomy. Factors to be weighed carefully by your veterinarian include the advantages of desensitization versus the disadvantages of potential neuroma regeneration.

physeal stapling An orthopedic procedure applied to crooked-legged foals, especially those with knocked knees. Under general anesthesia, stainless steel vitallium staples are surgically implanted and strategically placed over the epiphysal line of the knee to provide stabilization of the area. These staples remain in the leg for several weeks until leg growth and straightness of limb indicate the time for removal. Confirmed by radiographs, the staple-removal time is critical since the bone has a tendency to overcompensate and even go in the opposite direction if removal is delayed for any reason.

This corrective procedure has been very satisfactory in preventing a self-perpetuating limb deformity in young foals. Although 85 percent of knock-kneed foals correct themselves with nutrition, exercise, and growth, there are the other 15 percent that require stapling to prevent crippling or possible epiphyseal fractures.

roarer *See:* LARYNGEAL HEMIPLEGIA.

stringhalt *See:* LATERAL DIGITAL EXTENSOR TENOTOMY.

tarsorrhaphy The surgical repair of torn or lacerated eyelids. There seems to be a higher incidence of this type of injury in valuable animals or in those animals confined for the purpose of fattening and conditioning for exhibition or sale. The majority are sensitive, inquisitive animals who, given the opportunity, quickly find any exposed nail, sharp board, or broken wire on the stall surface or fence line. Concerted efforts should be made to examine thoroughly all confines and restricting structures and to remove sharp and protruding objects, preferably *before* turning horses into the area. Even then, a daily inspection is wise and prudent.

I have surgically reconstructed innumerable eyelids, ears, noses, and mouths during my many years of practice and cannot help but wonder why a horse is so vulnerable. It is not that these horses were retardees, nor were they on some kind of a self-destructive binge!

I believe the reason for these injuries lies with the horse's vision. The horse has a sophisticated and efficient farsighted mechanism, but its nearsighted mechanism is less than proficient. It cannot focus on objects near the head and particularly near the nose. On behalf of the horse, let me suggest that this fact may account for the host of injuries sustained at close range. I rest my case!

When presented an eyelid laceration in my clinic, I am always relieved when I can locate the upper eyelid *in toto*, no matter how badly mutilated the tissue. The border holding the eyelashes, the mucoepithelial line, is irreplaceable and carries a great bearing on the outcome of a surgical eyelid repair. This layer with its eyelashes superbly protects the eye, and the cornea specifically, from irritation, dust, debris, and drying. When the mucoepithelial border is destroyed or lost in an accident, the area can be reconstructed through plastic surgery but never fully restored to normal functioning.

I have witnessed unfortunate individuals who must live with eyelid defects. Wind, dust, and debris are constants in the average horse's environment. With loss of eyelid protection there is increased irritation of tender ocular tissue, and excessive compensatory tearing. Although not life-threatening to the horse, it is a very uncomfortable condition and certainly reflects upon those responsible! Let no eye or eyelid injury go neglected. It is well worth any added time or effort on the veterinary surgeon's part to attempt a full restoration of any eyelid laceration.

trephining The removal of a small disc of bone usually from an area over a sinus cavity in the face of a horse. The instrument used, called a trephine, is a cylindrical saw with a centrally located point and a T-shaped handle for manual control. Trephining is carried out under sedation and with a local anesthetic for opening and entering the air sinus cavity. This relatively simple procedure is used either for exploratory and diagnostic purposes or for treatment by flushing and cleansing the infected area. It is recommended for two conditions: in cases of sinusitis when conservative antibiotic therapy has failed, and in cases where a large molar must be extracted.

When a diseased upper tooth must be extracted, the method of repulsion through the sinus cavity above the tooth is the recommended and preferred approach as opposed to extraction. Trephinization through the sinus cavity permits access to the tooth roots below and secondarily allows drainage from the root of the tooth and from the adjacent sinus. Sinusitis and diseased teeth are commonly found in combination, and are seldom seen separately.

tumors *See:* CRYOGENICS, ELECTROSURGERY.

Viborg's triangle A triangular space located in the horse's jowl area, a well-known designated site for surgical intervention into the guttural pouch. When guttural pouches become infected and extended, quite often surgical drainage and flushing is the only alternative treatment.

The sides of Viborg's triangle are formed by the huge jugular vein above, the external maxillary vein below, and the arch of the mandible (lower jaw) in the front.

The parotid salivary gland is found directly under the skin in the center of the triangle, and equine surgeons must skillfully by-pass this vital gland to enter the distended guttural pouch.

Viborg's triangle also serves as a surgical site to relieve guttural pouches of trapped air. Foals occasionally are affected. *See:* GUTTURAL POUCHES.

Viborg's Triangle,
surgical approach
to the guttural pouch

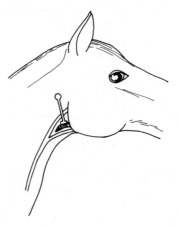

triangle boundaries: above, jugular vein; below, external maxillary vein; front, arch of
the mandible

PARASITES

anthelmintic A vermifuge or worm medicine powerful enough to destroy intestinal parasites. *See:* WORMING.

bots The larvae of the bot fly *Gastrophilus* that attach themselves to the gastric linings of the stomach. They remain in the stomach until maturity and then pass on through the intestinal tract into the manure pile where they complete their life cycle by developing into flies.

The bot fly emerges in late summer and attaches or glues its eggs to the horse's chin and leg hairs. After bot eggs gain entrance to the horse's mouth, they are swallowed and subsequently set up housekeeping for the winter months in the animal's stomach.

Horses hosting bot larvae in their stomachs show no external indication and are not necessarily unthrifty, but they are always subject to gastrointestinal upsets with sudden bouts of colic.

There is an infallible diagnostic clue to bot infestation: When you notice your horse take a few quick swallows of grain and then suddenly evidence gastrointestinal pain, drop down into the bedding with "crampy" symptoms, only to rise again quickly, apparently pain-free, and finish off its meal uneventfully, you have just witnessed a textbook case of bot infestation, with an apparent gastric rebellion. Not all horses with bots necessarily manifest this behavior, but when in evidence, it is diagnostic.

Tubing with a boticide (preferably Parvex Plus® [Upjohn]) should be done only *after* a truly killing frost. There is no point in worming to remove bot larvae if the bot fly is still buzzing around busily depositing fresh eggs.

The fertile eggs are very tenacious and require removal by manual methods: a razor, flame, or commercial comb designed for this specific purpose. Every egg that you remove and burn saves the host animal from this parasite's ravages.

Consult your veterinarian who will treat your horse with the boticide of choice. I would then dare to say that you will not see a repeat of the behavior just described.

Preventive measures:

1. Control the bot fly by breaking its life cycle. This requires: (a) tube worming to remove bot larvae from the stomach, and (b) manually removing all visible bot eggs deposited on the horse's hair.

2. Institute community co-operation by all owners of horses and farms.

Community co-operation can measurably reduce the bot fly population by control practices. Singular action prevents nothing, but a combined and concerted effort can conceivably eradicate bot infestation in a community. *See:* PARASITES (CHART, PAGE 172–173).

PARASITES (INTERNAL)
(ENDO PARASITES)

Common Name	Scientific Name	Worm Medicines	Brand Name
Bots	Gastrophilus intestinalis (common bot) G. haemorrhoidales (nose or red-tailed bot) G. nasalis (throat or chin bot)	carbon disulfide dichlorvos trichlorfon Parvex Plus	same Equigard Dyrex same
Roundworms	Ascaridis Parascaris equorum	piperazine salts pyrantel pamoate mebendazole Ripercol	same Strongid-T Telmin
Bloodworms	Large Strongyles Strongylus vulgaris (red worm) S. edentatus S. equinus Small Strongyles Strongyloides Poteriostomum Cylicobrachytus Craterostomum Oesophagodontus Cyathostomum Triodontophorus	mebendazole pyrantel pamoate cambendazole phenothiazine thiabendazole piperazine fenbendazole oxibendazole oxfendazole febantel	Telmin Strongid-T Camvet same Equizole same Panacur Anthelcide-EQ Benzelmin Rintal
Intestinal threadworm	Strongyloides westeri	Same as above	

PARASITES (INTERNAL)
(ENDO PARASITES)

Common Name	Scientific Name	Worm Medicines	Brand Name
Stomach worms	Habronema muscae H. majus Drashia megastoma	Same as above	
Minute stomach worm	Trichostrongylus axei	Same as above	
Pinworms	Oxyuris equi	Same as above	
Minute pinworms	Probstmayria vivipara	Same as above	
Tapeworms	Anaplocephala perfoliata A. magna	On recommendation of your veterinarian	
Lungworms	Dictyocaulus arnfeldi	levamisole phosphate (Levasole)	
Eye worm Liver fluke Hydatid tapeworm	Thelazia lacrimalis Fasciola hepatica Echinococcus	Veterinary consultation	

cerebrospinal nematodosis A rare nervous disorder of horses caused by parasitic larvae that invade the spinal cord creating varying degrees of inco-ordination. This entity simulates the classical symptoms of equine ataxia, or wobbles.

Endoparasites complete their reproductive cycle by migrating via the bloodstream throughout the body from their primary site, the gastrointestinal tract. Cerebrospinal nematodosis results when a bloodworm larva strays from the normal course of migration and enters the delicate spinal cord tissue, where its physical presence interferes with the transmission of nerve impulses. With the death of the worm, tissue damage is increased, adding to the severity of the neurologic symptoms.

Whatever the cause—congenital wobbles or an errant worm—the effect on the horse is devastating. Euthanasia is indicated for humane reasons. *See:* WOBBLES.

fleas Not commonly found on the horse, although they do lay eggs in cracks and crevices in the horse's environment. Conceivably they could infest a dirty stall and create havoc.

flies Although called "the housefly," *Musca domestica* often causes problems around the stable because it breeds in manure piles. Fly control could be better handled if everyone who kept horses would place a cover on the manure pile to help break the reproductive cycle of the fly.

The common housefly is a nonbiter, but it succeeds in spreading contamination mechanically; more importantly, it carries an intestinal parasite that does great damage to the horse when the fly is swallowed by the horse. *See:* HABRONEMIASIS.

Flies that are known to annoy horses include: housefly *(Musca domestica),* stablefly *(Stomoxys calcitrans),* horsefly *(Tabanus),* deerfly *(Chrysops),* greenhead fly *(Chloratabanus),* screw worm *(Callitroga hominivorax),* and blowflies *(Calliphora). See:* FLYING INSECTS (CHART, PAGE 175).

fungicides Agents that kill fungi. Examples of topical fungicides are: benzoic acid, cupric sulfate, diluted acetic acid, iodine (Weladol, Betadine), naphthaline, nitrofurazone, Nystatin, quaternary ammonium compounds, salicylic acid, and selenium sulfide.

Orally administered fungicides include: amphotericin, Nystatin, and griseofulvin (Fulvicin).

fungus infections Occur in two forms, external and internal. External infections appear on the skin and hair and usually respond to fungicidal agents. Ringworm, girth itch, and dermatomycosis are synonyms for the general *Microsporum* and *Trichophyton*. Well-known for causing external infections, both genera present a persistent skin problem in young horses, especially at race tracks. Ringworm is highly infectious and easily transmitted from horse to horse via tack, sponges, and grooming tools. The skin lesions commonly appear during the introductory phase of the horse's training schedule, and the resulting dermatitis with itchy sore skin areas has been known to interfere with training.

Treatment consists of early recognition with prompt application of fungicides and reduced physical exertion for a period adequate to the degree of infection. Isolate all equipment used on the affected horse and scrub well.

FLYING INSECTS

Common Name	Scientific Name	Clear Bite or Bloodsucking	Reproduction	Threat
Housefly	*Musca domestica*	Annoyance	Manure	Carrier of habronema (parasite)
Stablefly	*Stomoxys calcitrans*	Bloodsucking	Manure and urine-soaked bedding	Spreads anthrax, EIA, surra, tularemia
Horsefly	*Tabanus*	Bloodsucking	Lays eggs on bushes near water	Spreads anthrax, EIA, surra, tularemia
Deerfly	*Chrysops*	Bloodsucking	Marshy areas	Spreads anthrax, EIA, surra, tularemia
Greenhead fly	*Chloratabanus*	Bloodsucking	Near water	Spreads anthrax, EIA, surra, tularemia
Face fly	*Musca autumnalis*	Eats excretions around eyes and face	Lays eggs near manure	Traumatic accidents
Buffalo fly or Horn fly	*Haematobia exigua*	Biting	Lays eggs near water	Noted disease carrier
Black fly	*Simulium*	Bloodsucking, raises a wheal from toxin	Lays eggs near water	Noted disease carrier
Sand fly	*Simulium*	Biting, feeds on flesh	Lays eggs in marshy areas	Traumatic accidents
Mosquitoes	*Culex, Culiseta*	Biting, feeds on flesh	Lays eggs in marshy areas	Noted carriers of viral diseases
Screwworm flies	*Callitroga hominivorax*	Feed on flesh	Near Mexico; release of sterile males has virtually eradicated	Reportable disease
Blowflies	Calliphora	Feed on necrotic tissue	Near Mexico; release of sterile males has virtually eradicated	Reportable disease

fungus infections continued

Ringworm is also transmitted to people, causing similar skin lesions, so all who handle such horses must be careful to wash well and clean under the fingernails.

It is believed that horses thus affected develop a degree of immunity to this notorious fungus and seem to escape future bouts of mycotic skin diseases.

There is no vaccine available to prevent ringworm and its ravages. About 99 percent of race and show horses in the U.S. earn their own protective antibodies by suffering varying degrees of skin disease.

Unlike external fungal infections, which can be observed and treated, internal systemic fungal infections pose a solemn threat to the health of our future livestock. Aspergillosis is a prime example of an internal mycotic infection that easily establishes itself in the respiratory tract, is quite resistant to treatment, and can readily cause pneumonia. This fungal infection is a major concern to medical researchers and practitioners alike, who undoubtedly will not rest until an effective drug or vaccine is developed. *See:* ASPERGILLOSIS, FUNGUS INFECTIONS (CHART, PAGE 176).

FUNGUS INFECTIONS
MYCOTIC

Dermatomycosis (Skin Lesions)	Systemic Mycosis (Internal Lesions)
Commonly called Ringworm	Actinomycosis
Microsporum canis	*Actinomyces bovis*
M. gypseum	Aspergillosis
Trichophyton mentagraphytes	*Aspergillos nidulans*
T. equinum	*A. fumigatus*
	A. flavus
	Blastomycosis
	Blastomyces dermatities
	Coccidiomycosis
	Coccidioides immitis
	Cryptococcosis
	Cryptococcus neoformans
	Histoplasmosis
	Histoplasma capsulatum
	H. farciminosum
	Mycetoma
	Monosporium apiospermum
	Brachycladium speciferum
	Helminthosporium
	Phycomycosis
	Hyphomyces detruens
	Entomophthora coronata
	Rhinosporidiosis
	Rhinosporidium seeberi
	Sporotrichosis
	Sporotrichium scheneckii

habronemiasis (cutaneous habronemiasis)   A nonhealing "summer sore" on the horse, usually found during the warm and humid housefly and stablefly season.

Habronema muscae, Habronema majus, and *Draschia megastoma* are all internal parasites, normally found in the horse's stomach. Habronema is a roundworm that lives in the stomach and gains entrance via the housefly (*Musca domestica*). Although originally thought of as an internal parasite, habronema represents a great nuisance since it not only infests external "summer sores" on the horse's body and legs, but the larvae can also invade the horse's eye (perhaps during itching) and establish a severe irritation of the conjunctiva (conjunctivitis).

The reproductive cycle of the parasite habronema is completed through cooperation of the housefly. This is achieved when the fly larva, while in the manure, feeds on the eggs of habronema; later the fly carries the habronema larva to two possible sites: (1) when ingested by the horse, the housefly carries the parasite directly to its normal habitat, the equine stomach; (2) the housefly may also coincidentally deposit habronema larvae in contaminated wounds, resulting in the well-known and ugly condition called summer sore. Also called cutaneous habronemiasis, it is difficult to treat, and very worrisome for the horse.

Treatment calls for deworming for the stomach worm (habronema). Carbon disulfide is very effective; it is quite toxic, however, and should be used with caution by an experienced veterinarian.

For local external treatment, apply an organophosphate preparation (e.g., Ectoral, Dryex).

Any tiny prick or break in the horse's skin during the fly season is vulnerable to fly invasion and deposition of stomach-worm larvae. This immediately creates

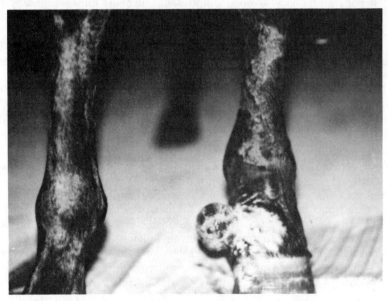

Habronemiasis (Summer Sores)

habronemiasis continued

irritation and contamination of the wound, to which the body responds by producing excessive granulation tissue. During the hot and humid months, when a break in the horse's skin occurs, especially on the limbs, immediately cover the area and keep it protected until healing takes place. This simple preventive action can avert the inevitable formation of scarring lesions, and will spare the horse considerable discomfort.

It has been my experience that once a deeply infested area becomes established on a horse's hide, even though it will dry and appear to heal when the weather changes and all insects disappear, the same unsightly lesion opens up again, just as annoying as ever, when the warm insect season comes around again.

Fly control is the only answer to this problem. By covering manure piles, it is possible to break an important link in the cycle of reproduction. Complement the covered manure pit with the use of screens on stall openings, a frequent spraying schedule, and a clean, tidy barn and premises. This will virtually eliminate all breeding areas for the housefly. With these efforts you can reduce, if not eradicate, the occurrence of resistant summer sores. *See:* CRYOGENICS.

insects   *See:* FLYING INSECTS (CHART, PAGE 175).

intestinal parasites   *See:* WORMING.

lung worms   Although no specific lung parasite has been isolated in the equine, the presence of such a parasite has long been suspected.

Interestingly, the use of an injectable cattle lungworm preparation, called Levasole, has been successful in the treatment of a cattle lungworm called *Dictyocaulus arnfeldi* and in nonspecific lung conditions in horses. Old horses affected with pulmonary alveolar emphysema (heaves) improve greatly after injections of Levasole (although its use in the equine has yet to be documented).

Ascarids, as found in foals and young adults, attack the lung tissue as they pass through during their reproductive cycle; although they are not lung inhabitants or lung parasites *per se,* they do cause great damage to lung tissue and encourage the coestablishment of infection.

Piperazine salts have been the standard treatment for ascariasis in foals. In addition, an anthelmintic combining piperazine and levimisole phosphate (Ripercol) has been developed specifically to rid the foal of all lung parasites.

mange (mites)   An itchy skin infestation of mites. Horses suffer from three types: sarcoptic, psoroptic, and chorioptic mites, each of which result in the development of mange. All three distinct types have separate characteristics and symptoms.

Sarcoptic mange *(Sarcoptes scabiei equi)* is the most serious and the most irritating and uncomfortable. It is also the most difficult to treat. In the early stages, intense itching occurs with multiple small elevations in the skin produced by the female mite as it burrows into the skin to lay its eggs. Lesions appear on the head, neck, and shoulders and soon develop into small hairless patches of skin. A clear discharge is produced at the burrow site; as it dries, it causes a crusty condition that adds to the itchy sensation. Self-mutilation, by rubbing, shortly results in large blood-tinged areas with thickened skin folds on the neck first and then all over the body.

MANGE

Type	Location	(Itch) Pruritis	Contagion	Burrow	Skin Surface	Dry	Moist	Treatment
Sarcoptic	Head, neck, shoulder, thin hair areas	Intense +	+	+	−	+	−	Dipping, spraying with miticide Lindane
Psoroptic	Mane, foretop, base of tail, heavy hair areas	+	+	−	+	−	+	Dipping, spraying with miticide Lindane
Chorioptic	Hind leg, feet, feathers on fetlock, abdomen	+	+	−	+	−	+	Dipping, spraying with miticide Lindane

mange continued

Diagnosis is achieved by skin scrapings and identification under microscopic examination. Psoroptic mange *(Psoroptes equi)* is the most contagious form of mange suffered by the horse. Psoroptic mites prefer areas of heavy hair, unlike sarcoptic mites which prefer areas of thin hair growth. The skin under the mane or foretop and at the base of the tail are the two most common sites of psoroptic mange, although the mites can develop any place on the hair-covered body. Broken or rubbed hairs are the first symptoms of psoroptic mite infestation.

Psoroptic mites characteristically live on the surface of the skin (they do not burrow), producing vesicles and small skin elevations. Scabs and crusts result that remain moist from the production of a clear serum. Hair loss, intense itching, and thickened skin areas result.

Diagnosis is confirmed by skin scraping and microscopic examination and identification.

Chorioptic mange *(Chorioptes equi),* or "foot mange," prefers to attack the hind feet and legs, especially the fetlocks of horses with heavy "feathering" (work horses).

The infested horse rubs its feet, but a more salient symptom is stamping the feet. This "stomping" action should alert the groom to a possible mange infestation hidden in the heavy hairs on the legs, commonly called "heel bug mite."

The chorioptic mite remains on the skin surface and produces moist vesicles and papules similar to psoroptic mange, but its location is a telltale sign in the diagnosis of chorioptic mange.

A secondary infection—such as the "grease" that occurs in work horses—can develop and add to the horse's misery.

Skin scrapings and microscopic identification help confirm the diagnosis.

Treatment for all three types of mange is very much the same, consisting of good nutrition and hygiene. A suitable miticide, such as Lindane® (a chlorinated hydrocarbon), employed in the form of dipping or spraying, can bring relief to the distressed animal. Also effective are diazinon and fenchlorphos applied two or three times at ten-day intervals. All animals on the premises must be treated simultaneously in order to control reinfestation and stamp out the persistent reservoir. Thorough treatment is essential, coupled with hygienic and sanitary cleansing of the entire area. The Lindane baths should be repeated in 12 to 14 days to kill any mites that may have survived the initial medication.

Mange is encountered in underweight and poorly cared for animals, and is invariably found in a generally substandard environment. I have fortunately seen but a few cases of mange in my practice. *See:* GREASE.

Onchocerca cervicalis A whitish, thread-like worm living within the large ligamentum nuchae located in the center of the horse's neck. Adult parasites range in size from 6 to 30 centimeters in length. Microfilariae are the causative agent and, although minute in size, are the migrating culprits that cause severe irritation and tissue damage.

Onchocerciasis is manifested by two conditions in the horse. Eye lesions are one form, and the other entity is seen as skin depigmentation and subcutaneous irritations over the head, neck, and body.

WORM MEDICINE GUIDE

Class	Trade Name	Generic Name	Large Strongyles	Small Strongyles	Bots	Ascarids	Pinworms	Thread Worms
benzimidazole	Telmin	mebendazole	X	X		X	X	
	Telmin B	mebendazole and trichlorton citrate	X	X	X	X	X	X
	Equizole A	piperazine thiabendazole citrate	X	X		X	X	
	Equizole B	thiabendazole trichlorfon	X	X	X	X	X	X
	Equizole	thiabendazole	X	X		X	X	X
	Camvet	cambendazole	X	X		X	X	X
	Panacur	fenbendazole	X	X		X	X	
	Anthelcide EQ	oxibendazole	X	X		X	X	X
levamisole	Ripercol	levamisole piperazine	X	X		X	X	
phenyl-guanidines	Rintal	febantel	X	X		X	X	
organo-phosphates	Equigel	dichlorvos	X	X	X	X		
	Equigard	dichlorvos	X	X	X	X	X	
	Combot	trichlorfon			X	X	X	
piperazine	Parvex Plus	piperazine carbon disulfide phenothiazine	X	X	X	X	X	
tetrahydro (pyrimidine)	Strongid-T	pyrantel pamoate	X	X		X	X	

Onchocerca cervicalis continued

The microfilariae of *Onchocerca cervicalis* also causes a uveitis in the eyes and has been thought by researchers to cause recurrent uveitis (moonblindness). Leptospirosis originally was believed to be the cause of recurrent uveitis. Some horses with a positive titre for leptospira have ocular onchocerciasis; however, most onchocerciasis cases are leptospira-negative.

Ocular symptoms are simply those of inflammation and all associated tissue changes. Eye treatment consists of local instillation of atropine sulfate and corticosteroids with diethylcarbamazine systemically.

In 1983 the FDA released an injectable drug that had been used extensively in Europe for many years in treating parasitic infections, both internal and external. It was touted as capable of totally purging the horse of every known internal and external parasite. And the drug, Ivermectin, was indeed effective against *Onchocerca cervicalis*. Itchy, moist lesions dried quickly, and irritation subsided within hours of injection.

The euphoria over this drug was short-lived, however. After it had been on the market about 18 months, its producer, Merck & Company, sent a letter to veterinarians serving notice of the discontinuation of injectable Ivermectin. The decision was based on a number of reported untoward reactions and subsequent deaths experienced in horses postinjection.

A paste form of Ivermectin continues to be available, but the veterinary profession still awaits the development of a miracle drug for use against parasites.

The microfilariae migrate subcutaneously from the adults' location in the neck region and eventually arrive at the ventral abdomen. Here they set up housekeeping.

Symptoms are sore, moist lesions causing great discomfort and pruritis. Skin irritations are classically found on the ventral midline abdominal area and become infected by secondary bacteria.

Warm insect weather seems to cause exacerbation, and with the first cool day of autumn, a sudden remission of generalized symptoms is noted.

parasites *(See:* PARASITES (CHART, PAGE 172).

piroplasmosis (babesiosis, equine piroplasmosis, biliary fever, equine malaria, horse tick fever, Texas fever)   Piroplasmosis is a tick-borne protozoal disease characterized by fever, anemia, and icterus (yellowing of ocular and oral membranes). This blood parasite disease is caused by two organisms, *Babesia caballi* and *B. equi* and requires *Dermacentor niteus* ticks as vectors for disease transmission.

For long this was considered a tropical disease, but in the late 1970s some cases turned up in Florida, Texas, the Virgin Islands, and Puerto Rico.

Diagnosis is confirmed by the complement-fixation laboratory test and permits a differential diagnosis from similar disease entities. Drugs are many, and treatment is complex, and even then it leaves much to be desired. I am certain that research will continue and with it will come a better method and treatment to rid the horse of this blood parasite forever.

Drugs effective against clinical piroplasmosis: Berenil, Diampron, Imidocarb, Ludobal, and Terramycin.

tick infestation There are two families of ticks that attack horses, the Ixodidae, commonly known as hard ticks, and the Argasidae, or soft ticks.

Ixodidae (hard ticks): of the genus Dermacenter—*D. venustus, D. occidentalis, D. variabilis, D. nitens, D. albipictus;* of the genus Amblyomma—*A. americanum, A. maculatum;* of the genus Ixodes—*I. scapularis, I. pacificus.*

Argasidne (soft ticks): *Otobius megnini.*

Hard ticks are classified by the presence of protective armor in the form of a dorsal scutum over the back and body. *D. venustus* is the famous Rocky Mountain spotted fever tick and the carrier of the western strain of equine encephalomyelitis.

Soft ticks lack the protective dorsal scutum. *O. megnini,* called the spinose ear tick, is the only soft tick known to attack horses and is a common nuisance in arid areas of the United States.

Spinose ear tick larvae crawl into the horse's ear and migrate to below the hairline in the external ear canal. There they feed on sensitive skin and remain for up to six months, causing a relentless irritation to the host horse. Symptoms are head-shaking, violent at times, with rubbing and itching. An abrupt change in disposition or tractability is evident, especially when a halter, rope, or bridle is placed even near the ear.

Diagnosis is confirmed by retrieving evidence of ticks deep in the ear canal. This is best accomplished by careful use of a long, flexible swab.

Treatment consists of the chemicals of choice. Five-percent Malathion is effective against these ear ticks, as are ear sprays and dusts (Lindane, Carbaryl, or Toxaphene). All are poison chemicals, so proceed with caution. Even better, avail yourself of the advice and supervision of a veterinarian trained in this field. Your horse will be the first to thank you!

trypanosomiasis *See under:* COMMON DISEASES.

verminous arteritis *See:* ILIAC ARTERY THROMBOSIS.

worming Procedure used in attempting to rid the horse of intestinal parasites. No service provides a greater health benefit to your horse than ridding it of worms.

A schedule of worming at precise intervals greatly enhances the efficiency of the procedure by interrupting the parasite's life cycle and reproductive proficiency. In contrast, worming at random or at erratic intervals is futile. It is costly to the owner and represents an insidiously dangerous threat to the horse's current and future health.

Although commonly thought of as basically intestinal parasites, the normal internal worm larvae migrate throughout all internal organs. Some travel via the circulatory system and others primarily invade tissue. All create destruction and irreparable tissue damage.

There are a multitude of parasites that attack the horse, but the three most common are bloodworms, roundworms, and bots.

Bot worms *(Gastrophilus)* are one of the most troublesome parasites affecting the horse. For a discussion, *see above:* BOTS.

Bloodworms *(Strongyles)* are notorious invaders and offenders in horses of all ages and groups, with no respect for station in life.

worming continued

Roundworms *(Parascaris equorum)* are unquestionably the worst enemy of a young foal's pulmonary system and gastrointestinal tract.

When in question as to what parasite is present, the veterinarian will run a fecal test to identify and determine how many parasitic larvae and eggs exist. The veterinarian can then determine which anthelmintic to administer and at what dosage.

It is considered normal and acceptable, even in a healthy horse that is wormed regularly and housed well with supervised pastures, to show a couple of parasitic eggs in a fecal examination. Constant reinfestation occurs by virtue of the horse's environment. When a fecal sample is entirely negative, please note this finding and repeat the laboratory test. If a horse shows a totally clean egg count, it is either sick or should be considered "suspect." (The obvious exception to the last statement is the horse that was just wormed 48 to 72 hours prior.)

Although the reliability of fecal tests is questionable, they are valid in resistant parasite cases, not necessarily for routine use. As the saying goes, a positive result is positive, but a negative result could be positive. *See:* FECAL TEST.

Worm medicines (anthelmintics) are intended to destroy horse parasites and are administered either by stomach tube, as commercial pastes placed on the tongue, or as powder preparations deftly hidden in the grain.

Stomach-tube worming is superior by far, although veterinary service is necessary for this method. It is even quite easy on the patient, contrary to the impression received by the average uninitiated owner. *See:* STOMACH TUBE.

Commercial anthelmintic pastes do kill worms, and no veterinary service is necessary with their use. *But use with caution:* Some pastes contain organophosphate chemicals. Although these cholinesterase-inhibiting drugs efficiently remove parasites, they do occasionally cause gastrointestinal upsets, especially in sensitive individuals. The organophosphate group of drugs was developed and subsequently advertised with great fanfare in horse journals. They are available under a variety of commercial names, but please, *first read the fine print* and be aware of the intimated warnings. These drugs also are incompatible and react adversely with the commonly used phenothiazine-derived tranquilizers. Chickens and pigeons that search through the droppings of treated horses to retrieve undigested grain are killed by the chemical.

There is no doubt that these worming compounds remove almost all parasites and their eggs, but while doing so, they threaten the health and environment of the host animal. I, personally, would rather see a few worms and not place my patient in jeopardy. Organophosphates are unsafe for use in horses, ecologically dangerous, and, in my opinion, their manufacture should be discontinued.

Palatable *powder form* worm medicines, placed on the grain, present a safer, although somewhat less effective, method of reducing internal parasites. The potency of the anthelmintics is compromised by the simultaneous ingestion of grain and its diluting effect.

Regardless of your choice of worming method, the particular drug selected for worming your horse is of equal importance. Determine, with your veterinarian, the anthelmintic that best fits your horse's needs. Age, sex, size, and role in life are essential factors, but especially important is the animal's environment. More than anything else, the horse's surroundings will dictate the drug, the method, and the frequency of worming.

Worming can be less frequent in a small private stable where there are roomy pastures and a minimum of horse traffic. On a commercial horse farm, where horses are crowded together, there must be frequent worming of all stock, since, with horses concentrated into small areas, reinfestation begins immediately after worming and continues unabated until the next scheduled treatment.

In the foal, worming should begin as early as four to six weeks of age, depending upon the environemnt, with treatment directed toward roundworm destruction. Worming should be repeated on a monthly regime during the first year of life. Worm medicine lethal to bloodworms should be incorporated with the second worming and continued thereafter. Yearlings are usually wormed every other month, and two-year-olds every third month. Adult horses, depending upon environment, require routine worming every four months, or three times annually.

Horses on pasture reinfest themselves with strongyles faster than those confined. Strongyles attack horses of all ages but prefer adults. Ascarids (roundworms) propagate very well in the straw and stall confines, but customarily affect horses under four years.

Some of the tried-and-true worm medicines available commercially are effective and yet quite safe to the horse. Although these drugs are not as efficient as the organophosphates, they are more desirable in several important respects, as discussed above.

For foals, usually ravaged by ascarids and strongyles, I prefer the prudent use of piperazine citrate employed with one of the many benzimidazoles. Adult horses respond quite well to benzimidazoles for use against strongyles, principally, as well as ascarids, pinworms, and threadworms.

Emphasis should be placed on the need to alternate anthelmintics to avoid engendering resistant parasites.

For treatment of bots, Parvex Plus has been a reliable drug, one which, if handled with respect, can be administered to all horses of all ages, even pregnant mares. As a rule, however, do not worm a mare closer than eight weeks from term. There may, of course, be times when, for greater reasons of health, this rule must be bent.

Overcrowding in the barn, with reduced hygiene measures, and/or overgrazing in the pastures are the two factors that allow parasites to gain control and to complete their life cycles for reinfestation of the horse.

A good rule of thumb is one horse per acre of pasture. These days, with land and fencing at a premium, this rule is often forgotten. Land is turned to other uses, and too many horses are turned into the pastures that remain. Parasitism with secondary malnutrition are the unfortunate consequences.

Better-run farms limit the number of horse residents and chain-drag the pasture to scatter manure droppings. Sunlight and drying destroy some of the parasitic eggs, but not all.

Parasites are "host specific" and thus they cannot complete their reproductive cycle in another animal. Larvae and eggs ingested by animals of

worming continued

another specie pass quickly and virtually untouched through the gastrointestinal tract, and are rendered useless and unable to reproduce.

Some astute farm owners, therefore, alternate cattle with horses in the paddocks and pastures every month or so. This effectively breaks the life cycle of the parasites and concurrently preserves the nutritive value of the pastures. Horses are considered "destructive grazers." Unlike cattle, they characteristically chew the grass very close to the ground, sometimes pulling the roots out. Rotating the grazing species helps the land to recover. This benefits not only the land, but the animals that live on it.

To win in the battle against the everpresent and sometimes even life-threatening internal parasite, try combining an intelligent farm manager, adequate land and buildings, good fences, and an interested veterinarian. I would then be willing to gamble that the worms would lose, at least for a while.

FEEDS AND FEEDING

amino acids The body develops its protein from amino acids. These are the basic building blocks of tissue construction.

Although there are many known in nature, there are ten essential amino acids required for normal tissue growth in animals. The body can generate some of these building blocks, but not at the rate required for growth, performance, and reproduction, so the animal's diet must contain these elements each day in order to satisfy its dietary requirements, hence the term "essential amino acids."

They are: arginine, histidine, isoleucine, leucine, lysine, methionine, phenylamine, threonime, tryptophan, and valine.

A word of caution about your horse's diet: Corn can not be fed alone because it lacks two of the essential amino acids. In order to round out your horse's diet, feed it a combination of alfalfa or clover hay with your other foodstuffs. The old-time corn diet can be fed, although I don't recommend it, but it must be supplemented by alfalfa.

In the world of competition horses, it is a well-known practice to give amino acids, in combination with an electrolytic solution before a race or event in order to promote better performance. Today's trend, however, is toward intravenous replacement of these elements after strenuous effort. Such replacement achieves quicker physiologic recovery and better preparation for the next effort.

apples In limited quantities, apples are a tasty treat for your horse. But since apples can cause the formation of gas by fermentation in the digestive tract, they should not be included in feeds or bran mashes. They are no substitute for carrots.

avocados A popular food for humans, but they are quite toxic for horses, especially when the stems and roots are eaten. Symptoms are depression, elevated body temperature, and lack of appetite. In lactating mares, severe mastitis develops. Keep horses away from avocado trees!

barley An important cereal grain that is superior to oats in total digestible nutrients and is slightly richer in protein than oats. Despite these facts, barley is not popular as a horse feed, probably because it must first be ground into a fine preparation (the hulls are quite thick). Horses are notorious for their dislike of powdery foods, which can lead to gastrointestinal disturbances.

Draft horses and mules can tolerate a larger percentage of barley in their diet. But, for the well-bred horse, I consider the disadvantages of barley to outweigh the advantages.

Ideally, barley bran, when combined with wheat bran as a mash, is an

barley continued

excellent source of nutrients. To aid in digestion, include 25 percent barley and feed cool mashes in summer and hot mashes in winter. *See:* BRAN MASH.

bedding There are many available forms for multiple purposes. Among the old-fashioned, standard beddings are:

Rye straw—This is the best possible straw bedding for horses. Although it is expensive, because of its bright, clean, shiny, coarse, long-stemmed characteristics, it is the straw of choice for fine horses.

Wheat straw—Coarse and stiff-stemmed, it serves as good bedding material because it is usually clean and free of dust and mold. Horses generally prefer to eat their hay rather than the wheat straw.

Barley straw—Somewhat palatable, but can cause colic if consumed in even moderate amounts.

Oat straw—Soft, with pliable stems, oat straw possesses some nutritive value, but it is seldom clean and free of mold. Usually it is chaffy and slightly darker than good rye straw. Oat straw can be dangerous if eaten freely; it has been known to cause colic. Its color is a good index for quality and cleanliness. When bright, it is clean; when dark, it may be dirty and possibly contain mold and dust.

Newer types of beddings ideal for obese animals or horses suffering from respiratory problems:

Peat moss—An excellent bedding that absorbs moisture well and serves as a good deodorant; it is very expensive, however. "Heavy" (bronchitic) and overweight horses do very well on it. Note that such horses love to eat their straw bedding (observed or not).

Peanut shells—These are sometimes used for bedding, although they are not highly absorptive and they attract flies because of their oily peanut residue.

Staz-Dri®—A commercial preparation made from sugar cane. It provides a fairly good straw substitute for either "heavy" or obese horses. Occasionally an individual animal will develop a taste for this type of bedding; when that happens, switch to something else!

Wood shavings or sawdust—Hardwood by-products, they can serve as bedding if clean, dry, and free of dust. Absorptive capacity is not comparable to that of straw, however.

bran mash Bran is derived from the coarse outer coatings or kernels of cereal grains—wheat, barley, rye, and other farinaceous (flour) grains. The kernels are separated by grinding and then sieving the grain. Bran was long considered a mere by-product of cereal grains, of no great value compared to the flour made from the grain. The outer darker brown layers of the cereal-grain kernels were discarded as nutritionally valueless. But time and experience have shown that bran is rich in protein and high in niacin, phosphorus, and fiber content; it has small amounts of vitamins A and D and calcium.

Bran, in the form of a bran mash, is an excellent bulk feed and a palatable and healthy menu change in any horse's diet. It provides not only bulk and fiber for the function of the gastrointestinal tract, but also has mild laxative properties for maintenance of idle animals or any animals subjected to stress or unscheduled exercise or dietary change.

Preferably, it should consist of equal parts of bran and oats or other concentrate of your choice (corn, sweet feed, etc). Wheat bran is popular, but barley and rye bran are equally nutritious.

To prepare a bran mash, place the oats in a clean metal pail and add boiling water slowly, stirring constantly until the grains of concentrate (oats, corn, etc.) soften and split open. (The concentrate requires cooking, the bran does not.) Now add the bran, stirring until the mixture is of a fluffy texture; it should not be wet and soggy. Cover the pail with a clean towel or burlap sack and allow it to steep until it has "cooked."

All horses in training, growing animals, broodmares, and retirees benefit from this delicious and nutritious treat. On cold evenings, especially, it provides warmth to the system.

The frequency of its use, whether served hot or cold, and the amount—these are questions to be answered according to the individual horse, its energy demands, health, and age. Mash is especially useful as a feed on idle days, during schedule changes, and before vanning or any anticipated stress. It can prevent tying-up, constipation, and even bouts of colic. Fed dry, it helps in cases of mild diarrhea. Any horse that is my patient or under my supervision receives a bran mash as a regular part of its diet. *See:* COOKED GRAIN.

brewer's dried yeast   *See:* VITAMINS.

cereal grains   Commonly called concentrates, they include oats, corn, wheat, barley, and rye. Their by-products include wheat bran, linseed meal, hominy, and corn gluten feed. Concentrates are feeds low in fiber and high in digestible nutrients yielding net energy: in contrast, the roughages (hay, fodder, straw, and silage are high in fiber and low in total digestible nutrients (TDN). Corn and wheat grains are highest, barley and rye average, and oats lowest in TDN.

Grains generally are low in protein, and the quality of the protein is poor because the grains contain minimal amounts of essential amino acids. This fact can seriously alter the nutritional balance of immature, pregnant, or competition animals.

Wheat bran supplies higher-quality protein than wheat grain. Corn oil meal from the center of the kernel has better protein than corn grain. Corn (shelled and ground from the ear), although high in total digestible nutrients, is an incomplete feed because it lacks two essential amino acids, lysine and tryptophan.

By feeding alfalfa hay with corn, however, you can achieve a balanced diet. *See:* AMINO ACIDS.

cherry tree   *See:* HYDROCYANIC ACID POISONING.

cooked grain   A superior method of preparing horse feed for the young and growing animal, the broodmare, and the hunting, showing, or racing horse. Cooking grain makes it more palatable and superior in providing intestinal bulk, thus it enhances the nutritional value of the grain.

Years ago, it was a common sight in well-run barns to see cookers started early in the day and steeped until late afternoon. Usually wood- or coal-powered, the large tanks would be watched by the head groom, who made sure that all the *cooked grain continued*

grain kernels were soft and split open. When the lid was lifted, eager neighs answered the escaping aroma. Barns where cooked feed was in the schedule always had fewer cases of colic, myositis, and gastrointestinal ailments.

Cooking feed required extra effort and time. I am sorry it has lost favor today. The quicker methods are satisfactory at best, but in no way comparable.

Here is an easy rule of thumb for feeding measures:

2-pound coffee can (1 quart) = 2 pounds of oats, or 1 quart
2-pound coffee can   = 2 pounds sweet feed, or 1 quart
2-pound coffee can   = 3 3/4 pounds of shelled corn, or 7 quarts

Remember, roughly speaking, "a pint's a pound the world around."

hay   Generally defined as roughage harvested for livestock consumption. Hay can range in grade from beautiful, green, leafy legume, glowing with nutritional value, to dried-out brown, or colorless sticks and stems of meadow grass, negligible in food value.

Among livestock people "hay," whether edible or not, seems to cover the complete gamut of roughage. Not so in the world of quality horses. These owners and breeders demand and usually pay well for "horse hay." And properly so, since it is not a simple task to make, bale, and deliver good hay. Even the most experienced farmer, equipped with modern hay-making machinery, looks upon this as a challenge requiring not merely skill, but favorable weather as well.

Cows, sheep, and goats thrive on all grades of hay, especially that rejected for horse use. Ruminants actually tolerate surprising amounts of mold, must, and dust in roughages. The situation is quite different for horses.

When considering roughage for your horse, there are two main types available: grass hay (timothy, bluegrass, and meadow grass) and legume hay (alfalfa and clover). Each has its particular advantages to meet the roughage needs of different horses.

For hay to be consumed safely by horses, it must meet these four cardinal specifications. It must be:

1. Leafy with few stems
2. Smooth and soft to the touch
3. Green in color
4. Clean, that is, free of mold, must, and dust

In the production of a hay crop, the key to making nutritious hay is not so much the type, but the age of the plants when they are harvested. A field of immature grass will yield enhanced nutrition and palatability, whereas a crop of mature grass will yield stems inferior in color, digestibility, and nutritional value.

When purchasing hay, be careful to avoid mature hay that is being passed off as immature lush hay—usually, as an added insult, at a premium price.

Old-time horsemen considered legume hay (alfalfa and clover) to be unsuitable as horse roughage. In preference to this "cow hay," they insisted on feeding horses the "true" horse hay, timothy. Today we know that these old-timers mistakenly believed that alfalfa would cause kidney disease and muscle disorders, and that clover would cause bloat in horses.

Let us bury this bit of folklore here and now!

No longer is the nutritional value of legume hay being lost to the horse world. I am happy to say that the use of quality alfalfa, popularly preferred to clover, is now well accepted in the better-run barns. Alfalfa that is grown on suitable and properly fertilized soil, harvested at the ideal time, and properly cured and stored is the nearest thing to an ideal "whole diet" available today, because it comes from the field and, if fed with discretion, it furnishes the horse with a superior balance of vitamins, minerals, and protein. Your horse's gastrointestinal performance will reflect far greater efficiency than it would on a diet confined to commercially produced pelleted feeds and supplemental additives. These preparations are aligned to standards established by business- and sales-oriented scientists. I grant that scientifically processed foods are quite adequate; however, the horse's gastrointestinal tract performs at maximum efficiency only when fed precisely what its absorptive and assimilative processes require. Expensive supplements and cereal grains fed in excessive amounts are not required so long as your horse's hay contains the right nutritional ingredients. (Frankly, I suspect that many of the supplements end up in the manure pile rather than being retained within the horse's system.)

Well-cured alfalfa is very palatable and is preferred by the majority of horses even when they are given the opportunity to select. I have, however, found that a high-grade timothy/legume hay mixture is easier for a performance horse to digest; it is preferred by some trainers. Strangely enough, some of the horses actually prefer the timothy/legume mixture when given the option.

The length of the timothy heads reveals the age of the hay at the time of harvesting and thus indicates its nutritional value. When examining timothy hay for purchase, reject any hay with timothy heads longer than 1½ inches.

Broodmares, young growing horses, and some athletic horses deserve vintage legume hay with all of its nutritional superiority. On breeding farms, the emphasis is on roughage; concentrates are secondary. But in performance diets, the opposite is true. Most athletes need the cereal grains to fill their nutritional needs.

I would conclude with a caution about the storage of hay.

All new hay, especially legume hay, contains a high moisture content and is put through a sweating, or curing, process before it is offered for consumption. This is the ominous period when spontaneous combustion can occur, and the threat of fire is ever-present to hay-making farmers who store new hay inside a barn, shed, or any enclosure.

Fire caused by spontaneous combustion is more likely to happen when carelessness and ignorance prevail. To prevent a disaster of this type, abide carefully by the following rules:

1. Stack bales in pillars, only two bales across. This allows air to circulate around each pillar and each bale.

2. Keep all barn doors, vents, and windows *open* constantly for five to six weeks.

3. Maintain constant air circulation.

kelp   Dried kelp or kelp meal is prepared from giant seaweeds found in the bottom of the ocean. Containing around 0.20 percent iodine and about 35 percent total mineral matter, kelp has interested nutritionists for years because

kelp continued

of its rich mineral content. To date, this seaweed has not proved any more beneficial than routine horse feeds. Kelp has been fed in its natural form and scientifically incorporated into conventional feeds, with no significant data forthcoming.

Some years ago I had in my practice an eccentric horse owner who had read some literature expounding the merits of kelp and was determined to feed it to his entire broodmare band. There were several mares in the group heavy in foal, and I became somewhat apprehensive about subjecting the mares to a drastic dietary change. But I could not dissuade the owner.

At great expense and trouble, the infamous seaweed arrived at the farm, packaged in huge sacks. Having purposely planned my call schedule so that I would be there at feeding time, I watched the foreman as he methodically measured and placed the kelp in each feed tub. The first four mares that were offered the new preparation promptly snorted and turned away to their hay, while the fifth mare decided to try it. She quickly emptied her mouth of all contents and went for the water bowl. All the mares refused to touch it!

My venturesome friend was greatly disheartened and ordered the remainder of the seaweed quickly discarded.

linseed meal   Ground flaxseed. A yellowish brown powder, high in protein and very rich in selenium. It is fed as an additive for improvement of skin and coat.

Linseed oil has been used as a laxative for horses. It is a harsh remedy, however. Use topically as a poultice for any hot, swollen, and painful condition (inflammation). *See:* POULTICE.

CAUTION: *Raw* linseed oil can be toxic if given orally. As a feed additive, use only rectified linseed oil.

methionine   An essential amino acid needed in the daily diet.

Some years ago, medical journals expounded the virtues of methionine and its oral use in cases of founder. It is believed to aid tissue integrity of the foot laminae and thus help prevent separation of the sensitive from the insensitve layers and consequent rotation of the os pedis. On the basis of this data, I have treated every laminitis case with massive doses of methionine via the stomach tube, and I must admit that I have seen some acute symptoms subside dramatically. *See:* LAMINITIS.

minerals   Essential minerals needed by the horse to maintain health are: calcium, phosphorus, chlorine, cobalt, copper, iodine, iron, magnesium, manganese, potassium, selenium, sulfur, and zinc, all of which are found in the normal adequate diet.

The old farmer's saying, "You can't take out what you don't put in" has stood the test of time. Although it may seem extravagant to constantly add minerals (fertilizer) to the soil, it does remain the only way, year after year, to continue farming the same soil.

A green, leafy, and properly cured legume hay cut from well-fertilized ground is an unparalleled food source, providing minerals in a form that can be properly assimilated into the horse's system. In contrast, the commercial vitamin and mineral products, although they are prepared in such a way as to mimic natural food grown on enriched soils, come in forms that are not efficiently digested or assimilated. These expensive supplements pass through the gastrointestinal tract, largely untouched, and end up in the manure pile.

Calcium and phosphorus are two very important minerals essential for a healthy skeletal system, sound teeth, and stable metabolic system. As with all the minerals in the body, their functioning is interrelated and depends on maintaining a critical balance. With calcium and phosphorus, research indicates that if an imbalance occurs, then neither mineral is utilized. A ratio of 2:1 of calcium to phosphorus is vital for a growing or immature colt and 3:1 in adult horses. It is easy to see how quickly this ratio could be thrown out of balance by the inadvertent feeding of additives or supplements. A deficiency can actually be created by providing an abundance of one mineral. Interestingly, when an imbalance in the ratio does occur, it is commonly the phosphorus and not the calcium (as everyone suspects) that is deficient.

Cereal grains (oats, wheat, barley, rye, and corn) are low in phosphorus and quite low in calcium. Corn is the poorest food in this regard.

Good legume hay is rich in calcium and low in phosphorus, but it supplies a high-quality protein and is rich in vitamins A and D. But, here again, phosphorus is undersupplied. A phosphorus deficiency not only affects bone development, but also has an influence on fertility.

The young growing animal, the reproducing broodmare, and the competition horse can all benefit by the addition of wheat bran to their already adequate diet. Wheat bran is high in protein, high in total digestible nutrients (close to the content of oats), and low in calcium, but it is the richest source of phosphorus known.

Prepared in equal parts with any cereal grain, moistened as a hot or cold bran mash, wheat bran provides bulk and fiber for the gastrointestinal tract. It provides a welcome warm meal in the winter. Not only is it palatable, but it is bulky and therefore satisfying. *See:* BRAN MASH.

Calcium deficiency occurs much less often than phosphorus deficiency, since there are many available dietary sources of calcium. Our cereal grains are low in calcium, but all legume grasses and hay contain high amounts. When broodmares suffer a dietary calcium deficiency, they quickly mobilize it from their own skeletal system and provide for the needs of the fetus. This cannot be repeated without stressing and literally destroying the matron. It is inexcusable when an owner fails to provide sufficient calcium to a pregnant mare.

Salt, or sodium chloride, is essential to life and equally as important as water intake. Mineralized salt blocks, containing all trace minerals, will meet the mineral requirements of the average horse in a normal environment.

Iodine deficiency results in goiter development in both young and old and is found in precise geographic areas. Here again, a mineralized salt lick is the answer.

Eclampsia, or lactation tetany, is thought to result from low calcium (hypocalcemia) or low magnesium (hypomagnesemia). Proper mineral intake is the best defense against this tragic development. *See:* ECLAMPSIA.

All plants provide phosphorus, sulfur, and potassium. Copper, manganese, zinc, and iron are found in good-quality hay.

Selenium deficiency seems to be increasing in incidence and is the cause of

minerals continued

muscle degeneration, or "white muscle disease," in newborn animals. Fertility is reduced in geographic areas of deficient soil; with the dietary addition of selenium, the pregnancy rate soars. Selenium is not found in mineralized salt licks and thus must be added to the diet. Linseed meal is ideal as a safe and natural source of selenium. Careful dosage must be met, however, as the required amount of selenium is so very close to the toxic dose, with no margin of safety. Consult your veterinarian.

Race horses and show horses that become stiff and sore during and after exercise respond very well to intramuscular injections of vitamin E and selenium. Usually, three injections are given ten days apart and then once monthly during extreme exertion.

molasses (black strap molasses)   When grain is crimped or crushed to make it more digestible, dust quite often is the undesirable result, since it represents a major insult to the horse's respiratory tract. Adding one part molasses to ten parts grain reduces dust and irritants and enhances palatability.

Rolled and crushed oats are to be avoided. Although basically designed to increase digestibility, this form of processing fails badly in the case of the horse. Most nourishment escapes during the processing and baggins procedure, and the feed is laden with dust, debris, and respiratory irritants.

"Crimped" oats are a much more efficient and more desirable food form, though second in choice to whole oats with all of the nutrition intact. Crimping slightly cracks the hull and kernel, preserving the nutritional contents. This processing simultaneously promotes mastication, digestion, and ultimate assimilation. No loss of nutrients and no dust!

If you have an old horse, feed him crimped oats. If your horse has a dental problem, have the problem corrected.

oats   An excellent cereal grain for light breeds and competition horses. By virtue of their hull, oat grains form a bulky and easily digested mass in the horse's stomach, unlike other, heavier grains. Although the nutritive value of barley, rye, corn, and wheat is higher than that of oats, these grains when fed alone have a tendency to form a consistency in the stomach that can cause colic in the horse. Combining these grains with molasses makes them more readily digestible, however, and feeds sweetened in this manner have gained great popularity over the years with all breeds, including some of the heavier types.

Oats as a cereal grain are low in protein and low in both phosphorus and calcium. They are, however, very palatable and supply needed energy for performance horses. Oats can be fed in a well-balanced diet by combining them with a good, clean, green alfalfa hay.

Clean, "plump" oats (Canadian grown) should weigh around 40 pounds per bushel. Locally grown oats (30 to 32 pounds per bushel) cannot compare and should be bypassed as horse feed.

pasture   Ground covered with grass for grazing animals. Pasture not only provides nutrition, but it allows the modern horse some relaxation and freedom to frolic and exercise while eating. If handled properly, a stand of good grass can provide the most economic feed for horses during certain months of the year, but not without hazard!

Every knowledgeable horseman has heard of "grass founder"; the danger lurks in every field of lush grass. Immature, actively growing grass is rich in protein early in the spring, and as summer progresses, the protein content gradually lessens, reaching a low ebb later in the summer as the grass matures.

When a working horse, one that is physically fit (race horse, fox hunter, carriage horse) and maintained on a high cereal-grain diet (carbohydrates), is suddenly turned out on a solid grass diet, there is an abrupt gastrointestinal change in protein intake. In the absence of dietary carbohydrates, this condition is thought to be the cause of grass founder.

Symptoms are classic, and once evident, they are difficult to reverse. The first step is to remove the horse from the pasture and place it in a large stall or small paddock free of grass.

Treatment for grass founder consists of small daily amounts of cereal grain with brown sugar added, as well as thyroid extract and daily doses of phenylbutazone.

Some individual horses with a breed predisposition are prime candidates for grass founder. Be on your guard with somewhat heavily muscled animals, easy-keepers, and aged horses, especially where there may be a borderline case of hypothyroidism.

I always advise the owner, in early spring, to turn out for one hour a day and to continue to feed daily one-eighth the amount of grain received during work. The one hour could be stretched to two hours daily after ten days. The horse could be turned out in a grass-free area for exercise; it must not be allowed to gorge itself on high-protein grass. In eastern Pennsylvania, for example, the "danger level" in the grass subsides around July 1 and at that time, the horses may have their grazing time extended.

To preserve your pasture and prevent the ravages of horse grazing, allocate one acre of pasture per horse and chain drag once a week to break up manure. This allows the heat and light of the sun to destroy parasite eggs, and encourages growth of grass in spotty areas. Pastures should be clipped or mown high frequently to prevent the growth of weeds that would otherwise strangle the desired grass.

For the safety of your horse, keep your fences in good repair. *See:* LAMINITIS.

pelleted feeds Feeds that have been commercially processed into compact pellets or small cubes. Solid grain, hay and grain ("complete feed"), and "hay cubes," containing hay only, are the common forms of pellets.

The advantages of pelleted feeds are many. Horses welcome their palatability and benefit from their dietary soundness. Dust and debris are virtually eliminated in these preparations, which is always desirable but especially so in cases of bronchitis and chronic alveolar emphysema (heaves). Antigens found in cereal grains (especially oats) and the invariable dust harbored in most baled hay are two great respiratory-tract hazards that are substantially reduced by the feeding of pelletized feeds. And, of course, these feeds take up far less storage space than hay and grain in their natural form.

The disadvantages of this form of feeding are numerous and warrant stating. It is impossible to monitor the quality of the grain and hay when it is mashed, dried, and compressed into cubes. The animal's gastrointestinal tract must make an adjustment to the dietary change from normal grain and roughage to the

pelleted feeds continued

dried, compressed form of feed. Colic is not uncommon in these animals. Constant munching or chewing on roughage is a normal behavior pattern in the equine, and a horse that is switched to a cube feed or pelleted diet may become discontent in the absence of incessant chewing on roughage.

phytin A compound present in cereal grains that actually inhibits the availability of calcium, magnesium, and phosphorus in the body.

Phytin is thought to interfere with the normal ratio of calcium and phosphorus. When young growing colts are fed large amounts of cereal grain rations, they then do not consume as much hay. Reduced hay consumption over a period of time could conceivably result in a mineral imbalance and nutritional deficiency.

Cereal grain, therefore should be limited in amount, and quality hay, with its ready source of calcium and phosphorus in proper proportion for optimum assimilation, should be available at all times.

A rule of thumb suggests that you not exceed 12 quarts of grain daily, but supply the best available clean, green, leafy alfalfa hay free-choice to growing weanlings and yearlings.

selenium *See:* LINSEED MEAL, MINERALS.

vitamins Dietary organic substances required in exceedingly minute and precise amounts for normal body function.

Vitamins are important nutrients found naturally in foodstuffs. Deficiencies in these nutrients can cause malnutrition, retarded growth, sex disorders, abortion, and assorted diseases. A deficiency disease can easily be caused by indiscriminate dietary changes. Young, growing animals, broodmares, and athletic horses are vulnerable to even subtle variations.

Once ingested, most vitamins can be stored quite well by the body. But outside the body, in their natural form, vitamins can lose their potency due to the action of sunlight, air, moisture, and temperature changes. The question of vitamin content and its maintenance during storage of cereal grains and roughages depends upon many factors. Time of year and stage of growth at time of harvest, environmental factors, and storage method and duration all affect the nutritional level.

Vitamins are divided into two groups, those soluble in fat, and those soluble in water. The fat-soluble vitamins, which include A, D, and E, hold the greatest potential for vitamin deficiencies in the horse.

The water-soluble vitamins, B and C, do not present as serious a concern. It has been documented in veterinary literature that the vitamin B complex is synthesized in the intestines and that vitamin C is synthesized in the horse's liver. The internal synthesis of vitamins can be assumed only in the presence of an adequate, balanced diet and a healthy individual, however.

Thiamine (vitamin B_1) was the first vitamin discovered, being identified in 1912 as a cure for beriberi.

Vitamin C (ascorbic acid) was identified next when it was found to cure scurvy, a disease that commonly afflicted sailors whose diets lacked the citrus fruits that are a primary source of vitamin C.

The fat-soluble vitamin A is essential for both animals and people. It occurs plentifully in nature, and yet lack of vitamin A in daily diets is commonly found in livestock, especially during the winter months.

The body produces vitamin A from carotene contained in plants (see chart, below), so animals should ingest adequate amounts of carotene-rich foods.

Around 3,000–5,000 I.U. per 100 pounds body weight has been determined as the daily minimum requirement of vitamin A, and fresh green hay or good pasture can more than meet this figure. Green color represents carotene content; hay that is stored for longer than one year, exposed to light and oxygen, is known to decrease dramatically in vitamin content. When forage is stored properly in barns, the nutritional loss is neither as rapid nor as great.

Cereal grains (concentrates) are notoriously low in vitamins A and D; the main sources in a horse's diet are leafy green hay and good pasture.

Internally, vitamin A is stored in the liver for periods of from six or seven weeks, thus a substandard diet can be tolerated for short periods in horses that have recently come off of good pasture.

Symptoms of deficiencies in vitamin A are poor fertility, anorexia, night blindness, excessive lacrimation (tearing down the face), reduced resistance to respiratory and other infections, poor hair coat, and poor hoof texture.

Dietary supplements can be used, but they also carry the danger of creating an imbalance of vitamins, and unless they are packaged in an available form, they may not be assimilated in the intestines. It is better to feed an improved quality of roughage (green and leafy) than to feed a commercial supplement—although an exception to this rule is the sick horse during recuperation.

Toxicity can result from overfeeding vitamin A. To add to the confusion, the symptoms of hypervitaminosis simulate those of a deficiency! Call your veterinarian when in doubt.

Broodmares require vitamin A for efficient fertility and maintenance of a healthy uterine endometrium. It has been determined by research that vitamin A acting alone does not produce an appreciable change in fertility problems. However, when combined with vitamin E, there have been detectable increases in conceptions and also in the number of pregnancies ending with delivery of a live foal.

The suggested ratio of vitamin E (alpha-tocopherol) is 1:1,000 of vitamin A.

Vitamin D does not represent a concern in the diet of horses. Sunlight and sun-cured forages provide all the vitamin D needed for our horse, the herbivore.

VITAMIN A (CAROTENE) CONTENT

Feedstuff	Carotene (MG per KG)
Alfalfa hay	33
Bermuda grass hay	36
Bluegrass pasture	386
Red clover	34
Timothy hay	11
Oats	0
Corn	2
Barley	0
Beet pulp	0

vitamins continued

Most plants contain ergosterol which is converted into vitamin D_2 (a percursor of vitamin D) by the action of ultraviolet rays from the sun after a plant is dead.

Another source of vitamin D occurs through exposure to sunlight. Ultraviolet rays supplied either artificially or by natural sunlight, activate the skin to manufacture vitamin D.

Ergosterol is abundant in yeast, and yeast irradiated with ultraviolet light provides a concentrated source of vitamin D_2. Irradiated brewer's yeast is a very popular method of supplementing the vitamin D dietary intake to horses during the long cold season with its short daily periods of sunlight. Daily minimum requirement is 300–500 I.U. per 100 pounds of body weight.

Vitamin D is intimately associated with the balance, absorption, and deposition of calcium and phosphorus. The three factors go hand in glove, and any slight deviation of one can upset the functioning of all three.

Vitamin D is the celebrated antirickets vitamin. Symptoms of vitamin D deficiency are calcium and phosphorus imbalance, resulting in calcification or decalcification of tissues, poor teeth, skeletal weakening, impaired joints, and enlarged ends of long bones resulting in deformities.

Since vitamin D is needed for assimilation of calcium and phosphorus, its dietary source is especially critical to the broodmare during periods of heavy demand, such as late in pregnancy and during lactation. No supplement is generally given, since sun-cured hay, preferably green legume hay, and sunlight provide natural sources of vitamin D.

Although vitamin E (alpha-tocopherol) has been called the antisterility vitamin, its use alone has not been scientifically substantiated. We need much more data on this vitamin. Breeding stock, young growing horses, and performance horses all clinically respond (e.g., glossier coat, improved appetite, weight gain) to the addition of vitamin E to feeds. Twenty I.U. per 100 pounds of body weight has been added daily as a rule-of-thumb measurement with no detectable unfavorable results. Ready available sources of vitamin E are cottonseed oil, some grains, and commercial wheat germ oil.

Research has indicated that both vitamin E and vitamin A in combination, when supplied orally or through injection, work synergistically to produce a favorable response. Broodmares received 100,000 I.U. of vitamin A and 100 I.U. of vitamin E daily for three months, beginning one month prior to the breeding season. The results were improved conception rates, decreased numbers of abortions, and an appreciable increase in the number of live foals carried to term and delivered successfully.

Vitamin E combines naturally with selenium, a trace mineral found in the soil and plants. Supplementation of this vitamin-mineral combination, either orally or by injection, has been helpful in the treatment of some muscle diseases in foals and in the well-known myositis in its various forms suffered by competition horses. A schedule of injections (I.M.) of vitamin E and selenium every other week for two months is recommended in these cases. Oral preparations of this vitamin-mineral combination are sometimes fed concurrently with the injections. Your veterinarian's advice should be heeded!

The B-complex vitamins, together with vitamin C, comprise the water-soluble group. B complex vitamins are synthesized inside the horse's intestinal tract (caecum and colon), and consequently they are abundantly available to horses that receive an adequate diet. They are also found in all quality hays and grains. No deficiency in this area can exist unless a gastrointestinal illness alters intestinal function and reduces its efficiency in the synthesis of vitamin B production. Also, a deficiency could possibly develop in the case of a very poor or a near-starvation diet.

Vitamin B_1 (thiamine) deficiency symptoms are nervousness, anorexia, bradycardia, hindquarter weakness, weight loss, and generalized weakness. The slang term "wash-out" describes a phenomenon that sometimes affects race horses upon entering the paddock before a race. The horse suddenly breaks out in a profuse black sweat, begins shaking, and literally "washes out." The great loss of fluids and electrolytes naturally weakens the animal and the race is lost! Along with management corrections and other treatments, massive doses of thiamine are administered with some degree of success. The intramuscular route is safer, since intravenous injections of thiamine have been reported to produce some unexplained reactions. Giving thiamine is a common practice at race tracks to supplement nervous and washy individual horses, although its value has not yet been documented. Both pre- and post-race injections yield inconsistent findings.

A thiamine deficiency is neither easy to identify nor easily differentiated. I would suspect a deficiency of the whole B complex, not just of one specific vitamin.

Vitamin B_1 is found in all quality hay and grain, so a deficiency is unlikely to occur unless the hay and grain are exposed to weather. Environmental conditions can cause a dramatic drop in B_1 content.

Ingestion of bracken fern *(Pteris aquilina)* or mare's tail *(Equisetum arvense)* can produce a thiamine deficiency. Both plants grow freely in pastures and are commonly baled into hay. *See:* PLANT POISONS.

The B complex is stored by the body in the liver. A good dietary supplement source of B complex is dried brewer's yeast. Three tablespoons daily on the grain can meet the daily minimum requirement.

Vitamin B_2, riboflavin, occurs abundantly in all hays and grains. Deficiencies should not arise in a normal environment.

For some time, an undersupply of riboflavin was thought to cause moonblindness (recurrent uveitis) in horses. Current thinking leans toward leptospirosis infection and/or the parasite *Onchocerca cervicalis* as partner offenders in this very old and frustrating disease of the horse's eye and vision.

Vitamin B_{12}, cyanocobalamine, is required for formation of hemoglobin. Here again, the horse forms some of its needed B_{12} in the large colon.

Use of injectable and oral preparations of B_{12} at race tracks is abused and represents a costly, unnecessary item in the majority of cases. B_{12} is thought to settle nervousness, increase appetite, and elevate the hemoglobin content. Although none of this has been proven satisfactorily, I am pleased with the effects of B_{12} when deemed necessary and used in moderation. I regard as criminal the random, promiscuous use of B_{12}, which is a suspected cause of hemorrhaging in race horses. *See:* EPISTAXIS.

Other B complex components are niacin, biotin, choline, folic acid,

vitamins continued

pantothenic acid, and pyridoxine. None of these components should ever present a deficiency problem in the presence of a good diet with accessibility to pasture.

Vitamin C, ascorbic acid, is a water-soluble vitamin abundantly available in the horse's diet. It is also synthesized with great efficiency by the horse's liver. Supplementation of ascorbic acid is a popular practice at race tracks. It is thought to aid in prevention and treatment of "bleeders." *See:* EPISTAXIS.

Vitamin C is also used as a dietary supplement in horses that have slow-healing and chronic wounds. Massive daily doses, used clinically as an adjunct with normal medical treatment of the infection, seem to aid in the healing process. Deep difficult wounds, such as fistulous tracts with networks of honeycomb pockets of infection, in some cases respond to supplemental dietary or injectable ascorbic acid.

water   An important constituent of living matter, essential for its physiologic processes. As a rule of thumb, the requirements are:

Average horse—8 gallons of water per day
Broodmares—10 gallons of water per day
Hardworking horses—15 gallons of water per day

Horse owners are guilty of neglect if they do not provide clean, fresh, and abundant drinking water for their horses, together with free-choice mineralized salt. Both are essential for life.

wheat germ oil   An oil specially processed from wheat germ, which is a natural source of tocopherols possessing vitamin E activity.

Vitamin E is thought to be essential in animals for reproduction, spermatogenesis, and development of the muscular, skeletal, and nervous systems.

On most breeding farms, wheat germ oil is fed to mares and stallions liberally on grain twice daily, starting one month before the beginning of breeding season.

Again, the value of this supplementation is difficult to assess, but I have never observed any untoward results for its use. My personal preference of a supplement for use on a breeding farm is wheat germ oil compound, consisting of vitamins A, D, and E. Each fluid ounce contains 20,000 U.S.P. units of vitamin A and 2,000 U.S.P. units of vitamin D in a wheat germ oil base. The general condition and coat finish of young horses seem to benefit from this preparation. If an animal is fed well, wormed and vaccinated properly, but still has a dull, rough coat, then 1 ounce of wheat germ oil compound fed twice daily over a period of one month should improve its overall condition.

I have found wheat germ oil compound to be very useful also when a yearling develops a splint formation on its legs of unknown etiology. In this case, double the dosage (2 ounces twice daily) and bandage the splint, keeping it warm and protected. Within six weeks, you may be pleasantly surprised.

Wheat germ oil compound has an odor like fish oil that causes most horses, especially the young ones, to turn away. To overcome this, rub the wheat germ oil all over and around the horse's mouth, then smear a coating of it all over and around the feed tub. Then watch them eat!

EMERGENCY SITUATIONS

anaphylaxis   An extreme reaction or hypersensitivity by the body to a foreign substance. Anaphylaxis is the most severe form of an allergic reaction recorded. Its rapid and dramatic onset is seen most often following an intravenous injection. Symptoms are increased respiration, increased heart rate, profuse sweating, anxious expression, dermatitis in the form of wheals and elevations with swellings, especially around the mouth and eyes. Some animals are so changed in appearance that they lose their characteristic shape and take on the appearance of a mulberry.

Bee stings are second only to drugs as the most common cause of anaphylactic reactions.

The dangerous presence of innumerable round swellings can interfere seriously with sight and breathing. *Immediate* medical attention is essential.

artificial respiration   A mechanical method by which air is allowed to enter the respiratory tract when normal breathing has ceased.

A thousand-pound horse does not lend itself well to manual artificial respiration and cardiopulmonary resuscitation (CPR), used so successfully for humans, although CPR and mouth-to-mouth resuscitation can be used quite well to save a foal!

If respiratory difficulty occurs, or if respiration ceases in a horse already in the hospital, modern sophisticated mechanical respirators can be utilized. However, if an adult horse is stricken by respiratory failure in any place other than a hospital, the situation is perilous.

As a heroic effort, under skilled supervision, the following procedure should be attempted:

The horse should be rolled up *onto its back* and steadied in that position. Two strong men will be needed for this. Two others should grasp the abdominal skin *and muscles* and—upon command—strongly *pull up* (creating an internal vacuum) and then release in synchronization. Repeat rhythmically and in unison. This permits the mass of abdominal contents to roll forward, pressing against the diaphragm. This, in turn, creates lung and heart compression and may stimulate normal breathing.

Under no circumstances should this be attempted by amateurs. And under no circumstances should anyone attempt to apply pressure to the rib cage, as in methods applied to humans. The only thing this technique will accomplish with a horse is fracture damage to the ribs.

bee stings   A true hazard, especially to grazing animals whose muzzles inadvertently enter a bees' nest. Toxic wasp and bee venoms act on the central nervous system. The closer to the face and head, the greater the danger. In a

bee stings continued

horse that has been sensitized previously to bee or wasp venom, one more sting may be fatal if it triggers an anaphylactic shock response. *See:* ANAPHYLAXIS.

A first-time encounter that results in many stings can cause respiratory distress which, if untreated, also may result in death.

First aid: Apply copious amounts of isopropyl (rubbing) alcohol; follow with a liberal application of sodium bicarbonate (baking soda) paste.

Your veterinarian may choose to treat with steroids or antihistamines, dictated by the severity of symptoms and the location of the stings.

If the reaction and tissue swellings begin to block oxygen intake, and if respiration becomes labored, then an emergency tracheostomy *must* be performed to save the animal's life. This is a true emergency and must be handled as such! Call your veterinarian!

bloat (gas colic) Abdominal distention from a buildup of intestinal gas, usually caused by fermentation or putrefaction of ingesta. The pain is acute, and unless treatment is immediate and effective, death may result.

Bloat is common in cattle, but when diagnosed in the horse, emergency measures are indicated and the prognosis is guarded. Pain from intestinal gas is so acute that restraint of the patient is essential to prevent self-inflicted damage and injury to the handler.

Treatment is specific. First, an injection of analgesic to reduce pain, followed by a relaxant (Dipyrone); then a stomach tube is introduced to allow the escape of stomach gas (to prevent the stomach wall from rupturing); then, through the stomach tube, the horse is given a colic mixture containing surface-reducing drugs and antiflatulant agents.

In extreme cases, when it can be determined that the caecum is bloated, trocharization is indicated.

This procedure produces dramatic relief in certain cases, but it must be performed by a veterinarian. *See:* COLIC, TROCHARIZATION.

burns Burns can result from a variety of causes: extreme heat, direct body contact with or inhalation of chemicals, electrical current, lightning, and, oddly enough, extreme cold or frostbite. Living tissue cells die and slough away while healing (this healing process is accompanied by an offensive odor).

Instantly following any burn (even though the local area has been treated), it is necessary to attend to the whole patient: All vital functions should be watched closely for any symptom of shock:

> Increased thirst
> Restlessness
> Coldness or clumsiness
> Weakness
> Increased pulse rate
> Ice-cold legs and feet
> Drop in blood pressure
> Paling of mouth or eye membranes

Large, surface burns are more serious than smaller, deeper burns. When an extensive area of protective skin is damaged or destroyed, there is loss of fluids and electrolytes (essential minerals), often followed by secondary infection. This poses a major threat.

All burns should be approached with caution; it is wise to have them assessed by a veterinarian, since their appearance can be misleading to an untrained eye. A burn may seem to be healing nicely, but ten days later, it may present sloughing with renewed tissue destruction. The situation is acute and vulnerable to secondary infection.

Treatment varies with the cause and degree of damage to the area. Burns have been classified into *five degrees:*

1. Painful redness of the skin, scorching
2. Formation of blisters
3. Destruction of the epidermis (outer layer) and exposure of nerve endings
4. Destruction of the dermis (entire skin thickness)
5. Actual charring of the soft tissue and the bony skeleton

Therapy for all burns includes:

1. Strictly controlled asepsis (cleanliness, hygiene)
2. Prevention of shock (veterinarian)
3. Control of infection (veterinarian)
4. Maintenance of patient's nutrition and comfort

First Aid:

1. Cleanse with mild soap and warm water, rinse with sterile saline water (1 teaspoon table salt in 1 quart previously boiled warm water), then bathe and coat the area with 1 tablespoon sodium bicarbonate (baking soda), dissolved in 1 pint warm water.
2. Saturate and cover well with butter, Desitin, A-D-E ointment, or any specific burn ointment.
3. Apply a light gauze dressing.

When a burn is chemically caused, determine whether it was by acid or alkali. Neutralize the chemical and flush well with quantities of water, then treat as for any burn.

To neutralize *acid* burns, flush well with clean water, apply sodium bicarbonate (1 tablespoon baking soda to 1 quart water).

To neutralize *alkali* burns (such as quicklime), flush well with clean water, apply a solution of vinegar and water, half and half.

Tannic acid (from brewed tea) is helpful when applied locally to an area burned by a corrosive chemical.

For *creosol* and *phenol* burns, neutralize and bathe with ethyl (grain) alcohol or castor oil.

Phosphorus burns should be immersed in water immediately. Avoid exposure to air.

Frostbite is the destruction of tissue caused by exposure to extreme cold. Initially the skin is pale with impaired circulation, followed by secondary symptoms of pain, swelling, heat, and redness.

Slight frostbite is treated by warming the affected area and covering with antiseptic ointment and sterile dressings.

burns continued

True frostbite is treated similarly and observed for a line of demarcation differentiating the dead cells from the live cells. The necrotic tissue is removed surgically to prevent infection; with healing, the adjacent healthy tissue characteristically shrinks somewhat.

Although frostbite is quite rare in my area of Pennsylvania, I have treated several cases involving ear tips, lips, and tails, all of which healed well once the dead areas were removed.

choke   The word describes the action. It is a reflex action to force a trapped mass of swallowed food to move either up or down, any place within the long esophagus.

Contrary to bovines, horses seldom choke, but when it happens, you are faced with an emergency situation. Neither the horse's temperament nor its sensitive esophageal tissues can tolerate a lodged mass of food for very long. Symptoms are anxious expression, extension of head and neck with desperate retching motions, and then panic, requiring immediate attention.

Choke is a common ailment in cattle and can be treated in a very satisfactory manner, at any time, even at the veterinarian's convenience, through the courtesy of the bovine's innate physiologic make-up. (This is an excellent illustration of the differences between the equine and the bovine. Their worlds are separate and distinct. Never borrow information from one and apply it to the other, because nothing fits and nothing applies!)

For the horse, choke is a serious condition. If not treated immediately, or if poorly treated, it can lead to death. The equine is affected quickly, panics, and becomes unmanageable, making treatment more difficult. The veterinarian's first concern is prompt removal of the lodged material before damage is sustained to the delicate lining of the esophagus. The condition can then be called severely serious, not fatal. Sedation and gentle massage to encourage disengagement of the trapped mass of food can be tried first. Additional sedation is followed by a stomach tube introduced carefully to deposit oil or other emollients adjacent to the mass. Then, further careful massage may, in some cases, correct the condition.

If these measures are unsuccessful, secondary tissue changes occur that cause swelling and pain, and the prognosis becomes grave.

The only choke cases that I have witnessed have been surgical patients recovering from general anesthesia. If a horse is permitted to eat hay or any bedding before the anesthetic drugs have dissipated well, choke is a real possibility and you can be thrown into an emergency situation in a few seconds. Until all the anesthetic drugs have completely cleared from the system, the horse's ability to swallow is quite inefficient. The animal develops a ravenous appetite before it is fully able to chew or swallow, and this presents a real hazard. To avoid this potential tragedy, someone must stand with the postsurgical patient for as long as necessary to keep the horse from trying to eat before it is physiologically able. It requires approximately one and a half hours after the surgical patient regains its feet and postural attitude for salivary flow and swallowing reflexes to safely function. By hand feeding one small stem of hay as a trial, carefully followed by a second small amount, one can be certain that full function and ability to masticate and swallow have returned.

I have often pondered over the innate picky eating preferences of the horse, compared to other species. Perhaps its reluctance to eat any but certain selected foods is responsible for the low incidence of choke among horses.

NOTE: Do not confuse choke, which occurs in the esophagus (passage to the stomach) with accidental aspiration (breathing in) of foodstuffs into the trachea (windpipe). Both are critical conditions and cause the horse to react with panicky, violent, self-destructive behavior. Call your veterinarian.

dehydration   A condition that results from excessive loss of body fluids, judged as a 20 percent loss of body weight. In my experience, dehydration is the constant companion of most disease conditions. It is associated foremost with diarrhea, fevers, hemorrhage, and sweating.

Simple dehydration is caused by lack of water intake (grown horses require ten to 12 gallons daily, more if they are exercising strenuously). If, for any reason, a horse stops drinking, if it cannot drink due to some bodily malfunction, or if water is not available, then it can readily suffer from simple dehydration.

Electrolyte imbalance inevitably accompanies dehydration. Fluid and electrolyte replacement, orally or intravenously, is the duty of the veterinarian, who must recognize the need and then determine the type, amount, and route of administration—being extremely careful as to the rate of flow!

No horse should ever be allowed to suffer from dehydration. When it occurs, it reflects on the quality of care and attention the horse is getting. Frequently the victims are animals that have been sent out to compete before they are sufficiently fit and able to meet the physical requirements or energy demands of the performance!

Keep a mineralized salt lick accessible to all horses to ensure electrolyte balance.

electric shock   Great concern is always shown for turned-out horses during thunder and lightning storms, and rightly so! I have answered many an early morning call and found a dead horse, usually under a tree, with evidence of charring on the body and seared grass on the wet ground nearby.

While we are aware that the hazards of lightning run high in pastured horses, I wonder if we are sufficiently conscious of another killer—the insidious and not-so-dramatic electrical outlet. Water is a marvelous conductor of electric current, so it is essential to keep stalls dry and to see that all wires, plugs, and sockets are covered and out of reach of a curious muzzle.

Death ensues spontaneously by electric shock. The nerves in the body and extremities conduct the electric current to the central nervous system, resulting in cardiac and respiratory arrest.

At the famous Devon Horse Show, one year the customary deluge of rain began, and because of poor drainage, some stalls flooded with rain water. Fine horses were standing in water over their pasterns and ankles. One young, inquisitive horse reached over the stall door and touched an electric socket with its nose. The shock killed the animal in less time than it takes to tell the story.

Check over all your electrical and grounding arrangements and be sure that this kind of tragic accident cannot happen in your barn.

euthanasia   The act of putting animals to sleep in a painless, humane fashion, then allowing them to slip into a quiet death. There are many drugs available for purposes of euthanasia, but an overdose of barbiturates intravenously is the unequalled method. Solutions of magnesium sulfate combined with strychnine sulfate or diluted hydrocyanic acid are inadequate, cruel, and fortunately outmoded.

The only times I have ever regretted being a veterinarian were those occasions when I was asked to put down a young or healthy animal. Owners do have that right, and it behooves us to provide this service.

fatigue   Exhaustion of a horse's strength caused by severe, overly extended, or prolonged exertion.

I, along with many others, believe that fatigue is the prime and basic cause of severe injury to both our young and older race horses today. The tendons and ligaments of the horse have a built-in compensatory mechanism that prevents damage during moderate or even semisevere exertion. When a horse is pushed to go beyond its preparedness level and beyond its "second wind," the tendons, ligaments, and muscles are stripped of the protective buffer zone. Exhaustion develops, damage occurs, and too often irreparable harm results.

A good race horse trainer will not permit this to happen!

fever   The elevation of body temperature above the established norm.

In the case of a slight fever of unknown etiology, call your veterinarian, who will determine the cause and treat the condition.

In an emergency situation, where the body temperature reaches 104° or over, while waiting for professional help, carry out the following measures:

1. Bathe or hose with tepid water or isopropyl alcohol and scrape dry
2. Place ice pack at base of skull
3. Administer cold-water enema
4. Place in a cool shelter
5. If chilled, cover with blankets
6. Stand in cool water to prevent founder

The veterinarian will probably administer fluids intravenously to reduce the fever, determine the cause and institute appropriate therapy. *See:* HEAT STROKE.

hemorrhage   A profuse flow of blood. Administer first aid while waiting for professional help. Apply direct pressure on the area. Use clean materials—a large wad of gauze or cotton is ideal. Direct pressure is the most effective and safest method of controlling hemorrhage if the location of blood loss permits. Cold is hemostatic, so if ice is available, crack or crush and place the ice in a bag or towel and hold directly against the bleeding area.

In minor weeping of blood, powders can be helpful since they aid in coagulation. Dusting powder, talcum, flour, powdered alum, or even—in an emergency—a handful of cobwebs, usually found at arm's length, can be held firmly against the leaking vessels. Old-timers sometimes used a large chew of tobacco to stanch the flow.

These suggestions may save a life while you are waiting for veterinary assistance. In any case, do something! Don't just stand there and allow the life-sustaining fluid to flow away uninterrupted while you are waiting for help.

In cases of severe hemorrhage, such as a ruptured or open vessel with uncontrollable blood loss, a tourniquet is the only salvation. Obviously, the use of a tourniquet is limited to the limbs, so if the loss of blood is located on the legs, bind a tourniquet around the leg above the bleeding area. This should reduce the loss of arterial blood from the heart, but it will not affect the leaking of venous blood from the wound or open area.

A tourniquet can be made from an old inner tube by cutting a piece several inches wide and 2 feet long. Proceed carefully! Observe the rate of flow and tighten only to effect control. Do not permit the tourniquet to remain in position for too long or tissue will be deprived of essential oxygen and die. Release ever so slightly every few minutes to allow a minute escape of blood and then retighten the tourniquet. Although the use of a tourniquet is often a lifesaving practice, in unskilled hands, a tourniquet can do considerable harm. *See:* EPISTAXIS, POSTPARTUM PROBLEMS, SILENT BLEEDER.

heat stroke (heat exhaustion, hyperthermia)   The usual causes of heat stroke in horses are: physical exertion beyond the animal's level of fitness; temperatures of 100° Fahrenheit and above; confinement in a small, hot, humid area; or standing in the sun at high temperatures. Inadequate water and salt intake also contribute to the development of heat stroke.

Under stress, a malfunction of the body's heat-regulating mechanism (hypothalamus) is believed to cause the high body temperature that characterizes heat stroke. With extremely high temperature, the peripheral skin vessels dilate and cause circulatory collapse. Once circulatory shock occurs, death usually ensues.

To treat, hose with tepid water all over the horse's body and place the feet in ice to help restore blood volume. Provide drinking water and ventilation. Place an emergency call to your veterinarian. The veterinarian will undoubtedly administer fluids intravenously and an injection to combat stress. Ideally, one liter of 10 percent saline and 5 percent dextrose, intravenously repeated every one-half hour for four doses, has been beneficial in some severe heat stroke victims.

Prevention is quite easy: Just keep your horse as cool and comfortable as you yourself like to be on extremely hot days!

inhalation therapy   Consists of an oxygen supply additional to atmospheric oxygen administered to the patient either through a mask or through tubes placed directly into the trachea. Oxygen flow is regulated at liters-per-minute and the prescribed rate depends upon the size, weight, age, and condition warranting the need for additional oxygen.

Inhalation therapy in the form of humidifiers, steamers, and some commercial aerosols can be helpful in temporary relief of respiratory distress or discomfort from any cause (e. g., allergic reaction, accumulated discharges from a respiratory infection, or a chronic breathing problem).

A small portable oxygen tank is part of the average equine practitioner's equipment today, and it does duty especially during the foaling season. Newborn foals are prone to suffer a delayed or sluggish respiratory response at birth and frequently they develop pneumonia and respiratory infections. At such times an oxygen unit, properly equipped with sterile disposable tubes and masks, is a vital and busy instrument. These foals respond well to oxygen supplementation.

I have found that a mask seems to terrify most horses, so when inhalation therapy is required, I use a small endotracheal tube inserted through the nose.

inhalation therapy continued

This method is much smoother and provokes much less resistance. The rate of oxygen flow can vary from one liter per minute in a foal to ten liters per minute for adult horses.

Antibiotic and expectorant aerosols are used in adult horses suffering excessive congestion and nasal discharge, usually as the result of a respiratory illness.

Medicated steam, administered through a large sac that covers the horse's nose or entire head, is very effective to clear, dry, and clean up a sinus drip or an upper respiratory infection.

A long time ago, when I was competing at horse shows every week, I owned and rode an open jumper with a chronic sinus condition and pulmonary alveolar emphysema. She was a small, courageous mare who had suffered a severe case of strangles at a young age and had not received the proper care and attention during her illness. The *Strep equi* continued for months to damage her respiratory tract, and as a result she sustained chronic sinusitis, pharyngitis, and intermittent guttural pouch drainage.

Religiously, each Saturday, I would place a mixture of camphor and eucalyptus oil in a small electric steamer and cover the entire apparatus with several huge and heavy feed sacks. Then I would coax my mare into position and cover her nose with the sacks up to a point just below her eyes (protecting the eyes from vapor). She would always complain by moaning softly, but after eight or ten good, deep whiffs, we would promptly load on the trailer and go off to the competition. I have never ridden a greater jumper in my life!

snakebite   In some of the remote areas of the United States, poisonous snakes present problems for grazing horses. Surprisingly, the number of snake bites reported each year continues to remain fairly high, in spite of our "built-up" environment.

Snakes become active during warm summer months while horses are actively grazing. The most common snakes in the United States are pit vipers, which include rattlesnakes, copperheads, and moccasins whose venom is destructive to tissue, causing large swellings that later slough away while healing.

Of this group, rattlesnakes are the largest and most aggressive, with the smaller, more secretive copperheads and moccasins responsible for fewer attacks.

Grazing horses are invariably bitten around the head, mainly because their noses are busy exploring at ground level. A large rattler can deposit a lethal volume of venom in one strike; the closer the site of the bite to the head, the more critical the case may be. The ensuing tissue swelling around the nasal cavity can threaten blockage and agitate the helpless horse. Remember, the horse can breathe only through the nasal canal, never through the mouth. When anything impairs nasal patency, the horse's life is in danger. Collapse follows suffocation.

Immediate veterinary attention is imperative:

1. Clear all airways if possible.
2. In severe cases where oxygen is critically reduced, a tracheostomy is required (by veterinarian).

3. Injections of cortisone or cortisone by-products are valuable to reduce inflammation and swelling.

4. Antivenom preparations, though expensive, are vital for survival in some snakebite cases; best as local injections into the bite areas.

5. Antitoxin against other serious bacteria will help defend against contaminants known to exist in poisonous snake venom.

6. Fluid therapy is given to restore lost fluids and electrolytes.

7. Antibiotic therapy is wise to prevent secondary infection. This is especially important during the sloughing stage.

8. Small incisions are carefully made in the swelling and suction applied. This must be performed shortly after the bite in order to be of any value.

9. A tourniquet may be applied if the bite is sustained on the limbs (*not* on the head).

Like their colleagues, the physicians, veterinarians in snake-infested country should keep a supply of antivenom handy. The quickness of treatment often decides the outcome!

transfusion There are two types of transfusions in horse practice: whole-blood transfusions and plasma transfusions.

A whole-blood transfusion is a lifesaving procedure but is not without its dangers. It is most useful in accident cases where large volumes of blood have been lost or in diseases that have left the patient exhausted and depleted of red blood cells (erythrocytes), white blood cells (leucocytes), and immune bodies (gamma globulins). Red blood cells are the main source of danger in a transfusion. They are coated with antigens that can react with incompatible and hostile antibodies floating in the serum of the recipient. If incompatible red blood cells are transfused, a severe and life-threatening situation can occur through an allergic or anaphylactic reaction. Please understand the dire importance of blood-typing and cross-matching of both the donor and recipient to ensure compatibility. Blood types A negative and Q negative have been established as universal donors and can be used with both safety and impunity.

Unlike whole-blood transfusions, plasma transfusions are free of circulating red blood cells and are desirable in equine practice. They can restore the circulating blood volume and supply clotting factors and lost immune globulins without the risk encountered in a whole-blood transfusion. Plasma is produced by the simple removal of the red blood cells, either by gravitation or centrifugation in the laboratory.

In foals suffering an immune deficiency, due either to congenital or hereditary factors, or to failure of passive transfer of maternal antibodies, a plasma transfusion (500 to 1,000 cc) can provide the antibodies and necessary immune globulins for survival.

trocharization The word *emergency* should always precede the word *trocharization*, especially in the horse. The procedure involves the insertion of a sharp, pointed instrument in order to effect the release of gas. Although it is almost routine in cow practice, the equine practitioner does not embark on trocharization unless it is absolutely a matter of life or death. Since horses are prone to peritonitis, the need must warrant the risk.

Most veterinarians carry a sterile pack ready for such an urgent situation. The reason for trocharization is a condition of bloat or gas buildup in the

trocharization continued

intestines—the caecum, principally. Site for trocharization is on the horse's right side over the paralumbar space, the hollow cavity immediately in front of the hip and just behind the last rib. This area is quickly clipped, shaved, and vigorously scrubbed and flushed. In the final seconds before the procedure, an iodine preparation with alcohol is applied, then dried with sterile sponges.

Equine practice uses a trochar specially designed for the horse. After a small amount of local anesthetic is injected at the site, the trochar is pushed through the thick, durable skin, subcuticular tissue, muscle layers, peritoneum, and ultimately, through the distended wall of the gas-filled caecum. A sudden burst of gas, odor, and moisture is released.

The trochar can be secured into place by gauze and tape wrapped around the abdomen. Antiflatulent drugs or surface-reducing agents (Cerusol) can be introduced through the trochar directly into the caecum. By this method, any additional production of flatulence or gas can escape over a period of hours; the trochar can later be removed at the discretion of the attending veterinarian.

After removal, tamed iodine (Lugol's Solution) should be applied to the skin area and covered with a taped-on sterile pack to keep out air-borne contaminants.

The horse's temperature should be taken twice daily for seven days and recorded on a chart for the convenience of your veterinarian. Tetanus Toxoid and daily antibiotics for a few days will probably suffice to protect your horse from possible peritonitis.

STABLE MEDICINE BOX

Absorbine   A commercially prepared liniment, primarily used on a horse's muscles and legs under bandages prior to competition or after hard use. *See:* LINIMENT.

alcohol   Ethyl alcohol, which is distilled from grains, fruits, and starches. Used internally as a soother of the stomach lining, nutrient, and sedative. For massage purposes it is applied externally. It serves also as an antiseptic for the hide and is a circulatory stimulant; 6 ounces of isopropyl (70 percent alcohol) in a pail of warm water produces a relaxing "brace" to wash down a competition horse. Alcohol also serves as a solvent for drugs in tincture form.

alum   Aluminum ammonium sulfate in dried or burned form is a major ingredient found in most astringent powders used to control bleeding or to inhibit excessive granulation of wounds (proud flesh).

aluminum acetate solution (Burow's Solution)   A colorless fluid containing 5 percent aluminum acetate used for its astringent and antiseptic properties. Applied as a wet dressing (10 parts of water) to soothe and cool inflamed tissue, swellings, and burns.

CAUTION: Keep dampened at all times or remove. Do not allow to dry while on the area or heat will be produced! *See:* WHITE LOTION TABLETS.

ammonia   A gaseous compound produced by bacterial action upon protein. It was discovered originally as rock salt resulting from camel dung deposits in Egypt.

Ammonium compounds serve a number of purposes, such as expectorants, acidifiers, antiseptics, disinfectants, and fungicidals.

Aromatic spirits of ammonia (smelling salts) is made of ammonia gas mixed with alcohol and certain aromatics. For use by human beings to prevent fainting, a crushed ampule can be placed in a tissue and held below the nostrils. Although it is valueless in horse care, I have carried a few ampules in the side pocket of my black bag since I began my practice. Although I have never needed the drug for my patient, I have not infrequently broken an ampule into a small towel and averted a human crisis. Often a faintheaded horse holder has needed attention before I could proceed with my equine patient.

anise (anisum)   This old-fashioned remedy is both aromatic and carminative (a gastric pacifier or stomach tonic). Oral administration helps ease colic or gastric distress: 5 drops of this oil placed on the tongue can often relieve a horse's distress in minor cases. Any amateur can administer this.

antiphlogistics   Substances that counteract fever and inflammation. In order to reduce inflammatory conditions, the application of poultices, wet dressings soaked in antiphlogistic agents, and "hosing" are recommended.

Antiphlogistics include: Bowie Mud®, Denver Mud®, Unna's paste®, bentonite powder, Antiphlogistine Paste®, and fuller's earth.

Don't forget to hose with tepid-to-cool water.

army whitewash   *See:* WHITEWASH.

arsenical solution (white arsenic, Fowler's Solution)   A white or transparent highly poisonous substance. It is toxic for human beings and lethal to most carnivores. Herbivores, such as horses, sheep, and cows, seem to tolerate minute amounts, but *do not* make the mistake of administering it to milking cows!

Contrary to the reaction of other animals, horses dramatically improve when Fowler's Solution is used to treat dermatitis and gastrointestinal disturbances. This drug is a superb stomachic and intestinal tonic in horses.

Used cautiously, Fowler's Solution can be added to your horse's daily ration of grain. Dosage: 8 to 10 drops on the grain each day for a thousand-pound animal. Daily minute amounts are palatable and will result in improved appetite, weight gain, and a glossy, healthy coat.

Although horses of any kind improve with this medicine, I routinely prescribe it for my geriatric cases and am always pleased with the results. *See:* STRYCHNINE.

asafetida   A gum resin from the root of *Ferula foetida*, it has been used in human medicine for many years as an antispasmodic, antiflatulant, and a central nervous system sedative.

Before the use of tranquilizers and modern sedatives became widespread, the average trainer, working with a high-strung, sometimes spoiled animal, had little to help him other than daily repetitious schooling and disciplinary tactics.

I remember one very neurotic filly from years back. Her future was doubtful; she seemed unable to cope with the routines of galloping and conditioning. Not only was it difficult to ride her from the barn to the track, but her behavior on the racing surface was so erratic that it endangered everyone. The frustrated trainer suddenly remembered what an old horseman had told him about such problem animals. That very day he visited the local drug store, purchased some asafetida and began his new daily routine.

Each morning I watched him soak a 1-inch gauze roll of bandage in the asafetida solution, then carefully wrap the entire bit. I then had the doubtful honor of riding this filly.

To my astonishment, she improved steadily. One afternoon I returned to the barn and found her with a chifney (a breaking, "pacifier" bit with three keys attached, used for babies) snapped to her halter. It was well wrapped with asafetida-saturated gauze. She was peaceful, but the gauze wrap could be smelled many feet away from her stall!

She made it to the big tracks and finally broke her maiden after seven second-place finishes. The hussy could run!

astringent (styptic)   An agent that causes constriction of tissues, arrests secretions, and produces tropical control of the specific area of bleeding. Examples: dried alum, potash alum, silver nitrate, copper sulfate, ferric chloride, lead acetate, tannic acid, zinc sulfate, and aluminum acetate solution (Burow's Solution).

ball A slang term for a large pill or bolus, about the size of a hickory nut, used to administer medicines, usually cathartics (laxatives), or anthelmentics (worm medicines). *See:* BALLING GUN.

balling gun A metal syringe about 18 inches long with a pocket at one end in which to load the medicinal ball (pill). At the other end is a strong plunger that is operated to propel the ball well into the horse's large oral cavity. It can be used without difficulty by an average-size individual.

The balling gun has been in use for years in spite of the hazards its use presents. Instead of swallowing the ball, the horse may chew it up, causing burning and irritation of the mucous membranes. Or the ball may accidentally lodge in the esophagus and even enter the windpipe (trachea), in which case the horse may choke, gag, and show great discomfort. In fact, inexpert use of the gun could cause fatal damage to the horse. The balling gun must be used carefully, with skill.

Fortunately, the stomach tube has replaced the dangerous and antiquated gun. Today this technique should be restricted to use by a veterinarian.

bandages There are many types of bandages, each of which serves a specific function. (For medical bandages, *see:* DRESSINGS.)

Some examples of bandages:

Standing bandages are used basically while the horse is in the stall at rest after application of a light brace or alcohol. Wound around the leg between knee and ankle in fore leg and between hock and ankle on hind leg, the bandage is comprised of flannel 6 inches wide and approximately 12 feet long (usually torn to preferred size) and rolled over 4 to 6 sheets of shipping cotton.

Shipping bandages are comprised of the same materials as the standing bandage, but their function is that of protecting the leg while the animal is being transported. This bandage should extend from just below the knee in the fore leg down over the coronary band. On the hind leg, it should begin just below the hock and extend down over the coronary band.

Run-down bandages are used during competition to provide protection for the tissues in the posterior underneath portion of the ankle, which can suffer burning due to excessive speed, stress, and overextension of the limb while on the track surface. This can occur with equal frequency in all four limbs.

Spider bandages, also called many-tailed bandages, are almost specifically used to bandage the knee where even pressure and protection are desired. The spider bandage serves well by preventing pressure-caused necrosis in tender areas, especially over the accessory carpal bone, located at the back of the knee.

Never bandage a horse's knee or hock with a conventional bandage.

Poultice bandage, see: POULTICE.

bentonite Derived from a clay found in the western United States, bentonite (U.S.P.) is used internally for treatment of diarrhea and externally for skin disorders. It is the most common ingredient in modern poultice powder mixtures. *See:* ANTIPHLOGISTICS, POULTICE.

blister A sac or collection of fluid beneath the epidermal layer of skin. In the human, it characteristically develops on a "soft" or unused hand after hard (and unaccustomed) work.

blister continued

In the equine, a blister can occur in this form, but it is indeed rare. *Blister,* in the horse world, is the term used to describe the application of a counterirritant. This is an agent or substance that, once applied externally, causes mild to severe inflammation of the skin in order to produce an acute inflammation where a chronic condition exists. Blisters are often applied to bucked shins, osselets, strained knees, flexor tendons, and suspensory ligaments.

The strength of the preparation, the method of application, and/or the use of bandages determine the degree of tissue response and the blister's overall effectiveness. Counterirritants, or blisters, range in strength from very mild (almost a brace) to quite severe.

Blisters consist of liquids, pastes, or internal injections, and their effects are determined by the contents and techniques of application. The standard ingredients are iodine, cantharides, croton oil, red mercury, camphor, creosote, acetic acid, turpentine, pine tar, boric acid, silver iodide, menthol, methyl salicylate, potassium iodide, chloroform, and mercuric chloride, each in a soothing and buffered base.

CAUTION: Before starting on a course of blistering, be sure to consult a professional for the well-known lists of *do*'s and *don'ts*! Use of a cradle, sedation, clipping, greasing tender areas well, and proper application of bandages (if required) are but a few aspects of this technique.

It is often said that the success of blistering is owed not so much to what blister was used or how it was applied, but to the enforced period of rest or the period of time the horse is allowed to remain away from the rigors that produced the condition primarily and the ensuing soreness.

Commercial blister preparations: Ball's Solution®, McTarnahan's®, Bone Radiol®, Harvey's Embrocation®, Lambert's Irish Reducine®, M.A.C.® Counter-irritant, McKays Blister®, Royal Embrocation®, and Savoss Liniment®.

Internal blisters are administered by veterinarians and usually consist of a tamed iodine preparation in a soothing base of sesame or peanut oil.

Blue Lotion   A very common and very popular antiseptic used to cover any and all abrasions or small irritated areas. Made of methylene blue dye in an alcohol base.

CAUTION: Blue Lotion is good to use on surface wounds, but *never* apply it to a wound of any depth. It has a drying tendency and can cause the surface to close prematurely. Also, do not use it near eyes, ears, mouth, anus, vulva, or prepuce.

boric acid (boracic acid)   A white or colorless crystal or powder, soluble in water. Best known for use in skin and ocular infections as a 2 to 3 percent solution (dissolve one teaspoon in one pint warm water).

If mixed with water of questionable purity or in a dirty container, the results of treatment are varied or inconsistent. For this reason, boric acid as an antiseptic has been judged unfairly. This old remedy has losts its popularity to the more modern, safe, and efficient eye-ointment preparations.

brace   A very mild liniment that gives tone to the body when applied externally. Brisk manual application increases general circulation and blood supply locally.

I am convinced that the benefit derived from the application of a brace is from the manual stimulation of the circulation and not at all from the ingredients of the brace. EXAMPLES: acetone, acetone-menthol-thymol, alcohol (ethyl of isopropyl), ammonia, camphor, chloroxylenol, menthol, oil of wintergreen (methylsalicylate), thymol, turpentine and glycerine, wormwood (oil of chenopodium).

Burow's Solution   *See:* ALUMINUM ACETATE SOLUTION.

cough medicine   *Ethylene diamine dihydroiodide* is a very popular antitussive and expectorant drug for horses with chronic cough, nasal discharge, or a general respiratory low-grade infection. Also used as an iodine supplement in geographic areas known to be iodine-deficient.

Dosage: young horse, 10 grains three times a day; adult horse, 20 grains three times a day. Schedule for feeding is ten days on, five days off, ten days on, until there is improvement.

If eyes begin to tear (signs of moisture on skin of face), or if the coat becomes rough, discontinue use of this powder and consult your veterinarian. Such symptoms are considered to be signs of "iodinism." *See:* EXPECTORANTS.

counterirritants (blisters; paints)   These are agents that cause skin irritation or inflammation and are designed to change a chronic state into an acute condition. Examples: black mustard, camphor, croton oil, iodine, menthol, red mercuric iodide, and turpentine. *See:* BLISTER.

Dairmol   A good antiseptic mild enough to use on skin, mucous membranes, and wounds. Its active ingredients are: potash soap, camphor, thymol, naphthalene, and ethyl alcohol.

Dairmol serves as a superb antiseptic for all gynecologic procedures, and makes a superior wet dressing for wounds or areas suspected of possible contamination.

Unexcelled as a deodorant, lubricant, and cleanser, Dairmol is almost guaranteed to be found in every equine practitioner's medicine bag.

Dakin's Solution   *See:* SODIUM HYPOCHLORITE SOLUTION.

diluted acetic acid   *See:* VINEGAR.

disinfectant for stalls   Carbolic acid is a good disinfectant for stalls, stables, and trailers. To disinfect after a disease process of fungal infection, mix one pint carbolic acid with one bucket limewash. First scrub stalls and floors with an iodine compound or Lysol. Allow to dry and then paint walls and ceilings with the carbolic acid/limewash mixture. *See:* WHITEWASH.

drenching   An old-fashioned, inefficient, and sometimes dangerous method of administering liquid medicines orally. When drenching, medicines should be diluted to prevent irritation to the delicate lining of the pharynx, larynx, and esophagus.

A dose syringe or long-necked plastic bottle is introduced into the interdental space (between the corner incisor and the first molar, where the bit fits) while the head is held high. Give no more than *4 fluid ounces* at one time, then quickly lower the head so that the horse can swallow.

Do not allow anyone to tie a horse's head up for drenching reasons! Because *drenching continued*

the soft palate cannot elevate itself while the head is in this "held-up" position, swallowing is impossible and aspiration of the fluid into the trachea and possibly into the lungs will result, with aspiration pneumonia as a possible consequence.

I have watched many a groom stretch and struggle to elevate a huge horse's head while attempting to give an oral drench. Usually these men are ex-jockeys, gentlemen riders, or just naturally short. The horse always has the last say.

I gave up the drench and the ball gun years ago and now always use my small, trusty, and gentle stomach tube. Its efficiency is unmatched!

Epson salts *See:* MAGNESIUM SULFATE.

expectorants Drugs that facilitate the liquefaction and expulsion of mucus from the respiratory tract. Examples: ammonium chloride, benzoin, ethylene diamine dihydroiodide, eucalyptus oil, glycerol guiacolate, creosote, pine tar, potassium iodide, and turpentine oil. One or more of these expectorants are found in most cough preparations.

Fowler's Solution *See:* ARSENICAL SOLUTION.

Furacion A synthetic nitrofuran highly effective against most bacteria commonly causing surface infections, including some that have become resistant to antibiotics.

Glauber's Salt *See:* SODIUM SULFATE.

glycerine A transparent trihydric alcohol obtained from fatty acids and as a by-product in soapmaking. It is useful in cosmetics and explosives, but its use in the horse as a leg sweat is unparalleled.

If previously warmed, glycerine can be massaged well into any soft-tissue swelling. Cover the area after massage with a small piece of sheet cotton, then follow with a layer of something impermeable (e.g., oiled silk, Saran Wrap), and finish off with a liberal cotton roll and a bandage.

Glycerine is mild, it softens and never threatens to scurf, and it produces a good, reliable, and safe sweat. You can mix equal parts of Listerine and glycerine and use in the same manner with equal results.

heavy liquid petrolatum *See:* LIQUID PETROLATUM.

iodine Used as an antiseptic and fungicide. A trace element, iodine comes as bluish black crystals, almost insoluble in water as a solution but highly soluble in alcohol as a tincture. A very popular ingredient as a counterirritant in paints, blisters, and even in injection form as an internal blister.

By combining potassium iodide progressively with iodine crystals, the solubility of iodine is increased to as much as 18 to 20 percent. This much stronger preparation is especially helpful when treating thrush or fungal infections in the feet.

In the Great Lakes and Rocky Mountain regions, dietary iodine deficiencies are responsible for goiter in livestock. Iodine deficiency also causes hairlessness and abortions. Iodides are fed daily on feeds, and sometimes Lugol's Solution is painted on the skin of goiter victims. An iodized salt lick, provided "free choice" to livestock, usually answers the vital need for this trace element.

A strong iodine solution (5 percent aqueous solution or Lugol's Solution) is a standard antiseptic for navel submersion in the newborn foal and is useful for postpartum flushing of the vagina and uterus.

Tincture of iodine (U.S.P.) is usually 2 percent and serves well as an antiseptic. Strong tincture of iodine (U.S.P.) (7 percent) is used as an effective topical skin treatment for dermatitis, ringworm (fungal), or any minor external irritation. The antidote is milk or eggs. *See:* COUGH MEDICINES, IODINATED CASEIN.

isopropyl alcohol (N.F.) Used as an antiseptic and for massage purposes to stimulate increased blood supply to the area. An important ingredient in all braces, liniments, and compounds used for cooling out, under wraps, or in mild paints. It is also an antipruritic, used to stop itch from minor skin irritations. Toxic if taken internally.

itch ointment Combine: ½ pound melted lard, 1 tablespoon sulfur, 1 tablespoon coal oil (kerosene), and 1 tablespoon Lysol. Apply to areas of pruritis once daily, or as needed.

kidney tablets *See:* METHENAMINE.

leg paint The formula is: 120 cc tincture of iodine (7 percent), 30 cc turpentine, 30 cc glycerine.

liniment A pharmacopoeial preparation consisting of a solution of a medicant either in alcohol, oil, or water. It is best applied by friction to the skin in the form of massage.

Liniments vary in strength from weak to borderline "blisters." The desired effect depends upon the dilation of capillaries, which is governed by the amount of vigorous massage applied.

Commercial preparations: Absorbine®, Bigeloil®, Kincades®, Tuttle's Elexer®, Vetrolin®, and White Liniment®.

Liniments can also serve as a brace for use after exercise. Alcohol or witch hazel, diluted in a pail of warm water, helps to soothe and relax sore, tense muscles and prevent stiffness. (Witch hazel only: 2 ounces to a gallon of water; alcohol only: 2 ounces to a gallon of water; equal parts witch hazel and alcohol; 2 ounces to a gallon of water.) Not only does this act as a body- and muscle-stimulant, but its antiseptic properties aid the skin and coat and contribute to overall sound hygiene.

CAUTION: Liniment has a tendency to dry the coat if used daily, so restrict its use to after strenuous exercise only.

Here are two standby stable remedies:

Soap liniment: 4 tablespoons soft soap, 2 tablespoons strong liquid ammonia, 4 pints water. Boil the water and dissolve the soap in the water. Cool the preparation and then add the ammonia.

Another: volatile oil, camphor, soap liniment; this combination has been used for years as a reliable preparation in varying proportions to suit the trainer's preference.

liquid petrolatum Heavy-grade white mineral oil; a colorless, oily liquid insoluble in water. Used as a lubricant and softening agent in constipation, gastrointestinal upset, flatulence (gas), and as an emollient in cases of diarrhea.

Heavy liquid petrolatum is the only proper type of mineral oil to use internally in the horse when treating colic or any intestinal disorder. A danger exists when a lighter-weight, less expensive product is substituted. This inferior product is sometimes absorbed through the intestinal wall, causing an assimilation inefficiency. Mineral oil should not be administered daily, on a continual low-dose basis. This also interferes with normal assimilation and *liquid petrolatum continued*

indirectly causes nutritional imbalances. A proper diet, including adequate roughage, together with normal exercise, in most cases precludes the need for lubricants placed in feeds. In conclusion, mineral oil should be administered only during illnesses or on the advice of your veterinarian.

magnesium sulfate (Epsom salts)   An active saline laxative, anti-inflammatory if applied locally on the skin, anesthetic if injected intravenously. Also used in euthanasia. (One liter of supersaturated magnesium sulfate, administered I.V. with a 14 or 16 g needle for rapid infusion, will effectively euthanize a thousand-pound animal. Although this is a readily available drug and quite inexpensive, I prefer the use of irreversible barbiturate solutions. They are very smooth, very humane, and effective.)

Although it is an old-fashioned remedy, Epsom salts is a very useful drug and I keep it handy at all times.

medicine chest   A well-stocked and well-maintained medicine box is essential in every barn, van, or trailer. Wherever the horse goes, a suitable medicine chest should follow. In the barn, please keep it high on the wall out of children's reach; for added insurance, keep it locked. Please consult your veterinarian before stocking the chest. The following list is not complete, but it may serve as an outline:

- 1 pint colic medicine (from veterinarian)
- 1 pint chill medicine (from veterinarian)
- 5 pounds Epsom salts (magnesium sulfate)
- 2 pounds Glauber's Salts (sodium sulfate)
- 1 pound table salt (sodium chloride)
- antibiotic ointment for wounds
- antiseptic ointment for minor abrasions
- topical antiseptic spray (Blue Vitriol)
- fly or insect spray
- poultice powder for swellings after hosing or soaking in a tub
- thrush medicine
- Vaseline® for general use
- caustic powder to prevent excessive granulation
- rubbing alcohol or witch hazel
- iodine (tincture or solution), consult your veterinarian
- large animal thermometer, at least 5 inches long (for safety's sake, tie a thin, strong string with a clothespin attached to the other end of the thermometer)
- sterile gauze dressing
- sterile gauze bandages
- tape (adhesive)
- section of rubber inner tube for use as a tourniquet

Injectables should be left to the judgment of your veterinarian. They require refrigeration and so have no rightful place in a medicine chest. Although sedatives are frequently required, they are best left in the hands of your veterinarian.

Respect drugs for their actions and possible reactions. If you treat your horse in the manner in which you would like to be treated, you will not use cheap, outdated, chemically degraded, or questionable preparations. Trust your veterinarian.

methenamine (kidney tablets)   Urinary antiseptic; a white crystalline powder, highly soluble in water.

Methenamine tablets are a convenient form of treatment for urinary tract infections in the horse. The large, white tablets, available over the counter, can readily be placed into the water pail. Dosage is usually one tablet in drinking water twice daily for seven to ten days.

CAUTION: If the horse fails to drink the entire pail of water, do not empty the contents left in the bottom of the pail; this drug concentrates in the residue, so just add some water to dilute the remainder and perhaps the horse will then finish the contents. (Grooms have a habit of throwing away any water left, cleaning the pails and refilling. Some horses will reluctantly drink to a precise level and then stop, especially when the water has been adulterated with a drug.)

I recommend this regime to be followed twice a year as a health-maintenance practice for competition horses, especially geldings.

Milk of Magnesia   A white aqueous suspension of approximately 8 percent magnesium hydroxide, used as an antacid, antidote, and laxative. Helpful in hyperacidity and flatulence in the gastrointestinal tract.

Constipation is a major problem in the newborn foal and warrants a watchful eye. I have relied upon Milk of Magnesia for routine treatment in foals during constipation, hyperacidity, impaction, and even diarrhea. The incorporation of a small amount of Milk of Magnesia in milk, medication, or any other substance can be beneficial and vital to the health of the neonate's gastrointestinal tract. An oral preparation, Milk of Magnesia should be administered with an oral syringe or via a stomach tube.

mineral oil   *See:* LIQUID PETROLATUM.

Naquasone (trichlormethiazide, dexamethasone)   Although the Naquasone boluses are large and difficult to swallow, this oral diuretic continues to maintain its popularity among horse trainers. Differing from other diuretics, it has little effect on acidity, and the steroid ingredient complements diuresis, resulting in remission of edematous ankles, tendons, knees, hocks, or any sundry swellings over the body surface.

Numotizine   An antiphlogistic agent; ideal for poulticing any inflamed area. Acts as a continuous moist pack for 12 hours or more. Relieves pain and reduces swelling and congestion. Contents: guaiacol, beechwood creosote, methyl salicylate, solution formaldehyde, polyols, and aluminum silicate.

olive oil   An emollient and cathartic, depending upon dosage.

A mild laxative if ingested in small amounts. Locally, very useful when applied daily to soften and remove skin encrustations and warts or to soothe any inflamed area.

I have found olive oil (it need not be a fine imported variety) to be effective when liberally applied to the stallion's or gelding's penis and entire sheath *after* a good scrubbing with Ivory soap and a thorough rinsing with plain water. Olive oil is a soothing emollient, maintains moisture, and prevents excessive drying and subsequent tenderness.

olive oil continued

I have often been handed a bottle of the finest olive oil, undoubtedly taken from the kitchen shelf, to be used on a patient. I accept it graciously, but I usually request that it *not* be returned to the cook's shelf, but be kept instead in the barn for future use! *See:* SHEATH CLEANSING.

paint   *See:* LEG PAINT.

paregoric (camphorated opium tincture)   An analgesic, hypnotic, and anti-spasmodic agent.

Paregoric was freely available "over the counter" at any drugstore until fairly recently when government regulations prohibited its use except with a doctor's prescription. Unaware of its habit-forming property, people had been innocently using drops of paregoric liquid for a wide range of pain-related conditions such as arthritis, rheumatoid discomfort, and gastrointestinal upset. Parents would massage an infant's gums with the drug during teething pain, and the quieting effect was welcomed by the tired parents, who could then sleep.

Abuses became rampant and misuses existed in all walks and stations of life. Tolerance to the drug built up in many users. Finally, through education and regulatory legislation, the preparation was removed from drugstore shelves.

Paregoric was helpful, in my practice, especially in equine pediatrics. It is basically a powerful antidiarrhetic to use while treating a systemic infection in a foal. Regulations curtailed its ready availability and presented additional paperwork and inconvenience for doctors when ordering drugs. I must agree, however, that controls in this case have been beneficial in preventing uninformed people from developing an addictive habit.

peroral treatment (per os)   Treatment by or through the mouth. Medicines can be administered in grain or drinking water as long as the horse will tolerate their presence. But administering oral medication can be difficult when the patient is a "cagey" old horse, a clever pony, or an elusive foal. The trick then is to mix an electuary. This consists of powdered medicine, incorporated with honey, corn syrup, or molasses. The sweet, sticky preparation is then placed on the tongue, cheeks, and lips, and usually goes down immediately.

Other per os methods include: stomach tube—administered by the veterinarian; drenching—using a large oral syringe; boluses—using a balling gun; capsules—given on feed or slipped up inside of the mouth between the cheeks and molar teeth; pills—same as capsules.

poultice   A moist, warm, and soft preparation applied thickly on the horse's foot or leg to reduce inflammation (heat, swelling, pain, and disuse). A poultice to a horse is comparable to chicken soup to a human.

There are many commercial poultices offered, such as Bowie Mud®, Antiphlogistine®, Numotazine®, and Phlogo®—all containing essentially the same ingredients.

Some of our old-fashioned poultices are quite effective and are still in use. One is bentonite powder or kaolin mixed with glycerine; another is flaxseed (linseed) poultice mixed with warm water. These mixtures are placed directly on the inflamed area, covered with freezer foil or plastic, then followed by a covering of cotton and a final sturdy bandage over all. The sustained warmth aids circulation and reduces discomfort somewhat. It should not be disturbed for at least 48 hours.

Although considered to be outmoded by some, I find the poulticing of legs and feet invaluable after shoe removal. Leg swellings, from any cause, or hot inflamed feet respond well to the poultice's cleansing, softening, and cooling action. I am convinced that the therapeutic value of a poultice is its ability to maintain heat and moisture while it is held into place by a dressing.

There are as many types of poultices and methods of application as there are reasons for their use. Old horsemen have their favorites and are secretive about their contents and methods of application.

If the drugstore is closed when I need a foot poulticed, I suggest a hot bran mash poultice or a linseed meal poultice, the ingredients of which can easily be found in most stables. I know of nothing more effective, if applied correctly.

To prepare either poultice, mix with hot water, make pasty, and apply over the area and bandage. If the inflamed area does not lend itself to bandaging, then cover with a piece of brown paper to hold it firm and prevent it from flaking as it dries due to the skin's inflammatory heat.

A cooling or astringent poultice can be made by adding one ounce of alum powder to six coagulated egg whites.

For a clay poultice, mix 4 parts kaolin to 1 part boric acid; add glycerine sufficient to make a pudding-like consistency. Add one ounce of thymol, methylsalicylate, or peppermint for fragrance and astringency.

I have found *Unna's paste* superb as an antiphlogistic preparation to cool hot and swollen areas on horses' legs. When incorporated into gauze bandages, it can also provide for leg support while exerting its anti-inflammatory action. The formula:

gelatine	150 grams
zinc oxide	150 grams
glycerine	350 cc
water	350 cc

Mix all ingredients and stir well, then place in a double boiler and cook until the mass has the consistency of glue. While warm, apply in a poultice-like fashion to the area. When the paste cools, it takes on a consistency like foam rubber. Unna's paste can be reheated at any time for future use.

For use as a supportive bandage in tendonitis, apply the paste to the leg and then, as you wrap the gauze bandage, incorporate the paste within the wraps of bandage material. Allow a half hour for it to cool, set, and dry before moving the horse. These rubbery supportive bandages can be removed simply by cutting with scissors.

protectives Inert drugs that form layers on the mucous membranes or skin and often absorb toxins and waste products. They include: albumin tannate, bismuth magma, bismuth subcarbonate, calamine, calcium carbonate, kaolin, pectin, petrolatum, talc, and zinc oxide.

sodium hypochlorite solution (Dakin's Solution) Greenish-yellow liquid with a chlorine odor. Used in a diluted 1:10 solution, called diluted sodium hypochlorite solution, for irrigation of wounds. This solution is an excellent antiseptic and germicide when applied to contaminated wounds in the form of a wet dressing. Although the popularity and effectiveness of antibiotics have overshadowed this preparation and its many uses, Dakin's Solution still serves

sodium hypochlorite solution continued

today as a respectable wet dressing for horses' wounds. Indeed, it makes an excellent wet dressing for any purpose.

sodium sulfate (Glauber's salt; salt cake)   A cathartic and antidote, named after the German chemist who first discovered the medicinal properties of sodium sulfate. It is an old remedy for the treatment of constipation in horses. Glauber's salt can be administered in drinking water, by oral syringe, or in solution through a stomach tube.

Sodium sulfate acts to hurry unwanted ingesta through the system; in cases of overeating, early treatment may prevent indigestion with subsequent founder. It is also useful in suspected poison cases, where it acts as both a cathartic and an antidote.

Glauber's salt is old-fashioned, but is a very important ingredient for every horse medicine box.

stomachics   Drugs that improve the appetite in horses by promoting the flow of gastric juices which in turn aid in digestion. Examples: alcohol, gentian, ginger, nux vomica, quinine, sodium arsenate, and strychnine.

sweat   The name "sweat" is descriptive of its action; that is, precisely to aid in the removal of swollen tissue, commonly a swollen edematous extremity.

Application of a sweat is indicated in any tissue swelling where fluids and electrolytes have left the capillaries and entered the interstitial cellular spaces. Swollen ankles and legs (the condition commonly called "stocked-up") are candidates for sweating, as are swollen tendons, tendon sheaths, and joint capsules.

All sweat preparations—whether commercial, prescription, or home-brewed—incorporate a glycerine or glycerine-type base with one of a variety of aromatic oils. The thick, soothing base softens and removes moisture from the superficial tissues and skin surface. Aromatic oils add color, fragrance, and antiseptic properties.

The secret of most sweats lies not in the ingredients, but in the *method* of application. Sweats apply easily and more efficiently when previously warmed. Massage and proper bandaging are essential for the success of the sweat action.

Firm dressings, properly applied, provide support to the lymphatic system, encouraging the return of an efficient venous circulation. A small, light piece of cotton should be placed next to the skin to absorb excessive moisture, followed by a piece of plastic, oiled silk, waxed paper, or Saran Wrap. A roll of cotton and the outside layer complete the bandage. If the sweat is effective, inner layers of the bandage will be soaked when the bandage is removed. Continue application on a daily basis until the layers are dry when unwrapped. Sweats alone without the firm support of the external bandage are quite negative and ineffective.

Sweats have the opposite properties and desired effects from that of leg braces, paints, and blisters, all of which encourage circulation to the area.

Examples of sweats—all good—are:

1. Alcohol, half and half with glycerine
2. Listerine (the mouth wash), applied as is
3. Glycerine, carbolic acid (phenol), and oil of wormwood

tightener (leg tightener)   A leg tightener simulates the action of a leg paint, although very mild in nature. The tissue responds after application with a very slight increase in circulation, so the tightener could be considered a weak counterirritant. The blood and all of its constituents promote healing and increased venous and lymphatic drainage in the localized area (usually the equine extremity). The formula:

> 4 ounces tincture of belladonna
> 2 ounces tannic acid powder
> 2 ounces menthol crystals
> 1 ounce camphor crystals
> alcohol, to make 1 pint of solution.

Unna's paste *See:* POULTICE.

vinegar An acid liquor made from wine, cider, or malt due to fermentation caused by the bacterial "mother of vinegar," *Mycoderma aceti* or *Acetobacter aceti*.

Vinegar contains around 5 percent acetic acid and is often substituted for diluted acetic acid (6 percent strength) in treatment of fungal infections.

Vinegar is often used in leg braces and body washes after strenuous physical exertion.

white liniment For use as a mild counterirritant and rubefacient to relieve muscle and joint soreness. The formula: camphor (3.0%), oil of turpentine (13.75%), ammonia water (1.5%), ammonium chloride (3.0%), soap (3.0), water (Q.S.A.D.).

white mineral oil (heavy grade) *See:* LIQUID PETROLATUM.

whitewash *Simple whitewash* is made by mixing 5 pounds of slaked lime in 30 gallons of warm water. Used to clean and disinfect fences, stalls, and other parts of the horse's environment.

Army whitewash is made by first dissolving 25 pounds of unslaked lime in 30 gallons of hot water; cover with a sack for a few minutes, until the lime goes into solution. Add 8 pounds of sodium chloride (table salt) dissolved in hot water. Cook 3 pounds of rice to a pasty consistency and mix with the lime and salt. Add a half pound of Spanish whiting. Dissolve 1 pound of glue and stir well into the mixture. Then add an additional 5 gallons of boiling water and stir to a smooth creamy paste. Allow to stand for several days. Stir again and apply as you would a paint.

witch hazel Made from the leaves of *Hamamelis virginiana*, a shrub or small tree that grows in damp, rocky soil in the eastern and central parts of North America. Applied externally to sore muscles and contusions. It is a common ingredient of many braces applied to the legs and back of the horse.

wound dressing powder There are many preparations available for dressing wounds; they are useful where granulation tissue formation is needed as well as antisepsis. A typical formulation is: urea (80%), iodoform (1%), sulfathiazole (2%), sulfanilamide (10%), in an inert base. Apply to wounds or abrasions as directed by your veterinarian—preferably under dressings or bandages. *See:* CAUSTIC POWDER.

yellow mercuric oxide A good ophthalmic ointment (1 to 2 percent) that can be used safely to calm eye irritation.

VETERINARY DRUGS

Acepromazine *See:* TRANQUILIZERS.

acetic acid A caustic agent or rubefacient (produces redness of the skin). Used to destroy warts and keloids (excessive amounts of fibrous tissue), and as a fungicide. (Vinegar contains 4 or 5 percent acetic acid.)

aconite The dried root of *Aconitum napellus* (monkshood or wolfsbane). For treatment of colic, 10 drops of tincture of aconite may be placed on the horse's tongue. Although most regard it as outmoded today, aconite used externally will relieve soreness or inflammation of the gums. It also reduces fever, acts as a diuretic, and can depress cardiac and respiratory rates.

activated charcoal An adsorbent black powder that is introduced either with grain, by drenching, or via a stomach tube for the purposes of adsorbing gases, odors, or toxic elements that have accidentally been ingested by the animal. Activated charcoal forms an effective barrier between toxic substances and the sensitive mucosal linings of the stomach and small intestines, the site of absorption into the horse's system.

Cyanide is the most prevalent poison that attacks herbivores, including horses. Unfortunately, this well-known poison adsorber is not effective against cyanide poisoning in the equine. *See:* POISONS.

alkaloids Organic, nitrogen-containing, bitter-tasting substances found in the leaves, bark, seeds, and other parts of plants. Found most frequently in poisonous plants, alkaloids often contain the active principle of a crude drug and are notably soluble in water.

aconite tincture	lobelia
areca	morphine
arecoline hydrobromide	nicotine sulfate
belladonna leaf	nux vomica
cocaine HCl	opium
codeine	pelocarpine
colocynth	physostigmine
curare	quinidine sulfate
diamorphine HCl	quinine
ergonovine maleate	rauwolfia
ergot	scopolamine hydrobromide
hyoscyamus	stramonium
ipecac	strychine

Antidotes are tannic acid and activated charcoal.

aloes A purgative or laxative derived from the dried leaves of plants of the genus *Aloe,* native to certain parts of Africa. Old-time horsemen would fill a gelatine capsule with aloes, grease the outside of the capsule, then use a balling gun to administer it orally.

The capsule is intended to dissolve in the stomach after releasing the cathartic, but it has been known—tragically—to disintegrate within the delicate lining of the espohageal area. Balls containing their bitter, irritating chemicals can rupture in the mouth and then be crushed by the horse's teeth, causing irritation of the tissues and destruction of the mucosa. An emergency call to your veterinarian must follow any such eventuality!

Thank goodness, the practice of balling horses (with all of its accompanying hair-raising stories) has lost favor with modern horsemen. They now choose to have their veterinarians use the stomach tube, which, when handled proficiently, has eliminated the balling gun and its dangers.

aminoglycosides (aminocyclitols) A specific group on antibiotics effective against both gram negative and gram positive bacteria and possessing other similar actions. They include: Amikacin®, Dihydrostreptomycin®, Gentamicin®, Kanamycin®, Neomycin®, Sisomysin®, Spectionomycin®, Streptomycin®, and Tobramycin®. *See:* ANTIBIOTICS.

In my practice alone, this new group of drugs has been responsible for saving many foals suffering with septicemia.

aminophylline Known as theophylline ethylenediamine, this drug is both a diuretic and respiratory stimulant. Horses with congestion of the lungs or pulmonary emphysema receive some relief following injections of aminophylline, and it often is combined wth appopriate antibiotics in special cases of infection.

ANTIBACTERIAL DRUGS

Nitrofurans	Nitrofurazone, Furaltadone, Furazolidone, Nitrofurantoin, Nifuraldezone
Sulfonamides	
Short Duration	Sulfathiazole, Sulfasoxazole (Gantrisin), Sulfamethiazole
Intermediate	Sulfapyridine, Sulfadiazine, Sulfamethazine, Sulfachloripyridazine, Sulfamerazine, Triplesulfas, Sulfamethoxypyridazine
Long Duration	Sulfamethylphenazole, Sulfabromomethazine, Sulfadimethoxine, Sulfaethoxpyridazine,
Enterics (gastrointestinal)	Sulfathalidine, Sulfaguanidine, Succinylsulfathiazole, Sulfaquinoxaline
Sulfonamide Potentiators	Trimethoprim, Diaveridine, Pyrimethamine, Ormetoprim

aminophylline continued

ANTIBIOTIC DRUGS

Penicillins	
Natural	Benzyl Penicillin (Penicillin G)
Semisynthetic	Penicillin V,
	Phenethicillin,
	Propicillin,
	Phenbenicillin
Isoxazolyl series	Oxacillin, Cloxacillin, Dicloxacillin,
	Flucloxacillin, Methicillin, Nafcillin,
	Ancillin, Quinacillin
Wide-spectrum	Ampicillin, Carbenicillin, Ticarcillin,
	Amoxicillin, Hetacillin, Pivampicillin,
	Cyclacillin, Talampicillin, Bacampicillin
Cephalosporins	
Oral route	Cephalexin, Cephoglycin, Cephradine,
	Cefadroxil
Parenteral route	Cephaloridine, Cephalothin, Cefamandole,
	Cephapirin, Cephazolin
Experimental	Cefoxitin, Cefatrizine, Cefazaflur,
	Cefuroxine
Bacitracin	Vancomycin
Polymyxins	Polymyxin B, Polymyxin E
Novobiocin	
Antifungal Agents	Nystatin, Amphotericin B
Chloramphenicol	Chloramycetin
Tetracylines	Chlortetracycline, Oxytetracycline,
	Tetracycline, Methacycline,
	Dimethylchlortetracycline, Doxycycline,
	Minocycline
Macrolides	Erythromycin, Carbomycin, Spiramycin,
	Tylosin, Oleandomycin
Lincosamides	Lincomycin, Clindamycin
Aminocyclitols	Spectinomycin
Aminoglycosides	Streptomycin, Kanamycin,
	Dihydrostreptomycin, Gentamicin,
	Neomycin, Amikacin,
	Tobramycin, Sisomycin

anticonvulsants Drugs used to prevent or arrest convulsions. Examples: diphenylhydantoin sodium (Dilantin), paramethadione (Paradione), primidone (Mysoline), and trimethadione (Tridione) above.

antifungal agents *See:* ANTIBIOTIC DRUGS (CHART).

antihistamines Antihistamines are a group of drugs with a specific action that is antagonistic to that of histamines. Histamine is an amine found in the skin and adjacent tissues. When these superficial tissues are injured, histamine is liberated, causing several responses: Vessels enlarge, blood pressure drops, and gastric secretions increase. When these symptoms are observed in concert, this is an allergic reaction.

Antihistamines (e.g., Benadryl, Phenergan) should be used only under veterinary supervision. *See:* ALLERGY, ANAPHYLAXIS.

anti-inflammatory drugs In the late 1940s, with the advent of steroids, the medical profession rejoiced at the miracle drug cortisone, believing it to be the ultimate answer to inflammatory problems, especially arthritis.

Today, in the mid-eighties, we are somewhat reluctant to consider using steroids unless specifically indicated. The immediate remissions and cosmetic wonders we hoped to achieve with steroids were persistently overshadowed by destructive and sometimes irreversible side effects.

In horses, the incidence of joint capsule disease and destruction as well as unexplained founder increased until cortisone was recognized as the culprit. It is still respectable in the practice of good medicine to use steroids *prudently* in cases of stress, shock, and debilitation. There is, however, a new group of drugs emerging, which show great promise and equal safety. These are the prostaglandin inhibitors. Unlike steroids, they provide both anti-inflammatory and analgesic action in the absence of undesired and dangerous side effects. Some are fed with grain, while others are injectable, but all are effective and carry a wide margin of safety.

Interestingly, one of our oldest and most reliable drugs, aspirin, is included in this latest, up-to-date group of drugs. It is only recently that we have come to understand how this drug, first popular around 1895, acts upon the body. It is now classified as one of the nonsteroidal, anti-inflammatory, prostaglandin inhibitor drugs.

Of the drugs in this classification, I prefer phenylbutazone, both I.V. and orally, to any other drug in this classification, despite its adverse publicity. In trained, humane hands, this drug is invaluable for the relief of aches and pains in our modern horse.

The anti-inflammatory drugs include:

Nonsteroidal

aspirin	naproxen
flunixin meglumine	phenylbutazone
indomethacin	salicylates
meclofenamic acid	

Steroidal

ACTH	prednisolone
cortisone	prednisone
methylprednisolone	

antimony trichloride *See:* BUTTER OF ANTIMONY.

antipruritics Agents used to relieve itching. Examples: alcohol, camphor, coal tar, menthol, phenol, witch hazel, as well as the modern anti-inflammatory drugs. *See:* ANTI-INFLAMMATORY DRUGS.

antipyretic An agent that tends to reduce fever. Injectable Dipyrone and Novin are superior antipyretics for the equine. Results are excellent when combined with fluid therapy. Prohibited for use in human medicine.

Injectable thiosalicylate is another useful horse antipyretic. Other examples: aspirin, ethylnitrate spirits, sodium salicylate, and, for external use, alcohol, tepid water. *See:* COLIC, HEAT STROKE.

areca (areca nut; betelnut) A botanical containing arecoline and other alkaloids. As a brown powder with an astringent, bitter taste, it was used as a worm medicine; now obsolete.

Arecoline hydrobromide is an alkaloid derived from areca. A white, bitter-tasting crystalline powder, it is a very strong cathartic and anthelmintic (worm medicine).

army anesthetic General anesthetic. Used intravenously to induce a slow, questionably safe, and prolonged anesthesia in horses. Each 500 cc contains: chloral hydrate (328 gr), pentobarbital (75 gr), magnesium sulfate (164 gr), and alcohol (9.5%), in an aqueous propylene glycol base.

atropine sulfate Both a poison and a salt of the alkaloid atropine. The actions of atropine are too dangerous when used in any manner other than for ophthalmic treatment under the strictest veterinarian control. No usage other than treatment of the eye will be discussed in this book.

In my opinion, atropine sulfate ophthalmic ointment (1–2 percent) is your veterinarian's first line of defense when a horse's eye is affected. This ointment or liquid has two actions: It causes the pupil to dilate, preventing the formation of adhesions that could bind the iris and pupil into immobility; secondly, atropine acts as a local anesthetic and so reduces the irritation that accompanies a painful ocular condition.

CAUTION: The effect of atropine on the pupil of the eye is to cause dilation and render the pupil motionless when subjected to light or other stimulus. Consequently, the eye is completely vulnerable to further tissue damage deeper within the globe.

If a decision is made to instill this mediction, your veterinarian must arrange for protective covering of the horse's eye, as well as a darkened environment during the recovery period.

Blinkers with a closed cup, or a cotton gauze bandage "hat" fashioned with ear holes to fit the head, will be effective. Many horses can continue to train in spite of an eye problem, as long as they are protected from light, air, and dust.

Never use atropine without supervision by your veterinarian and *always* provide adequate protection for the eye.

flunixin meglumine (Banamine) Indicated for the alleviation of inflammation and pain associated with musculoskeletal disorders in the horse. It is noted for its effectiveness in control of abdominal pain in colic cases.

Banamine is a potent, nonsteroidal, nonnarcotic analgesic drug with anti-inflammatory activity. Its action is believed to interfere with the ability of the prostaglandins to convey pain to the subject.

Banamine has been used in combination with phenylbutazone with some success at race tracks for alleviation of arthritic disorders and muscular pain.

CAUTION: This drug is so effective that its use can actually mask a serious abdominal problem that may require immediate attention. A consequent delay in treatment could result in loss of life. Therefore, a careful evaluation of the patient is of foremost importance before administering Banamine in abdominal cases.

Banamine is available in both the oral form for convenience, and in the supersafe injectable form, prepared for either I.V. or I.M. administration.

barbiturate   A salt of barbituric acid; a hypnotic, sedative, surgical anesthetic. Such compounds are derived from barbital. They are rapidly destroyed in the liver, then eliminated by the kidneys.

There are four main barbiturates in use today: pentobarbital sodium (Nembutal), secobarbital sodium (Seconal), thiamylal sodium (Surital), and thiopental sodium (Pentothal).

These four compounds all act in the same ways, although each drug is distinct from the others. They have gained popularity in modern practice, since they can be used in combination with other drugs to produce very safe and effective anesthesia for the equine patient.

Until as late as 1950, the horse surgeon had to rely upon a combination of barbiturates for surgical anesthesia for either minor or major procedures. The notorious "Army anesthetic," with its varying effects upon the patient, undeterminable range of dosage required, and unpredictable duration, posed danger for the patient, the surgeon, and the attending staff.

Today's anesthetics are wonderfully safe. With a trained anesthesiologist in attendance, horse surgeons now may concentrate upon refining their surgical skills, knowing that the risk associated with anesthesia has been reduced to the minimum.

Apart from their use as anesthesia, barbiturates serve in another distinct and irreversible action. When a veterinarian is faced with a suffering animal requiring euthanasia, barbiturate drugs can provide a smooth, quiet euthanasia. When using the barbiturates, therefore, skill and caution must be combined and dosages measured exactly for the purpose at hand.

braces   Steel and aluminum braces are available commercially for treatment of crooked legs in neonatal (newborn) foals with imbalances of tension in muscles and tendons. Such braces can be designed by your veterinarian and fashioned by a skilled blacksmith to meet the immediate need in a malformed leg.

Realize that such braces or splints require knowledge and skill in their proper application so as to avoid damaging soft tissue or distorting the development of growing bone. Braces are generally reputed to be more hazardous than helpful when prescribed and applied by an inexpert practitioner.

In the case of an adult horse that has suffered a fracture, after the necessary surgical repair, a steel brace is needed most often for exterior support and reinforcement of the plaster-of-paris or fiberglass cast material. An equine brace differs greatly from a human brace in its size, weight, tensile strength, and overall requirements. Judging these critical requirements should be entrusted

braces continued

only to an equine orthopedic surgeon, and construction of the brace only to a skilled blacksmith.

Butazolidin   *See:* PHENYLBUTAZONE.

butter of antimony (antimony trichloride)   A caustic preparation used to treat thrush infections in the foot; there are reports of its being used also on canker cases. Since its actions are escharotic (corrosive), caution must be used to avoid accidental application to healthy soft tissue. I would advise greasing the heel area with Vaseline before treating any diseased thrush area in the foot. There are thrush remedies available that are equally effective and less dangerous to use. *See:* THRUSH.

caustic powder   An overall term for preparations that are used to aid the healing of stubborn wounds. These powders both stimulate granulation of tissue and burn away excessive granulation tissue.

The secret lies in the contents, typically copper sulfate (50%) and boric acid (15%) in an inert base (35%). These ingredients are found in commercial powder preparations under many names. Look in your local tack shop or ask your veterinarian.

chlorhexidine (Nolvasan)   Antiseptic, disinfectant, bactericide, fungicide, and virucide; it is nontoxic, nonirritating, and not neutralized by body fluids.

Nolvasan solution is excellent as a wound cleanser and wet dressing, and as a preoperative scrub. The ointment serves well as a wound dressing.

croton oil   Originates from seeds of *Croton tiglium*, an East Indian shrub. It is the most drastic of all cathartics and, fortunately, is an obsolete drug today.

Not outdated, however, is its use in leg paints and blisters (counterirritants) to increase the severity of the reaction and enhance the effectiveness.

dexamethasone (Azium)   This preparation is one of the most commonly used steroids in general horse practice. The powder form is palatable and therefore easily administered. The injectable form is nonirritating to skeletal muscle and is easy to inject.

This steroid, unless overdosed, is harmless and does not carry the threat of causing idiopathic laminitis within two weeks of its use.

Azium is an anti-inflammatory drug successfully used for hot, painful swellings, nondescript dermatitis, and allergic reactions.

diluted acetic acid   A colorless liquid of 6 percent strength. An effective fungicide, it is also used for wart removal. Vinegar contains 4 percent acetic acid and is sometimes used in the barn as a substitute.

Recommended strength for application of the skin is 8 fluid ounces per one pint of warm water. *See:* VINEGAR, WARTS.

Dipyrone   *See:* METHAMPYRONE.

D-S-S (Cerusol)   A 5 percent water-miscible solution of dioctyl sodium sulfasuccinate. This preparation is commonly used via the stomach tube to treat cases of constipation or impaction (8 ounces per gallon of water). It can be used also as an enema (4 ounces per gallon of water).

Cerusol softens exudates in the ear canal. Instill several drops into the ear, wait several minutes, massage gently, and then swab clean with cotton-tipped applicator. Follow this with a solution of alcohol (10 ml), glycerine (90 ml), salicylic acid (sufficient quantity), boric acid (sufficient quantity), tannic acid (sufficient quantity); warm and apply in ear canal as drops, then massage gently.

electuary   An old-fashioned medicine preparation that melts in the mouth. Powdered medicine is incorporated with honey, corn syrup, or molasses. The sweet, sticky preparation is then rubbed or placed on the animal's tongue, lips, and teeth.

emollient   A substance that soothes or softens the skin or mucous membranes.

Intestinal emollients are invaluable in treating any horse with colic, a sluggish or chilled intestine, low-grade impaction, or intestinal mucosa irritated from toxic foodstuff. Emollients can allay irritation of intestinal mucosa in cases of protracted diarrhea.

Examples: heavy-grade mineral oil (U.S.P.); glycerine, olive oil, linseed oil, and Cerusol (dioctyl sodium sulfosuccinate solution, or D-S-S).

furosemide (Lasix®)   An effective diuretic possessing a wide range of actions and administered either orally or by injection. Lasix is useful in reducing tissue swelling, especially edematous areas, for example, hind leg and abdominal areas associated with wounds or trauma.

This drug can cause loss of body fluids and electrolytes, but especially loss of potassium, as well as lowered blood pressure. The promiscuous use of this potent diuretic can result in generalized weakening of the animal.

It has been documented that bleeding in race horses has been greatly inhibited by the prudent use and careful dosage of Lasix prior to competition. A relentless program of post-race examination and recordkeeping has contributed greatly to our knowledge. However, to this point, the multifaceted conditions responsible for internal hemorrhage in race horses have not yet been uncovered, let alone answered. *See:* EPISTAXIS.

hemostatics   Agents that arrest bleeding. Examples: alum (topical) epinephrine (injected), ferric chloride (topical), malonic acid (injected), oxalic acid (injected), oxytocin (injected), posterior pituitary injection, and trichloracetic acid (topical), vitamin K (injected).

heparin   An anticoagulant used to prevent formation of thromboses inside of the blood vessels and blood clotting inside of the tubing during transfusions.

Its use is contraindicated in cases of liver disease; hemorrhage occurs as the result of overdosage.

In recent years a controversial use of heparin has come to the forefront of veterinary medicine. Daily oral administration of heparin has resulted in claims of improved soundness in cases of navicular disease, even in horses literally crippled by the disease. I would give this treatment careful consideration before advocating its use, however. *See:* NAVICULAR DISEASE.

hyaluronic acid (sodium hyaluronate)   A substance extracted from rooster combs and highly purified for precise aseptic injection. It is believed to act by altering joint fluid pH in some way that encourages healing and regeneration of articular cartilage.

HA built its reputation in Europe where it was used for competition horses suffering from both early and chronic arthritic symptoms. In November 1984 it was approved and released by the Food and Drug Administration for legal *hyaluronic acid continued*

therapeutic use in the United States. This was good news for the racing establishment and especially for those stiff and sore equine campaigners afflicted with osteoarthritis.

Commonly referred to as "acid" on the barns and backstretches, hyaluronic acid (Hylartin, Adequan, Healon) was the first real breakthrough in lameness therapy in almost 20 years. Data from Europe and scattered information gathered in the U.S. have indicated that this intra-articular joint therapy is indeed effective in the treatment of a variety of arthritic and other joint maladies.

CAUTION: The use of hyaluronic acid is strictly contraindicated in any infection of the joint, even if only suspected.

During the years when the drug was illegal for use in the U.S., a black market for it existed at every track in the country. Several hundred dollars would be exchanged for a 2-cc vial. I found it distressing not to be able to help a horse that might benefit from an injection of HA, and yet the thought of an illicit purchase of questionable purity and unclear labeling was repugnant. Fortunately, such conflicts are behind us now. *See:* ARTHRITIS, OSTEOARTHRITIS.

iodinated casein   Formed by treating milk casein with iodine. When fed orally, iodinated casein simulates the action of thyroxine, a hormone produced by the thyroid gland that regulates metabolic rate in the body.

Iodinated casein, which comes in a palatable powder form, is commonly prescribed in cases of hypothyroidism, obesity, chronic low-grade laminitis, reduced libido in the stallion, and infertility in some mares. All these entities just listed are symptoms of hypothyroidism. Your veterinarian will suggest a protein-bound iodine test for the evaluation of thyroid acivity.

Dairy farmers feed iodinated casein to their fat old cows to improve milk production. *See:* HYPOTHYROIDISM, LAMINITIS.

Lasix   *See:* FUROSEMIDE.

lidocaine hydrochloride (Xylocaine Hydrochloride)   White powder soluble in water; injected near nerves to desensitize leg areas for diagnostic purposes in examining for soundness. Also injected by local infiltration to numb the area for lancing or treatment purposes.

OILS

Name	Use
Almond	Emollient.
Anise	Aromatic carminative and flavor.
Betula (wintergreen oil, methyl salicylate)	Antirheumatic; antipyretic (fever). Methyl salicylate is commonly found in leg braces, body washes, and many ointment preparations.
Camphorated (camphor liniment)	Mild counterirritant (external use only). At weaning time, apply camphorated oil to the broodmare's udder twice daily.

OILS

Name	Use
Castor	Cathartic. Saturate any cluster of warts on a young horse's muzzle twice daily. Watch for spontaneous remission.
Chenopodium (wormseed oil)	Anthelmintic worm medicine; ingredient in sweats and leg braces.
Cinnamon (cassia oil)	Aromatic flavor and carminative.
Clove	Externally—counterirritant (local analgesic). Internally—carminative ingredient of liniments and leg braces.
Cod liver	Oral source of vitamins A and D.
Corn	Feed orally to improve poor coats. Rich in unsaturated fatty acids.
Cottonseed	Substitute for olive oil.
Croton	Cathartic internally. Externally—counterirritant. A good ingredient that increases efficacy when carefully added to an external blister or an internal counterirritant.
Fennel	Aromatic carminative—used with purgatives to prevent griping.
Harlem	Old-fashioned diuretic, irritant. Was commonly used to treat any pain manifested by the horse, urinary or gastrointestinal. Fortunately it has been outmoded by superior drugs.
Lavender	Aromatic and flavoring agent.
Lemon	Flavoring agent.
Linseed (flaxseed oil)	Internally—cathartic. Raw linseed oil, if used internally as a cathartic, contains a toxic element. Rectified linseed oil is strongly recommended. Externally—poultices and emollient liniments.
Mineral (white mineral oil)	Emollient—constipation. See: MINERAL OIL.
Nutmeg (myristica oil)	Aromatic flavor and carminitive.
Olive	Emollient, laxative, and nutrient. Apply generously to the pepuce, sheath, and penis of a stallion or gelding immediately following a good cleansing with white soap, cotton, and water. Prevents excessive drying, scaling, and soreness.
Orange	Aromatic flavor and stomachic.

OILS

Name	Use
Peach (persic oil)	Similar to almond oil emollient.
Peanut (arachis oil)	Ingredient in liniments, ointments, and soaps. Slows absorption and reduces irritation when added to injectable internal blisters. If injected, it can produce a fibrosis or scar formation.
Peppermint	Aromatic flavoring and carminative.
Pimento	Flavoring agent and carminative.
Pine	Veterinary insecticides and disinfectants.
Pine needle	Inhalation medicant for respiratory inflammation.
Rosemary	Carminative and rubefacient.
Sassafras	Counterirritant, rubefacient.
Sesame	Emollient vehicle and substitute for olive oil.
Spearmint	Flavoring agent.
Sweet (baby oil, glycerine)	Emollient and solvent. Safe and effective for cleansing ears or any delicate area or orifice.
Tar	Internally—expectorant. Externally—antiseptic irritant, skin diseases.
birch tar	Expectorant, dermatitis.
juniper tar (cade oil)	Aromatic and dermatitis.
pine tar	Internally—expectorant. Externally—antiseptic and dermatitis.
Turpentine	Internally—use rectified. Superb ingredient found in all colic mixtures and many leg paints and blisters. Turpentine combined with camphor in a vaporizer or nebulizer provides effective treatment for respiratory disease, especially chronic pharyngitis. Antibiotics may be added, if indicated. This strong expectorant will establish drainage of the inflamed respiratory mucosa. Externally (turpentine oil)—rubefacient, counterirritant.

Over the years I have found multiple uses and applications, both culinary and medicinal, for these fascinating oils.

phenylbutazone (Butazolidin)   A nonhormonal anti-inflammatory agent. It is a white crystalline solid, soluble in water, and odorless.

Phenylbutazone is indicated for the treatment of acute inflammatory conditions, including musculoskeletal (arthritic) ailments. It is available in both tablet and injectable form.

Overdosage of tablets can cause intestinal irritation with possible ulcer formation, and phlebitis (inflammation of a vein) can occur at the intravenous site if the drug is carelessly administered.

I have found Butazolidin a safe drug to use in treating any inflammatory condition, acute or chronic. Its action is that of a super aspirin with no side effects. If used prudently, it can serve both the horse and the owner well.

Unlike Butazolidin, the corticosteroids, also used as anti-inflammatory agents, carry the potential for hazardous side effects to the equine patient.

Promazine   *See:* TRANQUILIZERS.

prostaglandins   Naturally occurring compounds found in all mammalian tissues and thought to originate from fatty acids.

Prostaglandins cause a variety of effects on the body. They are the mediators of pain. They also act directly on the pituitary gland, which reacts by releasing multiple hormones that affect the reproductive system and result in changes (for example, induced estrus, abortion, and shortened intervals between estrus periods).

An injection of prostaglandin causes increased blood pressure, decreased rectal temperature, and stimulation of smooth-muscle tissue.

When an indication exists for the use of prostaglandin, please warn the farm manager or uninitiated owner to expect some side effects to the injection. Within approximately 15 minutes of the injection, the mare will proceed to break out into a black sweat and continue to perspire profusely for 15 minutes or so. In some cases, the water pours from the abdominal midline. Subsequently, overt symptoms subside as quickly as they occur and with no discernible discomfort to the mare.

Prostaglandins are very useful to the equine gynecoloist in treating broodmares that are visiting breeding farms for the explicit purpose of returning home pregnant. I must, however, stress that a thorough gynecologic examination is recommended prior to any consideration of using this substance; so many physiologic processes are vulnerable to its use that the decision should be reserved to the veterinary professional.

reserpine (Serpasil)   A crystalline alkaloid of rauwolfia that acts to depress sympathetic nerve function, causing lowered blood pressure and decreased heart rate. It also has sedative and tranquilizing properties.

Rauwolfia compounds are characterized by slow onset of symptoms and sustained effects. Depression may persist for several months after withdrawal from the drug.

This drug was used and unfortunately abused by show horse people for years until the authorities finally developed a test for its presence. Well-bred, spirited Thoroughbreds would hack without restraint under the influence of reserpine.

When faced with a "rogue" to break and train, I can then see legitimate use

reserpine continued

for this drug, but keep in mind that it is a dangerous drug that has caused accidents, especially when used in jumping horses.

Rompun *See:* XYLAZINE.

salicylates Analgesic and antipyretic; used in aches, pains, arthritis discomfort, and frequently for sore muscles. Examples: acetylsalicylic acid, methyl salicylate, phenyl salicylate, and salicylic acid.

sodium bromide A sedative and hypnotic used in convulsions and in nervous animals to induce sleep. In the past it has been used in an unsafe and unethical way.

I first saw the words *Sodium Bromide* on a soiled label stuck on a dusty old bottle in a horse dealer's cluttered barn. Being about 12 years old at the time and full of curiosity about horses and horse medicines, I quickly memorized the name. The dealer was expecting a potential customer and was grooming his horse's coat to a high gloss in readiness. I watched as the old man took a rusty oral syringe, plunged it into the bottle marked Sodium Bromide and drew up close to 4 ounces. Next he went to the horse and thrust the nozzle of the syringe through the side of the horse's dental space and up into the oral cavity. Then he massaged the animal's throat, while the horse managed to spit some of the liquid out. This operation completed, the old man promptly hid the bottle and syringe in a closet back in the tack room. In a few minutes he returned, took the horse from the stall, crosstied him in the aisle, and continued his last-minute polishing. The buyer arrived and requested to ride the horse.

With this, the horse staggered out of the barn, crossing his legs intermittently and actually stumbling once. I was frightened and concerned that the horse might fall, possibly injuring both rider and horse. I watched as the man rode him around the ring many times and finally returned to the barn still in one piece. Thank goodness he did not decide to jump the horse.

The purchase was made on the spot. A van arrived shortly after the horse was loaded, and out the lane they went!

With this I scurried home to look up the meaning of the words *sodium bromide* in my veterinary book.

sodium oleate (Osteum) An injectable preparation used to stimulate bone-cell formation in the fracture line. Osteum is considered by some to be osteogenic (promoting bone healing).

CAUTION: This drug is very irritating to soft tissue, and should be used *only by professionals*. In one case I recall, a young filly was injected for bucked shins (periostitis). Some of the drug accidentally entered the tendon sheath of the extensor tendon at the point where it traverses the front of the shin area. A few days later, the filly could not support weight and an infection developed. Eventually, all soft tissue on her shin area sloughed off. Needless to say, she lost the remainder of the racing season: it was a year before she could return to training.

Drugs and their actions are lifesaving in some cases and very helpful in the restoration of health in other cases, but *any drug* can be dangerous in the wrong hands, no matter how well intentioned they may be!

Sparine *See:* TRANQUILIZERS.

strychnine sulfate A respiratory stimulant and a powerful stomachic in the horse. Its favorable actions include dramatic improvement in appetite, coat, and increased gastrointestinal tone and proficiency.

Although strychine is curiously beneficial to herbivores (horses and cattle), it is, however, lethally toxic to most carnivores (cats and dogs). Great care should be stressed on precise dosage even in the horse, since strychnine is an alkaloid and a basically poisonous substance.

Strychnine sulfate combined with arsenic trioxide in a palatable licorice powder base is one of the finest tonics for horses of all ages. Horse doctors know it as a standby remedy for many of the problems faced in older horses—unthriftiness, depressed appetite, poor hair coat, diarrhea, gastrointestinal flatulence.

A mixture of powdered strychnine and arsenic is not only a reliable geriatric preparation, but also a very helpful tonic during convalescence from any protracted or debilitating illness.

terpin hydrate An expectorant, helpful in respiratory conditions, especially in chronic forms of bronchitis.

thimerosal (Merthiolate) A cream-colored crystalline powder slightly soluble in water; a good antiseptic, effective against bacteria and fungi. It is used to disinfect skin-tissue surfaces prior to surgery, and is also useful on minor skin abrasions. In alcohol (1:1,000), as a tincture for intact skin; in aqueous solution (1:1,000), for wounds and denuded areas.

thyroxin The active iodine compound found in the thyroid gland. This hormone has various actions, but primarily it regulates the body's basal metabolic rate. Useful in cases of hypothyroidism, cretinism, obesity, and dullness. Thyroid extract is available in tablet and powder form. *See:* HYPOTHYROIDISM.

thymol Fungicide and antiseptic; useful in skin infections or dermatitis of fungal origin.

tincture of benzoin Stimulant expectorant used in inhalation therapy (nebulization) in cases of laryngitis, pharyngitis, and bronchitis. Also, a good ingredient in sweat preparations for leg ailments.

tranquilizers (ataratics) Defined as drugs that cause tranquility by calming, soothing, and quieting without depression. We use tranquilizers in equine medicine primarily to reduce anxiety and fear in our patients.

The two most reliable and dependable tranquilizers to date, with the widest margin of safety, are promazine (Sparine) and acetylpromazine (Aceromazine). They are both phenothiazine derivatives and have a prominent effect upon the cardiovascular system. They produce a perceptible drop in blood pressure and an increase in heart rate. Not only do these tranquilizers serve well as a preanesthetic agent and later again in the recovery room, but they are very useful when chemical quieting is needed for minor procedures, such as sheath cleaning, clipping, hauling, grooming, breaking, or treating painful areas.

It is important to bear in mind that although a tranquilized horse may act sleepy and mild, the tranquilizer drug has no effect on pain perception. Thus, a very dopey looking animal can respond suddenly to a minor stimulus with a strong and excitable reaction. The combination of tranquilizers and narcotics

tranquilizers continued

produces a marvelous state of tranquility *and* analgesia. The equine practitioner is truly grateful for this advance in medical knowledge.

Oral administration of tranquilizers in granular or powdered form is convenient for the owner, but the effects are somewhat inconsistent or less predictable. Usually, the injectable route is preferable; it is much safer, more reliable, and quite predictable.

CAUTION: Great care must be taken with the intravenous injection of the phenothiaizine-derived drugs. Do not allow the needle tip accidentally to enter the carotid artery, which is situated dangerously close to the jugular vein. An intracarotid-artery injection results in collapse, convulsions, and death. A small needle, anything smaller than 20-gauge, presents an added hazard since it does not permit the warning surge of red blood backwards into the syringe that is so characteristically seen when a needle of larger size has entered the artery rather than the vein.

ANOTHER WARNING TO HEED IS THIS: Never allow the use of a phenothiazine tranquilizer in an animal known to have received a dose of organic phosphate worm medicine. It has been documented that these tranquilizers can strengthen or lengthen the effects of organic phosphates whether for worming or as an insecticide. To prevent a hidden danger in the form of drug incompatibility, inform the veterinarian of the animal's history of worm medication.

Turcapsol   Colic mixture for relief of pain; retards fermentation and stimulates peristalsis. It contains salicylic acid, menthyl salcylate, camphor, and oil of turpentine in a diluent of oleoresins of capsicum and ginger.

Dosage: 1 to 3 fluid ounces via stomach tube or drench.

turpentine oil (spirits of turpentine)   Counterirritant, rubefacient, expectorant, and carminative. It is a colorless liquid, soluble in alcohol, and volatile.

Turpentine is a very important ingredient in liniments, braces, and mild blisters for the treatment of muscle and leg soreness in horses.

Rectified turpentine oil (N.F.) is used for internal purposes, such as colic mixtures, cough medicines, and stomachics (tonics).

Turpentine also can be incorporated with boiling water as an inhalant for bronchitis, heaves, or any respiratory congestion. *See:* INHALATION THERAPY.

White Lotion Tablets   These tablets contain zinc and potassium sulfate, and are popularly used to make astringent cold-water dressings for treating hot, sore, and inflamed leg areas.

Dissolve several tablets in 1 gallon of hot water, allow to cool, and submerge leg dressings until thoroughly saturated. The cooling, astringent action of White Lotion Tablets will reduce inflammation over a period of 12 to 24 hours. Apply the dressings wet over the swollen areas and every few hours—without fail—add solution.

CAUTION: Under no circumstances allow the bandage to dry on the horse's leg. Maintain constant supervision, with liberal application of fresh solution, to maintain wetness. The severity of the injury, the weather, climate, and temperature are all factors to keep in mind. If bandages inadvertently dry, this drug perversely creates heat and in some cases burns or blisters the patient.

White Lotion has taken a back seat to some of the newer astringent preparations, most of which can be left in place indefinitely with safety. *See:* POULTICE.

xylazine (Rompun) A thiazine compound used as a nonnarcotic sedative, analgesic, and muscle relaxant. This drug is very useful to the equine practitioner when treating nervous, fractious horses and can even be used while in the barn for minor surgical procedures.

For major surgery requiring a general anesthetic, its preanesthetic properties are unexcelled, and when used in combination with the inhalation anesthetic Halothane, it can also then provide a smooth recovery. When a thousand-pound animal is put under general anesthesia, the type of recovery it makes from the anesthesia can and often does decide the success or failure of the case, regardless of the surgical expertise. Induction time is rapid, desired effect is of short duration, and awakening is often abrupt.

Rompun is a very expensive, yet very popular, sedative. Practitioners dealing with rogue horses are sometimes heard to call it "the equalizer."

yucca A genus of plants growing in Mexico and southwestern United States, also called soap root. Their roots contain mucilage and saponaceous matter. Yucca is a reliable diuretic.

I have used yucca board for splint material in young foals with fractures or a need for extra support. Yucca board is flexible, yet when combined with the materials commonly used in bandages and casts, it provides adequate support for light-weight foals.

zinc chloride A white crystalline powder, soluble in water, used as a caustic and astringent. Local and topical use only in ulcers and fistulas.

zinc oxide A white powder, insoluble in water, used for its protective and astringent properties. In ointment or powder form, it is used for wounds and dermatitis.

zinc undecylenate A white powder used in ringworm infections and other forms of dermatitis.

DIAGNOSTIC PROCEDURES AND LABORATORY TESTS

acupuncture (stylostixis)   Puncturing with long, fine needles for diagnostic or therapeutic purposes. Detailed charts developed in China for use in humans. This precise information has been extrapolated for use in veterinary medicine. Show meridians to follow for treatment of specific disease entities.

The art of acupuncture has made great strides in the United States in recent years and is now being used fairly extensively for both local (regional) anesthesia and muscular disorders. Although great and exciting claims of phenomenal cures are reported in veterinary circles, the comfort that acupuncture provides appears to be of short duration. It has not been studied long enough in the U.S. to provide a compilation of data suitable for scientific analysis.

AGID   Agar-gel immunodiffusion laboratory test for the presence of EIA (equine infectious anemia), commonly known as the Coggins test. *See:* INFECTIOUS ANEMIA.

arthroscopy   Procedure for examining and assessing the internal status of a joint in the body. The arthroscope is a small, delicate, rod-shaped instrument equipped with a fiberoptic light source, enabling exploration of the joint space in its entirety.

When joint injury or disease is suspect and there are unanswered questions remaining after conventional diagnostic procedures and radiographs, then arthroscopic intervention is indicated.

Under a local anesthetic, an arthroscope can be introduced into the joint cavity. Based on the findings, a decision to treat conservatively or embark on surgical repair can be determined. This phenomenal instrument requires a mere 5 mm incision and one mattress suture for closure. *See:* ARTHROSCOPIC SURGERY.

biopsy   Gross visible and microscopic examination of tissues or cells removed from a living patient for the purpose of diagnosis or prognosis of disease or the confirmation of normal conditions.

There are several types of biopsies:

1. Aspiration or needle biopsy, a method by which a minute amount of tissue for examination is withdrawn through a hypodermic needle

2. Endoscopic biopsy, in which a tissue sample is obtained through or under the guidance of an endoscope (a long, flexible tube used for internal viewing of tissue and organs)

3. Punch biopsy, a method in which a cylindrical piece of tissue is removed by means of a special instrument introduced directly into an organ

fecal test Used to obtain information concerning the parasitic load affecting the horse, to evaluate the worm medicine used, or to assess the parasite control program to be instituted by the farm manager.

Bits of manure are collected, identified, and sent for laboratory examination. The feces are ground, soaked in a supersaturated sugar solution, and centrifuged for the purpose of concentrating the parasitic eggs. A drop of the concentrate is then placed on a slide and examined under a microscope. The type and number of ova (eggs) are recorded and this information is passed on to the doctor.

mallein test *See:* GLANDERS.

nerve block Use of a local anesthetic for diagnostic purposes. The anesthetic, usually 2 percent procaine hydrochloride, is injected into a nerve branch known to innervate a precise area. A definitive diagnosis can then be determined by the response of the horse to the local or regional desensitization.

In lameness diagnosis, the veterinary clinician customarily begins at the foot and systematically works up the leg until a conclusion can be established.

paracentesis (tapping) The passage of a needle or trocar into a cavity for the purpose of removing fluid or material for examination and analysis. Paracentesis is used in treatment, diagnosis, and prognostication.

Paracentesis can be performed on many areas of the body (abdomen, eye, thorax, etc.). The type most commonly peformed is abdominal paracentesis, which veterinarians carry out in intractable colic cases to determine the severity of the illness and the general condition of the intestines. The results can indicate the need for immediate surgical intervention or continued conservative treatment.

To perform an abdominal paracentesis, the veterinarian will determine a midline point between the umbilicus and the xyphoid cartilage situated on the end of the sternum. Aseptic preparation of the inconvenient and out-of-sight location on the standing horse consists of clipping, scrubbing, and shaving. Then a specially designed, shielded trocar is used to penetrate the muscles and retrieve the contents for both clinical (on-the-spot) and laboratory examination. *See:* COLIC.

PREVENTIVE MEDICINE
Boosters
Immunoglobulins
Quarantine
Teeth
Vaccination
Worming Program

boosters *See:* VACCINATION.

immunoglobulins *See:* VACCINATION.

quarantine If you run a healthy and happy barn, beware of the "newcomer." In spite of health certificates and apparent good physical appearance, horses can carry, incubate, and explode with an infectious disease within hours or days of arrival. Every good horse farm, therefore, should have a shed or some kind of quarantine shelter well isolated from the main barn and paddocks.

Place every new member into isolation for at least 18 days or whatever time duration your veterinarian deems necessary. Keep separate all utensils, both grooming and stable, as well as the clothing and boots of farm personnel. Request from the owner a current negative Coggins test for equine infectious anemia (EIA) and a negative fecal examination with a record of a recent worming. Be sure the horse has received a tetanus booster along with boosters for influenza, rhinopneumonitis, and *Strep equi*. Depending upon your geographic location and the time of year, question your veterinarian about the advisability of an equine encephalomyelitis vaccination.

teeth A horse's teeth continue to grow throughout its entire lifetime. This single fact distinguishes the equine from other species, and explains why horses so frequently need dental care.

Anatomically, the upper jaw (maxilla) of the horse is wider than the lower jaw (mandible), and thus the teeth and the entire dental arcade meet unevenly. This results in the formation of a ledge on the unopposed areas—the upper outside and lower inside surfaces. Rows of sharp projections form which, if allowed to grow unabated, can restrict jaw movement. This directly affects the efficiency of mastication.

Horses chew normally by moving their jaws laterally in a grinding and sliding motion. Formation of overgrown tooth edges can greatly interfere with grinding grain or other ingesta by limiting the range of jaw movement during chewing. Cheeks can be irritated and, in some cases, actually punctured by upper outside tooth edges. The tongue suffers equally from lower inside fang formation. Thus we see how these sharp and rigid tooth edges have the potential for damaging the horse's health and its ability to perform.

Painful conditions of the mouth are reflected in the horse by such behavior as resentment of the bit, head-shaking, and excessive salivation.

The answer to this ceaseless dental growth is a procedure called "floating," which means simply rasping away all unwanted tooth edges with the primary objective of leaving a smooth, functional, and comfortable dental arcade. A long-handled, specially designed instrument with a short dental rasp in the form of a blade is skillfully employed to smooth off all sharp points on the outside upper and inside lower edges of the molars. In addition, a conscientious horse dentist will use a so-called S-blade to round off all corner edges, especially those teeth exposed to the bit during exercise.

All the incisors (12) and the first three molars above and below (12) shed temporary teeth and then erupt permanent teeth. Only the last three molars above and below (12) have no temporary teeth; they erupt once as permanent teeth.

As the first three molars are pushed up from underneath by growth of the permanent molars, they are simultaneously worn down by opposing tooth pressure and a characteristic "cap" develops. When ready to shed, the cap has taken on the appearance of a plate-like structure, thin but wide, just barely covering the emerging permanent tooth. Natural shedding normally occurs in young horses during their late two-year-old or early three-year-old period. Caps often drop into the feed tub, having been removed in the way nature intended, by the grinding action of the molars.

A cap can, however, fail to shed, become sore, infected, and embedded in the gum tissue. A retained cap can result in an irritated, half-sick horse until the dentist lifts away and frees the fragmented piece of tooth.

Floating the teeth can be done as frequently as every four months in a sensitive performance horse. In an idle or retired horse, a once-a-year inspection is adequate.

It requires much practice to become skilled in floating teeth, not to mention the strength, dexterity, patience, and kindness that are needed, especially in working with high-strung horses. The jaw area of the horse, with its powerful muscles and large molar (grinding) teeth, is very dangerous to approach. It is my opinion that floating teeth is a job for a horse dentist, someone who is trained in the practice and who does it as a livelihood; it is not a job for a veterinarian, who is a doctor trained to treat and minister to the horse's medical needs.

Dental formulas have never ceased to confuse, so I have devised my own method of clarification.

At maturity, usually around five years of age, all horses have a "full mouth," indicating that all permanent teeth have erupted and are in proper position.

Normal mares have 36 teeth; normal male horses have 40. The difference is in the tusher teeth, sometimes called canine or bridle teeth. Males possess four tusher teeth (see below), while mares have none. If the wolf teeth (see the following page) are counted as premolars, then each sex has two additional teeth.

teeth continued

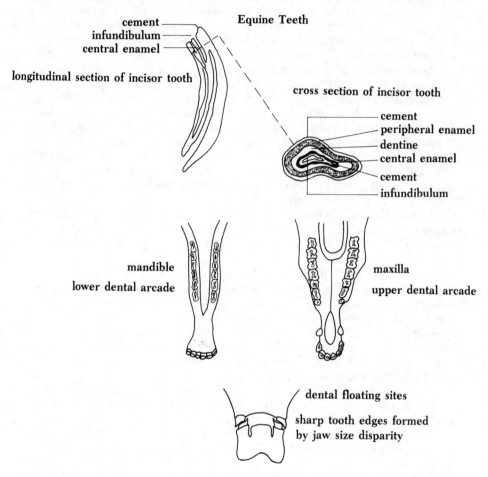

Equine Teeth

cement
infundibulum
central enamel

longitudinal section of incisor tooth

cross section of incisor tooth

cement
peripheral enamel
dentine
central enamel
cement
infundibulum

mandible
lower dental arcade

maxilla
upper dental arcade

dental floating sites
sharp tooth edges formed
by jaw size disparity

Bastard Root of Tooth, root of inferior molar protrudes below lower jaw

　　　An adult horse possesses 12 front teeth called incisors, six above and six below. The incisors' only purpose is prehensile, for grasping or biting, not for chewing or mastication. As the incisors grasp the food, the powerful, muscular tongue propels it back into the horse's mouth, that dark, out-of-sight place where amateur hands should never venture. Here is where the molars reside—six above and six below on each side—for a total of 24 grinders. This is also the site of mastication and early digestive enzyme action through the jaw movement and the flow of saliva.

　　　To complete the description of the dental arcade, most horses have a rudimentary vestige of the first premolar; called a wolf tooth, it is found nestled against the front surface of the upper molar on each side. These small, single-rooted teeth are a painful nuisance, especially when the bit inadvertently presses against them; they are best extracted, since they serve no known purpose. Wolf teeth, contrary to the belief of some, occur equally in both sexes.

A roomy interdental space is found between the incisors in the front of the mouth and the large powerful molars in the back. The bit fits well in this unrestricted area.

The only teeth found in the interdental space are the tushers, the so-called male teeth. A tusher can be found, one above and one below, on each side of the horse's mouth. Sharp, pointed, and well spaced from each other in the interdental space, their function is still a mystery.

Common signs of a dental problem while riding or driving are head-shaking, resentment of the bit, and excessive salivation. At rest or while eating, symptoms are head-tilting, peculiar chewing motion, pausing during mastication, and dropping small bits of half-chewed food back into the feed tub. Loss of body condition in spite of good stable management is another sign.

A "hay dunker," a horse that consistently submerges each mouthful of hay into the water bowl or pail before chewing and swallowing, is ready for a visit from the dentist.

Since horses' teeth do not decay or form cavities like those seen in all other domestic animals, an odor on the breath is a definite indication of either gum disease, sinusitis, or any one of a variety of tumors that may be found in the head and jaw region. The closely associated teeth then begin to loosen and suffer secondary to these diseases. A regularly scheduled dental check-up is equally as important as a parasite and vaccination program, and should be carried out semiannually in any conscientious program of active horse care.

vaccination Any vaccination program you follow is only as efficient as the biologics that are used. Your veterinarian utilizes vaccines from reputable drug houses, knowing that they have been accurately labeled (expiration dates and recommended dosage) and properly handled and stored (protected from extreme temperatures, lack of refrigeration, exposure to sunlight, and other circumstances that could cause them to degrade). Keeping these factors in mind, it is then possible to design a routine vaccination program. Rely on your veterinarian to determine dosage and to devise an individualized health-mainte-nance schedule for your horses and your geographic location.

Unfortunately, there is another class of drugs, those that are ordered by mail or purchased "under the counter" at cut-rate prices. Frequently these preparations are outdated, improperly labeled, and degraded due to improper storage. Instead of affording protection, they invite tragedy! Even when all the variables are under the control of professionals—as with the drugs from reputable companies—the margin of safety is narrow. Therefore, please do not walk a tightrope and jeopardize the health and security of your animals. Put trust in your veterinarian and in first-rate products.

Horses and horse owners are fortunate today in having available a variety of ethical vaccines and bacterins. Although the present list is somewhat limited, it represents great progress and foretells the future development of exciting new biologics that will offer even greater protection from disease and illness for our friend, the horse.

I recall the toll that diseases took but a short 20 years ago, both on the large

vaccination continued

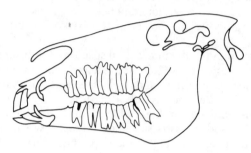

Horse Skull, dental arcade

breeding farms and on the farms of the "little" breeders. Today it is rare that a horse farm population is decimated by an epidemic. I say this not to lull the horse owner into a sense of false security, but rather to encourage a conscientious awareness of the need for a complete prophylactic medical program.

I would like to offer at this point a vaccination schedule for a mare being sent to a breeding farm, following her through gestation and parturition. The schedule then picks up her foal, and carries it through its first year of recommended protective vaccinations.

Each farm has its own immunization requirements, depending largely upon the knowledge and experience of the farm manager and the specific problems indigenous to the geographic location of the farm.

As a responsible owner, do not merely meet the farm requirements, but provide your animal with all available protection. Breeding farms are primarily concerned about infectious or contagious diseases, those that affect the well-being of a community of horses. You, as a horse owner, should be concerned with your mare's individual total protection. Send her to her breeding date as well immunized as you, your veterinarian, and modern science can ensure.

Give your veterinarian four to six weeks' advance notice of your plans. I must assume that your mare has been properly wormed against all parasites and has had blood drawn and submitted to the laboratory for the Coggins test for equine infectious anemia (EIA) and equine viral arteritis (EVA).

Begin with influenza vaccine (Flu Vac), rhinopneumonitis vaccine (Pneumobort K), and tetanus vaccine (Tetanus Toxoid), which can be administered simultaneously and, to ensure safety, in separate injection sites. Let me caution you that there are some highly advertised vaccines on the market today that combine three or four protective agents into one simple injection. This form of immunization is designed for convenience, expediency, and lower costs, and most likely it will be the method in the future. But before I, for one, blindly accept this "biologic package" for my patients, I want to see scientific documentation of additional experimentation and refinement of the drugs. Until then, I will continue the same regime of individual vaccinations, each in a separate site.

Allow one month's time to pass before the mare leaves, then give a booster of the three initial vaccinations. We have learned that the first influenza injection actually produces very few antibodies but acts as a preconditioner for the second, or booster, injection, which reacts dramatically to produce a strong defensive response.

An equine encephalomyelitis vaccination (bivalent) and Venezuelan equine encephalitis vaccination can be given during the second week of the program. Then the *Strep equi* bacterin, to prevent strangles, may be injected during the third week. Dosage and site should be judged carefully by your veterinarian. Remember, however, that you as the owner, have every right to insist on your horse receiving this muscle-irritating bacterin in the one proven location. The large gluteal muscle mass encompassing the major bulk of the hindquarters can quite well tolerate this testy bacterin. Seldom does a vaccination reaction develop in this location when reasonable precautions are followed, that is, cleansing well prior to injection and use of aseptic sterile equipment. I have seen horses suffer acute inflammatory reactions with subsequent severe muscle damage from the bacterin being injected into the neck, chest, or anywhere other than the muscles of the hindquarters. Deaths have been reported from careless use.

Strep equi bacterin is the only prophylactic drug available against the disease strangles and, although its use requires care and skill, it does provide some antibody protection against this dreaded disease. I think all would agree that this biologic belongs in the hands of the professional.

The boosters for influenza, rhinopneumonitis, and Tetanus Toxoid should be repeated in the fourth week.

Rabies vaccine and its prescribed use for horses is not substantiated, so this is a decision to be made by your veterinarian, based partly on the incidence of the disease in your area.

When sending your mare to the breeding farm, it is essential that you send, along with her other health records, written records of all the vaccinations she has received, including the dates. This information made available to the farm personnel could avert a mistake.

When your mare returns home pregnant, she should receive a rhinopneumonitis vaccine, namely, Pneumobort K (Fort Dodge Laboratory) killed vaccine, on the fifth month from the date of her last cover. This killed vaccine is safe for use in pregnant mares and should be repeated without fail on the seventh month of pregnancy and again on the ninth month.

One month prior to due date, it is advisable that the mare receive an injection of Tetanus Toxoid to stimulate the formation of tetanus antibodies in the colostrum (the first milk) to protect the newborn foal.

At the time of parturition, Tetanux Toxoid can be administered to the dam if it was not given at ten months, and the newborn foal should receive 1,500 I.U. of tetanus antitoxin along with the other routine injections, just to be certain that protection exists.

This is a highly controversial subject! Many practitioners believe that a tetanus antitoxin injection for the foal is an unnecessary precaution. I personally feel that it is better to be safe than sorry. It has been my finding that some mares fail to produce protective antibodies, and/or that some foals are unable to ingest, *vaccination continued*

assimilate, or even receive or benefit from the antibodies that are available. After considering the fact that several paths are open to failure, with no human way to recognize where the inefficiency lies—other than through tragedy—I therefore justify my routine 1,500 I.U. tetanus antitoxin injection to all newborn foals.

Also, all foals should receive the benefit of a recently developed zinc sulfate test for the detection of an unnecessary loss of an immune-deficient or immune-defective foal. This simple, on-the-spot screening test alerts the practitioner that an immune response is lacking in the foal. An immediate serum transfusion from an adult horse can supply the vital antibodies and in most cases save the foal's life.

Foals cannot produce their own antibodies before four months of age, and thus they live precariously with the help of maternal preformed antibodies. Although it has been documented that young foals respond poorly to antigens before four months of age, there are practitioners who insist on assaulting the foal's body with constant biologic injections during this early period. This is disconcerting if not actually damaging to the foal.

When the foal is 16 weeks of age, vaccines against influenza (Flu Vac), rhinopneumonitis (Pneumobort K or any other vaccine against rhinopneumonitis virus), and tetanus (Tetanus Toxoid) should be administered. In two weeks *Strep equi* bacterin (against strangles) should be given. The influenza rhinopneumonitis, and tetanus antitoxin vaccinations should be repeated, as boosters, in one month from the initial vaccinations to ensure immunity.

Advisability as to the use of equine encephalomyelitis vaccine in sucklings and weanlings will be decided subject to disease incidence, geographic location, and the discretion of your veterinarian.

You may have noticed that Pneumobort K vaccine is recommended for the foal as well as the broodmare. This could cause confusion without further explanation. *See:* RHINOPNEUMONITIS.

During their first three months, foals are vulnerable to a disease called Corynebacterium equi, for which there is no vaccine or bacterin. This bacterial disease causes the notorious "foal pneumonia" and is responsible for a high mortality rate in young foals. Fortunately, we do have effective antibiotics. If treatment is begun early and maintained with intensive efforts, some foals live.

After the initial vaccinations received during the fourth month, your foal will then require boosters of influenza and rhinopneumonitis every second or third month through the first year.

Tetanus Toxoid is required as an annual booster, unless otherwise indicated by lacerations or puncture wounds (especially in the foot area).

The number of vaccinations and the frequency of boosters depend greatly upon local disease incidence or prevalence, environmental conditions, weather changes, and most of all on the degree of exposure to or contact with strange horses, including new members added to the equine group and fellow competitors at horse shows, the race track, or other venues.

Please take the time, consult with your veterinarian, and design an annual schedule to prevent problems, maintain health, and promote productivity.

worming program   *See under:* PARASITES.

PREPARING A MARE FOR DEPARTURE

First Week	Influenza vaccine (Flu Vac, Fort Dodge Lab.)	Rhinopneumonitis vaccine (Pneumobort K, Fort Dodge Lab.)	Tetanus vaccine (Tetanus Toxoid, Fort Dodge Lab.)
	All three can be administered at one time.		
Second Week	Equine encephalomyelitis bivalent vaccine (Eastern & Western, Fort Dodge Lab.)	Equine encephalitis Venezuelan vaccine (optional use)	
Third Week	Strep equi bacterin (Strangles Bacterin, Fort Dodge Lab.)		
Fourth Week	Repeat the three initial vaccines given the first week: influenza, rhinopneumonitis, Tetanus Toxoid.		

PREGNANT MARE

* 5 months into gestation (count from date of last cover)	Rhinopneumonitis vaccine (killed) (Pneumobort K, Fort Dodge Lab.)
* 7 months	Repeat
* 9 months	Repeat
* 10 months	Tetanus Toxoid (Fort Dodge Lab.)

NEWBORN FOAL THROUGH FIRST YEAR OF LIFE

* At birth	1,500 I.U. Tetanus antitoxin. Repeat tetanus antitoxin if infection or delayed healing of navel cord occurs or in any puncture wound occurs especially low on the legs or in the feet.
* 4 months of age (16 weeks)	Influenza vaccine Tetanus vaccine (Flu Vac, Fort Dodge Lab.) (Tetanus Toxoid, Fort Dodge Lab.)
* 4½ months of age (18 weeks)	Rhinopneumonitis vaccine (Pneumobort K, Fort Dodge Lab.)
* 5 months of age (20 weeks)	Repeat the two original vaccines that now act as a booster (influenza and Tetanus Toxiod).
* 5½ months of age (22 weeks)	Repeat the rhinopneumonitis vaccine that now acts as a booster.

* Strep Equi bacterin and encephalitis vaccines can be administered in the foal anytime after 4 months as the prevalence of or exposure to disease dictates.

* Influenza and rhinopneumonitis vaccines should be repeated every third month during the yearling year.

* An annual Tetanus Toxiod booster suffices. When injury or infection develops, a booster is indicated.

POISONS

botulism A highly fatal food poisoning that affects both human beings and horses. *Clostridium botulinum* is the spore-forming micro-organism responsible for the disease. Resistant to most disinfectants, it requires warmth, moisture, and reduced oxygen in order to grow, sporulate, and produce its lethal neurotoxins. One small spoonful of toxin can kill a thousand-pound horse (a minute amount can kill a human).

The micro-organisms and its toxin are frequently found in neglected stalls, especially in corners under feed boxes and below water pails. This environment fulfills the botulism bug's need to propagate. If you see a green sprout growing in a dirty stall, you can be almost certain that the botulism micro-organism is also present, growing and producing its paralyzing endotoxin, since the sprout and *C. botulinum* require the exact same environment in which to grow and prosper.

Symptoms of botulism are:

1. Inability or difficulty swallowing with intermittent discharge of ingesta from the nostrils

2. Water-pail level remains constant—although the horse is attempting to drink

3. Dirty water in pail

4. Boluses of packed ingesta lodged between molars and cheeks, and small, moist boluses found in the feed tub

5. Progressive dehydration, weakness, and muscle flaccidity

6. Death

The nasal discharge consists of an admixture of soft grain particles and water. Normal body temperature, pink mucous membranes (oral and nasal), normal pulse, and normal respiratory rate are all curiously maintained until just before death.

Small, well-chewed boluses of hay and grain mixture can be found lodged in and around the molars, on the stall floor, or among the usually uneaten contents of the feed tub.

Dirty water in the pail is a prime clue that botulism is present. The water line is not lowered as the horse attempts to drink, because any water taken into the mouth pours out the nostrils and back into the pail. Once paralysis of the tongue and pharynx becomes established, the animal cannot eat or drink. This condition is irreversible.

The affected horse is hungry and seems normal though anxious early in the disease, but it grows steadily weaker until death arrives. Although the animal is *botulism continued*

completely conscious and mentally aware until the end, death comes through starvation and respiratory paralysis caused by the deadly toxin. This is a cruel disease!

Treatment consists of supportive therapy via tube feedings and intravenous fluid therapy. No effective or successful treatment is known, however. Prevention is the only cure.

To repeat the cautions I mentioned earlier:

1. Keep all stalls, including the corner areas, clean, dry, and well aired.
2. Clean up and remove all spoiled foods.
3. Avoid any source of contaminated food stuffs.
4. Keep your horse's total living environment clean and free of any decomposing or contaminated materials.
5. Feed only clean grains and clean hay.

Avoid mold-containing hay, feed mixtures, and grains. Moldy substances and the botulism toxins are death-dealing partners found together in spoiled hay or grain. Mold (fungi) causes a different disease with some symptoms similar to botulism. *See:* MOLDY CORN POISONING; MYCOTOXICOSIS.

You should be aware that people can contract the same lethal botulism toxin after eating canned goods that have been improperly prepared. Such food could contain contaminants or preformed toxins sealed into cans not subjected to proper temperature controls established for the processing plants by the Public Health Department.

Recent information has related *C. botulinum* infection to the mysterious "shaker foal syndrome." This research raises hope for better treatment and even a cure. Perhaps a vaccine or bacterin will be developed to prevent this ambiguous lethal disease of the newborn foal. *See:* SHAKER FOAL SYNDROME.

bracken fern poisoning   Bracken fern is a plant common to woodlands in the United States. The genus *Pteridium* is identified as the cause of poisoning in grazing animals. Bracken fern is not very palatable, but because it is green in color, it is more apt to be consumed in the fall and winter months in the absence of normal green pasture.

It is a poison with an insidious onset; animals have been known to graze on bracken fern for as long as 30 days before showing clinical symptoms. The effects of this poison are confined to the central nervous system in the horse, evidenced by inco-ordination, weakness, and staggering. If bracken fern is included in baled hay, it can cause toxicity in the stabled horse.

Treatment consists of thiamine hydrochloride injected (I.M.) at daily doses of 500 to 1000 milligrams.

Prognosis is usually poor because the amount ingested is unknown, and the time elapsed between ingestion and clinical symptomology precludes effective emergency poison measures.

hydrocyanic acid poisoning (prussic acid plant poisoning)   Prussic acid, a salt of hydrocyanic acid, is found in certain plants in the form of glycosides. A minute amount of this poison can cause death in a thousand-pound horse if it is ingested during certain circumstances. The poison element combines with the hemoglobin in the red blood cells (erythrocytes) and renders it inactive. In essence, no oxygen is carried to the tissues.

Precise conditions must exist to change a relatively nontoxic glycoside into a highly toxic prussic acid morsel for an unsuspecting horse. Young growing plants present a greater hazard to livestock because their glycoside content is higher than in mature plants.

If there is any abrupt halt in plant growth—caused, for example, by frost, drought, mowing, wilting, trimming, cleaning up—the harmless glycoside is chemically changed to the prussic acid. One wilted, crushed, green leaf (full of prussic acid) can, if ingested, kill a horse. The incidence of poisonings or deaths increases greatly after sudden wind and rain storms. Limbs are blown down and are damaged, thus prussic acid is produced.

Common plants that contain glycosides and are prime candidates for poisoning livestock are: black cherry tree, choke cherry tree, wild cherry tree, Christmasberry, Johnson grass, sorghum grass, and sudan grass.

Symptoms of poisoning are: weakness, blue gums (cyanotic membranes), heavy respiration, and collapse.

First aid calls for drenching with molasses and water as soon as the condition is recognized as prussic acid poisoning.

You can forestall poisoning by feeding corn or grain sorghums prior to turning the horse out to graze. Starch forms glucose in the gastrointestinal tract and helps prevent poisoning.

Although treatment is not too successful, call your veterinarian immediately. If the animal survives until the veterinarian comes, intravenous injections of sodium thiosulfate and nitrite combined with blood transfusions and oxygen therapy can be attempted.

The prognosis is guarded to poor.

Prevention is best. Remove all wild cherry trees from your premises. They are a common and constant threat, and have no place on a horse farm. Horses have been lost after a simple trimming or cleaning up of a downed limb by eating a few leaves that were missed by the rake.

I have treated many cases of prussic acid poisoning and have not been able to save many lives.

Be aware of the following common plants can be sources of poison: *See:* PLANT POISONS (CHART, PAGE 254–255).

metal poisoning *See:* CHEMICAL POISONS (CHART, PAGE 256–257).

moldy corn poisoning *See:* ENCEPHALOMALACIA.

mycotoxicosis *See:* ENCEPHALOMALACIA.

prussic acid *See:* HYDROCYANIC ACID POISONING.

PLANT POISONS

Species	Common Name	Symptoms	Location of Toxic Element	Geographic Location	Treatment
Amsinckia intermedia	Fiddleneck, tarweed, fireweed, buckthorn, yellow-burr weed	Liver degeneration	Common weed found in wheat; seeds contain toxic element (pyrrolozidine alkaloids)	Western U.S.A.	
Aspergillus fungi	Moldy corn poisoning, corn-stalk poisoning	Brain malacia, inability to eat or drink	Corn (mold)		Supportive
Astragalus oxtropis	Locoweed	Convulsive staggers, high-stepping gait	Leaves (alkaloid)	Western states	No treatment
Astragalus stanleya, Xylorrhiza oenopsis	Prince's plume, woody aster, golden weeds	Central nervous system disturbances, dark fluid feces	Plant (selenium)	Western states	No treatment
Centaurea solstitialis	Yellow star, thistle, Russian knapweed, sunflower family	Brain malacia, difficult swallowing, chewing and spitting, "wooden mouth"	Leaves and heads	Western states, California	Supportive, no treatment
Crotalaria spectabilis	Rattle box, rattle weed	Liver damage	Pyrrolozidine alkaloids	Southeastern states	
Equisteum	Horsetail, scouring rush	Liver damage	Meadow hay		Thiamine hydrochloride (1,000 mg)
Heliotropium	Not in the U.S.A.	Liver damage	Similar to senecio	Australia	
Lathyrus hirsutus	Caley pea, rough pea, singetary pea	Paralysis of hind legs	Baled hay		No treatment
Lupines	Lupines	Liver, diarrhea, and walking	Leaves (alkaloid)		No treatment

Scientific name	Common name	Symptoms	Toxic part	Location	Treatment
Nerium oleander	Oleander poisoning	Profuse diarrhea, irregular heart beat	Lawn clippings, leaves bailed in hay	California and southern U.S.A	
Nicotiana	Wild or tree tobacco poisoning	Central nervous system paralysis	Plant (alkaloid neonicotine)	Western states	No treatment
Persea americana	Avocado	Mastitis, reduced lactation	Stalks, leaves, & bark, fruit; pruning remnants	Tropical America; Florida and Southern California	
Pteridium	Bracken fern poisoning	Central nervous system disturbances, inco-ordination, staggering	Leaves	U.S.A. woodlands	Thiamine hydrochloride (1,000 mg)
Ricinus communis	Castor bean poisoning, castor oil plant, palma christi	Severe diarrhea	Seeds	California	
Senecio jacobaea	Ragwort, groundsel, willie, walking disease, Walla-Walla walking disease, winton disease	Liver damage	Pyrrolozidine alkaloids	Western and Mid-western U.S.A., Pacific Northwest, New Zealand	
Setaria galuca	Yellow bristle grass	Awns embedded in tongue and lips causing ulcers	Mechanical irritation	Western states	Cautery and debridement
Solanaceae	Nicotine	Central nervous system paralysis	Plant	Western states	
Sorghum	Sudan grass	Cystitis, bladder paralysis	Grass		No treatment

CHEMICAL POISONS

Poison	Source	Symptoms	Rx and Comments
Antu	Rodenticide	Nervousness, depression, death	No effective antidote
Arsenic	Insecticides, herbicides, rodenticides, wood preservatives, medicines	Acute: gastrointestinal upset Chronic: loss of weight at necropsy, resistive to tissue decomposition	Remove source and administer BAL (British AntiLewite)
Aldrin, Dieldrin, endrin, isodrin	Herbicide (chlorinated hydrocarbon)	Convulsions and colic	Too dangerous to use
Benzene hexachloride (BHC), lindane	Parasiticides, dips, sprays (chlorinated hydrocarbon)	Convulsions and colic	BHC is dangerous in milking and meat animals, as it is eliminated in milk and stored in fat. Protect feed and water source. Rx: sedation and calcium gluconate
DDT, chlordane	Parasiticides dips, dusts and sprays (chlorinated hydrocarbons)	Convulsions and colic	Use is outlawed; secreted in milk, low concentrations contaminate feed and water; tissue residues accumulate. Rx: calcium gluconate
Fluoroacetate (1080)	Rodenticides	Convulsions and diarrhea	Occurs in rodent eradication
Heptachlor	Parasiticides field, crop, spray or dust (chlorinated hydrocarbon)	Convulsions and diarrhea	Too poisonous in mammals to use
Lead	Insecticides, paints, medicines industrial fall-out gases and fumes	Chronic stiffness and weakness, central nervous system symptoms, difficult breathing with roaring; lead sulfide gumline	Rx: calcium intravenous, supportive treatment
Methoxychlor	Parasiticides (chlorinated hydrocarbon)	Convulsions and diarrhea	Least toxic of all effective chlorinated hydrocarbon insecticides; essentially nontoxic, noncumulative, and not eliminated in milk.

Poison	Source	Symptoms	Treatment
Organic phosphates	Insecticides, orchard and field sprays, pesticides	Colic, perspiration, profuse salivation, pupil constriction, muscular weakness	Rx: atropine intravenous with antidote 2-PAM (2-pyridine-aldoxime-methioide) every 3 hours
Phenol	Wood preservatives	Acute: Convulsions, paralysis, fatal Chronic: dermatitis, burns, central nervous system symptoms	Remove source, supportive treatment
Phosphorus	Fireworks storage	Colic, convulsions, garlic breath	Rx: supportive therapy
Zinc phosphide	Rodenticides (rat poison)	Colic (fatal), internal bowel hemorrhages	Rx: no effective treatment
Selenium (alkali disease)	Cereal grains (oats, corn wheat) and forage grown on soil with high selenium content	Chronic: unthriftiness, hoof changes, hair loss, internal lesions; kidney liver and spleen disorders	Rx: remove from source, supportive therapy
Strychnine	Pesticides, rodenticides, medicines	Central nervous system symptoms, convulsions	Rx: sedation, supportive therapy
Thallium	Rodenticides	Tremors, depression, paralysis, intestinal hemorrhaging	Rx: No satisfactory treatment
Toxaphene (camphene)	Parasiticides (ticks and mites) (chlorinated hydrocarbon)	Liver damage, central nervous system symptoms	Rx: calcium gluconate, effective against ticks and mites and safe when used cautiously; do not use in young or old horses.
Barium chloride	Rodenticide	Gastrointestinal	Rx: supportive therapy
Warfarin	Rodenticide	Shock and hemorrhage	Rx: whole-blood transfusions, vitamin K

TOXIC GASES

Gas	Source	Treatment
Carbon monoxide	Fuel gas, motor fumes, manure pit	Remove to open air, oxygen therapy, sedate, if necessary
Carbon disulfide	Solvent, fumigant used for lice and mites	Remove to open air, supportive therapy; dangerous fire hazard
Hydrocyanide	Fumigant	Remove to open air. Rx: dextrose and trypan blue sodium thiosulate (i.v. preparation)
Hydrogen disulfide	Manure pit	Fresh air, oxygen therapy
Ammonia	Fertilizer tanks, refrigerants	Remove to open air, supportive treatment; danger from leakage from tanks adjacent to stables
Nitrous dioxide	Silo gas	Remove to open air, avoid pulmonary edema, oxygen therapy
Ozone	Generators	Remove to open air, oxygen therapy
Sulfur dioxide	Fumigant, solvent	Respiratory irritant; remove to open air, protect eyes, oxygen therapy

VICES

aerophagia A wind-swallowing vice, constantly confused with cribbing and windsucking, each a separate entity. A horse can swallow air by simply elevating and extending its head and neck into the air. It does not require a ledge, fence, or solid object to aid in this vice, therefore physical destruction is not in evidence.

An aerophagic horse is much less obnoxious than a cribber, but it can suffer equally from gastrointestinal disturbances. If you stand by the stall quietly, you can readily distinguish the somewhat subdued sound made as air passes into the esophagus and down into the small and distended stomach.

I have had aerophagic patients in my hospital ward for days before they were recognized as wind-swallowers. I think you would agree an offensive and destructive cribber would be identified immediately. *See:* CRIBBING, WINDSUCKING.

bolt Slang term for rapid gulping of large mouthfuls of grain; can and often does result in colic pain and symptoms.

To prevent this vice, place a large salt block in the feed tub, or use large clean rocks. This allows the grain kernels to fall down and around the objects and prevents the horse from taking large mouthfuls in quick succession.

When feeding mashes, the large rocks are preferred to prevent gulping; salt blocks disintegrate into the mash and can act as a toxic agent—although most horses will reject an overly salty meal.

copraphagy The eating of manure; a foal can develop this vice in any circumstances. I have noted that foals with excellent nutrition and all-over good environment sometimes acquire this undesirable and distressing habit. Because manure is literally loaded with parasitic ova and irritants, consumption readily causes enteritis and intractable diarrhea.

Although it is a somewhat impractical suggestion, the manual removal of all manure from the stall before it can be ingested seems to be the only solution to copraphagy, aside from one's hope that the habit will eventually be broken, perhaps with maturity and/or a change in environment.

cribbing This vice requires a ledge, stall door, window base, feed tub, or any fence rail that the horse can grasp by the front teeth or rest upon. It requires positioning the head and neck precisely so that air can be pulled into the esophagus and swallowed, thereby entering the stomach.

This is an acquired habit usually learned at a young age and augmented or imprinted by seeing and hearing a "cribber" in the pasture or neighboring stall. Lengthy confinement, inadequate roughage, or (we suspect) boredom causes this habit. I have wondered, too, about hereditary predisposition. Long hours of practice are needed to perfect the act of cribbing, since a horse is a strict

cribbing continued

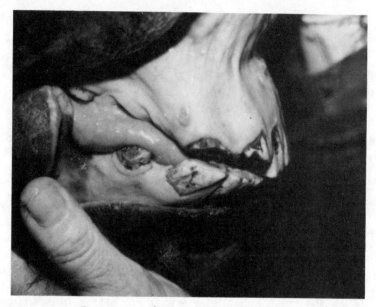

Destruction of Incisors Through Cribbing

nose-breather and is quite unable to breathe through the mouth; for air to enter through the mouth and be admitted into the esophagus, the horse must create a vacuum. Unlike the cribber, the aerophagic horse does this simply by elevating the head and nose and less air is swallowed with less gastrointestinal distress.

In explaining the mechanics of cribbing, it has been suggested that the horse grasps an object with the incisor teeth, preferably at head level, and then, by pressing downward with arched neck and open mouth, causes the elongated soft palate to be pulled upward. This achieves a momentary open airway for the air to be swallowed, accompanied by the all-too-familiar "gulp" or grunt associated with cribbing.

An owner is seriously at fault for allowing a young horse to be in a barn or paddock or on the premises of a cribber, for it will undoubtedly mimic the cribbing behavior.

Telltale evidence of this vice includes eroded incisors, the mark of a cribbing strap around the horse's neck, and ugly destruction of stalls, ledges, and fences. The horse suffers gastrointestinal distress in all its variations (colic, flatulence, irritation from splinters). Cribbing intermittently while eating grain induces choking, coughing, and various forms of indigestion.

Prognosis is guarded to very poor. Corrective measures may be attempted—cribbing straps, fluted bits, gallons of bitter-tasting chemicals, or even a radical, somewhat destructive, surgical procedure introduced in the late 1920s (Forsell's operation, the transection of two of the muscles used in swallowing)—but none has proved really satisfactory.

It is my opinion that once a cribber develops this habit of swallowing air, it is incurable and the long-suffering owner must endure its results for the life of the horse.

When I observe a cribber in action, the facial expression and relentless drive to overcome all efforts to inhibit the act simulate the almost desperate actions of a human being in the grip of narcotics addiction!

Do not confuse cribbing with woodchewing aerophagia or with the distinct and unique broodmare problem of windsucking. *See:* AEROPHAGIA, WINDSUCKING.

horsebites   The severity of an animal bite varies from animal to animal, of course. Carnivores inflict a puncture wound, then usually tear or lacerate the flesh as they retract their fangs or as the victim pulls away. This kind of wound usually becomes infected because the teeth and gums of dogs or cats are teeming with bacteria and in effect inoculate the traumatized tissue.

A horsebite is quite different from that of a carnivore. The head and neck of the average horse together weigh several hundred pounds; when used as a weapon, they inflict a terrible blow resulting in a large bruise, contusion, or hematoma in muscle tissue. Sometimes the skin is broken, but rarely to any significant degree compared to a carnivore's bite.

A horse's bite can be as traumatic and damaging as a kick! Both biting and kicking are serious vices!

rolling   The first symptom of colic or of any intestinal pain; in itself rolling constitutes a danger. After summoning the veterinarian, make every effort to keep the animal up on its feet. Rolling not only can cause external injury, but it can predispose or encourage a twisted intestine. By walking your animal, you are protecting it from self-inflicted injuries.

The veterinarian will administer a painkilling drug and relieve the animal somewhat. A diagnosis will then be forthcoming with appropriate treatment to follow.

Inexplicably, some horses take pleasure in habitually rolling in their stalls, and they may on occasion become cast. To rise, a horse needs its feet underneath its body, so being cast in a stall corner or against a wall with all four feet elevated, being quite unable to roll backwards, presents a serious problem. The horse might have to wait until morning for help to arrive. Injuries and illness can result.

To assist a horse in this situation, loop a rope around the fore and hind pasterns and give a hardy pull to help the animal roll over. It will then promptly rise.

A piece of gear called a "roller" can prevent these emergencies. It is a wide (1- to 6-inch) leather bellyband with a sturdy high ring at the vertebral column level that prevents rolling in the majority of cases. The roller allows the horse to recline and rest but *not* roll over.

wind swallowing   *See:* AEROPHAGIA.

windsucking   *See under:* BREEDNG.

LITTLE-KNOWN FACTS

Every day we learn something new to help raise our standards of horse care. At the same time, many of the old standby remedies of former times are simply forgotten. Other facts—perhaps because they are so obvious—don't seem to register with the majority of horse people, despite their crucial importance for the well-being of the horse (see, for example, the entry below on the subject of knots).

To conclude this book, then, I have collected some of these generally nonclassifiable bits of information. They are intended both to intrigue and instruct.

belch To eructate, or raise gas from the stomach. The equine lacks the ability to eructate and suffers all the consequences. What it swallows remains in its gastrointestinal tract and must pass through! The horse also is a notoriously selective eater, very fussy about what it allows even to enter its mouth. Is there perhaps an association here?

Contrary to what is documented, however, a horse *can* belch, but only under two very special circumstances.

I have observed in numberless cases, that within three minutes after removing a stomach tube from a horse, there is a belching of gas and semisolid material up through the esophagus. Perhaps the tube passing through the esophagus creates a transient reduction in tissue tone, permitting this unrecorded phenomenon.

The second condition when a horse is able to eructate is a grave and sad time. Eructation, with vomiting of the stomach contents, unequivocally means rupture of the stomach; death ensues within two hours. *See:* PERITONITIS.

bile Yellowish brown or green secretion of the liver that empties into the duodenum where it aids in digestion and peristalsis. Proper amount and flow of bile is necessary to maintain intestinal health.

The horse is unique in that it has no gall bladder in which to store bile; its liver produces a continuous flow of bile. Perhaps this is why horses prefer to eat small quantities of food continuously as opposed to the large meals interspersed with fasting periods that are preferred by carnivores (including the human being).

bishoping A fraudulent method of altering the teeth with a rasp and stain for the purpose of falsifying age. A common practice in the early part of the century when horses were still the major means of transportation. *See:* TEETH.

blacksmith   A smith who works in iron and makes iron utensils. Not to be confused with a skilled horseshoer, plater, or farrier. *See:* FARRIER.

black teeth   Stained teeth often found in horses shipped from the states west of the Mississippi River. It is believed that the stain comes from grazing on soil that is either deficient or overly rich in minerals. It is difficult if not impossible to remove. Stained teeth are not a health problem, only a cosmetic one.

bleeding   As a young person, I observed old-timers employ two crude practices that went by the name of "bleeding."

The first was used by unscrupulous horse dealers to quiet a horse just prior to showing the animal to a prospective buyer. The dealer inserted a large needle, or trochar, into the horse's jugular vein and "let" a large quantity of blood in order to temporarily weaken the animal. This made the rogue or bad actor seem quite placid, even calm enough for a trial ride and subsequent purchase.

In our day bloodletting has been replaced by tranquilizing. A small quantity of the proper drug, administered with a quick, small needle, is all that is needed to produce a quiet animal.

Another, very different, procedure, called "bleeding" was used when a horse foundered and the os pedis, the bone of the foot, began to break away from the toe-wall area. This is caused by the pooling of blood in the foot, with consequent changes in foot tissue.

Old-time farriers were able to prevent the irreversible movement of the os pedis by means of a radical cutting technique. Brute strength was required of these smiths to hold one fore foot and force the horse to bear its body weight on the opposite, exquisitely painful foot. As quickly and deftly as possible, the smith slashed deeply into the foot one-half inch in front of the apex of the frog. He would repeat this as many times as necessary until the foot was rid of the accumulated blood supply.

An iodine-soaked cotton swab was laid loosely over the cut area and the foot was bound in burlap sacks tied with baling twine.

Crude and cruel as this procedure seems to us today, it was often successful in preventing the crippling for which founder is so notorious. *See:* FOUNDER.

brine   Water saturated in salt. A supersaturated salt solution is commonly used to preserve raw fish.

While still a very young girl, I discovered that fish brine has an almost miraculous curative power for bowed tendons. I had purchased an aged gelding with two large bows in front. His steeplechase future was dubious, but his racing record was impressive, despite his huge, abused legs.

I began to research all the known treatments and remedies for so-called broken-down horses. The search went on and on, and I made no appreciable progress. Then, one day, a dear old horseman friend, who happened to be Jewish, came into my barn. I showed him my poor-legged, retired steeplechaser, explaining that I wanted to help it, but couldn't find anything that seemed a possible remedy.

His eyes opened wide and he beamed at me.

"Go to your local delicatessen and ask for a barrel of fish brine," he said. It specifically had to be mackerel brine. I was to bring home the barrel of brine, minus the fish, of course. "Saturate at least four sturdy leg bandages and apply

brine continued

daily," he instructed. "Remove just before exercise. Then replace immediately after exercise!"

I couldn't believe it, but I followed his advice. For three dollars a barrel, I smelled up the barn for weeks on end. And every day my old racer stood in the vile-smelling bandages. Three barrels of fish brine later, I noticed that his legs seemed smaller in size. Each day they were firmer and slimmer. And each day they more and more resembled pieces of petrified wood, not legs belonging to a live animal! The brine was "curing" his soft, mushy tendons.

After several months my broken-down champion returned to the races and performed creditably over the large brush jumps at Delaware Park. Never again did he show any sign of tendonitis or any inclination to re-bow. Believe me! *See:* BOWED TENDONS, TENDONITIS.

farrier   The correct term for a master horseshoer. A farrier is equally proficient in designing a shoe at the forge and anvil as he is in dressing and balancing a foot while crouched under the horse. Only through years of hard work, dedication, and time spent as an apprentice working with a skilled farrier is it possible to achieve such knowledge and dexterity. There are no short courses or shortcuts in learning how to shoe a horse properly.

The *plater* and the *horseshoer* are less skilled individuals. The former works mostly at race tracks. They apply aluminum or steel racing plates that come in a variety of sizes with features to suit different horses and conditions (e.g., toe grabs, block heels for elevation, mud stickers for an "off" track). If one size doesn't fit, another will. The shoes are applied cold and adjusted with the aid of a hammer and small portable anvil.

Horseshoers usually use steel "keg" shoes, also made ready-to-fit in all sizes. The foot is shaped to the nearest size of shoe available. These shoes suit the average pleasure horse owner who depends upon the local horseshoer to keep his animal ready for weekend riding.

A farrier takes his craft very seriously. He will watch a horse walk, observe the foot as it lands upon the ground surface, examine the old shoes for evidence of uneven or telltale wear, and then, with this information in mind, proceed to dress and balance each foot. He will wait for yet another walk to reassure himself that the foot is level when it meets the ground surface. By this time, he will have decided the size, shape, and total design of the appropriate shoe. The farrier will then go to the anvil and forge and proceed to make the shoe. He will make as many fittings as necessary to determine needed adjustments and will then apply the shoe. The job is not completed until he has watched the horse move with the new shoes and has done all necessary fine-tuning of the fit.

By taking this much time and trouble, the farrier can prevent much future trouble. Good farriers are a dying breed. Let us preserve and encourage the few that remain. *See:* FOOT.

glass eye (blue eye, wall eye)   An eye with a nearly white iris and a slightly blue corpora nigra (an area positioned centrally on the upper border of the pupillary opening and comprised of several small black masses).

The iris is responsible for the color of the eye, and is usually brown in color. Heterochromia, a variety of iris colors, is not common in the horse, but when

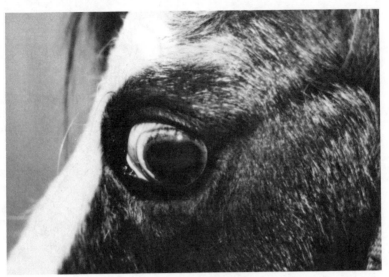

Glass Eye, or Blue Eye Heterochromia

found it is associated with paint horses (piebald, skewbald) and palomino horses. A heterochromic iris can be a combination of the colors white, brown, and blue.

Different colors of the iris have no bearing on vision; they represent only an aesthetic consideration—although this could affect the salability of a horse depending upon the purpose for which it is needed.

An old wives' tale has it that glass-eyed horses are temperamentally unreliable and that their vision is defective. Nothing could be further from the truth. During years of vetting horses for sales purposes, I have found that eyes with color variations, upon ophthalmoscopic examination, prove exceptionally sound and somewhat above average.

injections Administering drugs by injection enhances the action of drugs and provides a more controlled, accurate, and effective means of treatment. In contrast, oral administration of drugs is quite unpredictable because the stability of drugs in this form is affected by time and environmental factors, and because they interact with various influences in the gastrointestinal tract.

knots There are two essential knots for every horseman to master. One, perhaps the most important, is the *bowline*. Although best known around sailors and sailboats, the bowline is the safest knot for use with a horse when a neck rope is required either alone or in combination with a halter. This knot produces a loop that will never tighten down when pulled upon.

The other useful knot is a modified *slip knot,* used at the far end of the rope or shank when tying a horse. It is specifically designed to prevent the horse from releasing itself and yet it is impossible to tighten down and is always ready for emergency release. This knot has been called the "horseman's knot."

For my personal observations of the disasters that result when horses are improperly tied, I urge you to learn and use these knots, no matter how hurried you may be! *See:* BOWLINE KNOT, SLIP KNOT (ILLUSTRATIONS).

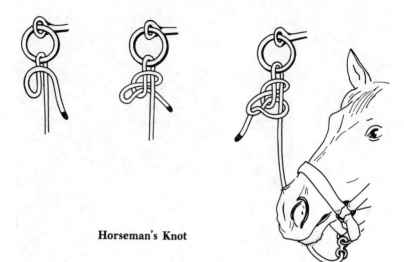

Horseman's Knot

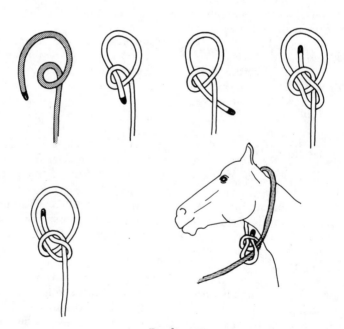

Bowline Knot

sheath cleaning At least twice a month clean the sheath of your gelding or stallion. Use warm water, white soap, and disposable cotton. Do not use barn sponges; they can transmit infection.

Be sure to clean the gummy substance, called smegma, from the little pouches on the end of the penis just above the urethral opening on down the entire inner surface of the sheath. If ignored, they become foul-smelling. Clean thoroughly around the preputial cavity. Rinse well with clean warm water. Then apply a generous coating of olive oil to the entire area. The oil prevents soreness and dryness and maintains the moisture necessary for good hygiene.

signs of the zodiac Many horsemen attach great importance to the phases of the moon. For example, one of the most widespread customs is to castrate animals in "the sign of the knees to the feet." It is claimed that the swelling will "run into the ground" and that recovery will be smooth.

If the operation is performed when the moon is "in the sign of the head or neck," belief has it that great swelling with develop. If surgery is performed "in the sign of the heart," the patient may bleed to death, while blood poisoning will surely develop if the operation is performed in the "sign of the bowels."

Another belief is that both mother and foal will survive much better if weaning is done "in the sign of the breast."

sling An apparatus specifically designed to elevate a recumbent horse onto its feet and provide intermittent weight support when needed. In certain situations, a sling can be a great help, *provided* it is applied correctly and managed properly. For its successful use, however, the patient's primary condition warranting the need for elevation as well as the horse's temperament bear more heavily than any concerted effort on the success and ultimate outcome.

The horse differs from other creatures by virtue of its size, weight, and temperament. A horse does not lend itself to the pressures and confines of a supportive sling with its array of straps, ropes, and chains. What is more, few people are experienced in the operation of a horse sling and, as shocking as it may be, in the wrong hands—no matter how conscientious—a sling can directly cause the death of a horse.

Once an animal is raised onto its feet by the use of a sling, the apparatus can remain in place to lend support in an *intermittent* fashion. The horse must not be allowed to hang in the sling, otherwise it will surely die. Vital respiration and circulation will be immediately impaired by profound pressure, with both systems eventually compromised. I would like to emphasize that a sling, therefore, is useful only to assist in rising and assist in standing; it is never to serve as total support. If a horse cannot support its own weight once elevated onto its feet, it should then be lowered back down into the straw to rest comfortably, perhaps to try again later.

It seems that slings are no longer manufactured; a good horse sling today has become a valuable and rare possession, one that every equine practitioner would like to own.

A useful and safe sling would include a durable wide bellyband with easily adjustable front and back panels allowing for critical balance of the animal while in suspension. All supports converge centrally over the animal's back to meet a

sling continued

single tree equipped with a swivel and chain attached to a chain hoist that is secured to the ceiling rafters.

A common error when suspending a block and tackle from the ceiling is the miscalculation of the distance needed for the horse's head and body once the animal is upright. To avoid undue stress by unnecessary handling of a sick and weak animal, be certain to place the hoist high enough, even if it requires making a hole in the ceiling for adequate elevation. This forethought can avoid wasting costly time, but more important, it can prevent undue handling with subsequent exhaustion of the patient.

In conclusion, it is easy to understand the hazards involved in the use of a poorly constructed sling or *any* sling in inexperienced hands. In an emergency, it is almost better to wait and avail yourself of advice from those experienced in the use of a sling than to pursue this adventure alone.

With all my warnings, you may find the use of a sling to be very rewarding, especially if you have a cooperative horse.

stay apparatus   Comprises a specific group of ligaments and some tendons in both the fore and hind limbs of the horse.

Fore leg, beginning distally and progressing proximally:

1. Group of sesamoid ligaments (ankle and pastern)
2. Large singular suspensory ligament (cannon bone)
3. Inferior carpal check ligament (below knee)
4. Superior radial check ligament (above knee)
5. Biceps brachii tendon and extensor carpi radialis tendon (shoulder and fore arm)
6. Serratus ventralis muscle (ribs and scapula)

Hind leg, beginning distally and progressing proximally:

1. Group of sesamoid ligaments (ankle and pastern)
2. Large singular suspensory ligament (cannon bone)
3. Inferior (tarsal) check ligament (below hock)
4. Gastroncemius muscle (gaskin area)
5. Peroneus tertius muscle (gaskin area)

This noteworthy apparatus of complex and interwoven checks and balances reduces concussive shock and prevents overextension of the limb, especially the distal joints of the long, vulnerable equine leg.

The stay apparatus is directly responsible for the horse's unique ability to sleep while in a standing position.

stomach tube (nasogastric tube)   An essential and integral part of the horse doctor's veterinary equipment. A stomach tube is a specifically designed tube made of plastic (polyethylene), approximately 8 feet long, from three-eighths to one-half inch outside diameter, and preferably soft in texture. In the proper hands, a stomach tube is the most humane and satisfactory instrument used in large-animal practice. Not only can the tube carrying bitter drugs by-pass all taste buds, it also obviates the need for swallowing large quantities of fluids (horses resist and spit out when drenched), and it introduces the needed medicines directly into the stomach with no question of a doubt. And it does all this with great ease on the part of the patient. Among its many applications are:

1. Administration of routine anthelmintics (worm medicine)
2. Administration of large quantities of fluid, perhaps bitter-tasting, in the treatment of colic symptoms
3. Allowing escape of trapped gas and stomach contents that might otherwise lead to rupture of the stomach

Since it requires a knowledge of anatomy, together with practice and skill to properly pass a stomach tube, tubing should be left to your veterinarian. Many unfortunate horses have suffered nose bleeds and various other traumatic injuries from inexpert use of a stomach tube; the most dreadful of all accidents is the introduction of the tube into the lungs rather than the stomach.

To sum up the value I place upon the stomach tube and its merit in horse practice: If I had to select one single instrument with which to practice, I would choose the stomach tube.

swallowing The ability to swallow is an important diagnostic sign in the differentiation of several diseases. Dysphagia, or difficulty in swallowing, occurs from a painful or inflamed throat, mechanical obstruction, or a central nervous system disorder, usually a toxicity.

To me, the symptom of reluctance to swallow in a horse is grave and alerts me to suspect some serious condition affecting the central nervous system: paresis associated with botulism or mycotoxicosis (moldy corn poisoning), tetanus, rabies, or some toxicity.

Once paralysis appears clinical in the pharynx, larynx, and tongue area, it is, in my opinion, irreversible. *See:* BOTULISM, MOLDY CORN POISONING.

tonsils The tonsil tissue of the horse differs greatly from that of other species. It consists of vast numbers of whitish nodules, looking much like tapioca pudding, evenly distributed on the roof of the pharynx. This tissue is credited with performing normal tonsil functions.

It is believed by some that the nodules vary in number, size, shape, and color consistent with changes in the immune response of young horses. The roughened pharyngeal surface gradually smoothes with acclimatization and antibody formation; the pharyngeal surfaces of older immune horses are smooth and glistening in appearance.

Thanks to the inception and clinical use of the fiberoptic endoscope, the otherwise hidden upper respiratory tract can be well explored and studied. *See:* RESPIRATORY TRACT.

vertebral formula This refers to the five areas of the spine, the chain of small bones (vertebrae) that extends from the skull to the end of the tail. From head to tail, the equine spinal column comprises between 51 and 57 vertebrae in groups designated cervical, thoracic, lumbar, sacral, and coccygeal. The "vertebral formula" is $C_7T_{18}L_6S_5Cy_{15-21}$.

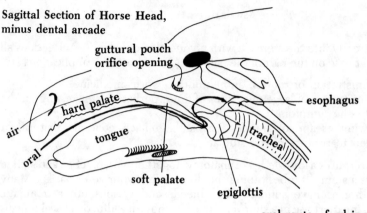

Sagittal Section of Horse Head,
minus dental arcade

guttural pouch
orifice opening

hard palate

esophagus

air

trachea

oral

tongue

soft palate

epiglottis

oral route—food ingestion
respiratory route—air inhalation
(please note that routes intersect)

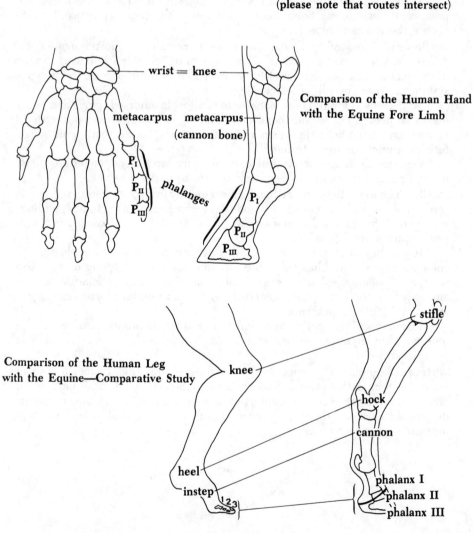

wrist = knee

Comparison of the Human Hand
with the Equine Fore Limb

metacarpus   metacarpus
(cannon bone)

P_I

P_{II}

phalanges

P_I

P_{III}

P_{II}

P_{III}

Comparison of the Human Leg
with the Equine—Comparative Study

stifle

knee

hock

cannon

heel

instep

1 2 3

phalanx I

phalanx II

phalanx III

Index

Abdomen, 19, 25, 26, 30, 32, 34, 47, 59, 126, 132, 153, 154
  cavity, 50, 153
  hernia, 165
  muscle, 22, 51, 139, 140
  pain, 5, 17–18, 229
Abortion, 11, 16, 43, 57–59, 62, 70, 125–127, 136, 144, 154, 196, 198, 216, 235
Abscess, 9, 16, 45, 61–62, 87, 122, 153
Absorbine, 211
Acetic acid, 224, 230–231
Achilles tendon, 102
Acidemia, 144
Acidifiers, 227
Acidophilus milk, 65
Acidosis, 18, 126
Actinobacillus, 25, 26, 50, 144, 153, 155
Acupuncture, 240
Additives. *See* Supplements
Adenoviral infection, 145
Adhesions, 54, 88, 89, 113, 114
Adrenal gland, 20, 22
Aerophagia, 259–261
African horse sickness, 9–10
Afterbirth, 134, 136
Agalactia, 126–127, 146
Age and disorders, 25, 34; *see also* specific ailments
AGID test. *See* Coggins test
Agglutination, 150
Aggressive behavior, 53, 160
Air, 3, 4, 79
  flow, 54, 84, 124
  guttural pouches, 28, 29
  pollution, 52
  sacs, 50, 51
Alcohol, 51, 113, 123, 202, 211, 217, 222
Alfalfa, 49, 52, 187, 189–191, 194, 196, 197
Alkaloids, 224–225, 228

Allanator's chorion, 136
Allergy, 10, 52, 53, 68, 201, 226, 230
Aloes, 225
Aluminum acetate solution, 211, 213
Alveoli, 50, 51
Amino acids, 187, 189, 192
Aminocyclitols, 225
Aminoglycosides, 225
Aminophylline, 225
Ammonia, 211, 226
Amnion, 127, 136
Amnionic membrane, 11
Amniotic membrane, 127, 136
  fluid, 127, 132
Amorphus globosus, 127, 136
Analgesics, 19, 33, 45, 67, 153, 202, 220, 236, 238, 239, 261
Anaphylaxis, 201–202
Anascarca, 132
Anemia, 39, 149–151; *see also* Equine infectious anemia
Anesthesia, 131, 161, 229
  epidural, 143
  general, 42, 58, 95, 159, 204, 228, 229, 239
  local, 82–83, 90, 106, 241
Animals, wild, 53
Anise, 211, 226
Anisium, 211, 227
Ankles, 49, 73–74, 81–82, 110–113, 167, 213, 219, 268; *see also* Joints and Lesions
Ankylosis, 74, 95
Antibiotics, 226; *see also* specific ailments or diseases
Antibodies, 2, 35, 43, 61, 62, 127, 142, 146, 147, 149–150, 152, 209, 248, 269
Anorexia, 197, 199
Anthelementics. *See* Worming medicine
Anthrax, 10–11

Antibacterial drugs, 225
Anticonvulsants. *See* Convulsions
Antidiarrhetics. *See* Diarrhea
Antidotes, 217, 219, 222, 225
Antihistamines, 10, 52, 53, 69, 140, 202, 226–227
Anti-inflammatories, 37, 80, 95, 100, 113, 218, 227–228, 230, 235
Antiflatulents. *See* Gas
Antimony trichloride, 230
Antiphlogistics, 212, 219, 221, 227; *see also* Cooling agents
Antipruritics, 217, 228
Antipyretics, 228, 236
Antiseptics, 61, 211, 214–217, 219, 221–223, 227, 230, 237
Antispasmodics, 212, 220
Anus, 45, 140, 141, 160, 214
Anxiety, 22, 48, 201
Appetite, 33, 43, 50, 53, 64, 126, 187, 212, 222, 237
Apple ankle. *See* Epiphysitis
Arbovirus, 11, 22–23
Army
  anesthetic, 228, 229
  white wash, 223
Arthritis, 74, 82, 89, 220, 227, 229, 232, 235, 236; *see also* Osteoarthritis
Arthroscopy, 93, 157, 240
Artificial insemination, 127, 129
Artificial respiration, 201
Artificial vagina, 129–130
Arytenoid cartilage, 41, 42, 56
Asafetida, 212
Ascariasis, 145
Ascarids, 51, 52, 178, 185
Aseptic injection, 232
Aspergillosis, 11–12, 29
Aspiration biopsy, 30, 240
Aspirin, 76, 93, 94, 113